Stereotactic Body Radiation and Stereotactic Ablative Radiotherapy Therapy for Cancers

Stereotactic Body Radiation and Stereotactic Ablative Radiotherapy Therapy for Cancers

Guest Editors

Sam Beddar
Michael D. Chuong

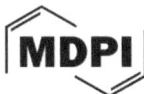

Basel • Beijing • Wuhan • Barcelona • Belgrade • Novi Sad • Cluj • Manchester

Guest Editors

Sam Beddar
Department of Radiation Physics
University of Texas MD Anderson Cancer Center
Houston
United States

Michael D. Chuong
Department of Radiation Oncology
Miami Cancer Institute
Miami
United States

Editorial Office
MDPI AG
Grosspeteranlage 5
4052 Basel, Switzerland

This is a reprint of the Special Issue, published open access by the journal *Cancers* (ISSN 2072-6694), freely accessible at: www.mdpi.com/journal/cancers/special_issues/SBRT_Cancers.

For citation purposes, cite each article independently as indicated on the article page online and using the guide below:

Lastname, A.A.; Lastname, B.B. Article Title. *Journal Name* **Year**, *Volume Number*, Page Range.

ISBN 978-3-7258-3574-4 (Hbk)
ISBN 978-3-7258-3573-7 (PDF)
https://doi.org/10.3390/books978-3-7258-3573-7

© 2025 by the authors. Articles in this book are Open Access and distributed under the Creative Commons Attribution (CC BY) license. The book as a whole is distributed by MDPI under the terms and conditions of the Creative Commons Attribution-NonCommercial-NoDerivs (CC BY-NC-ND) license (https://creativecommons.org/licenses/by-nc-nd/4.0/).

Contents

About the Editors vii

Youssef Ghannam, Adrien Laville, Youlia Kirova, Igor Latorzeff, Antonin Levy and Yuedan Zhou et al.
Radiotherapy of the Primary Disease for Synchronous Metastatic Cancer: A Systematic Review
Reprinted from: *Cancers* 2022, *14*, 5929, https://doi.org/10.3390/cancers14235929 1

John Michael Bryant, Joseph Weygand, Emily Keit, Ruben Cruz-Chamorro, Maria L. Sandoval and Ibrahim M. Oraiqat et al.
Stereotactic Magnetic Resonance-Guided Adaptive and Non-Adaptive Radiotherapy on Combination MR-Linear Accelerators: Current Practice and Future Directions
Reprinted from: *Cancers* 2023, *15*, 2081, https://doi.org/10.3390/cancers15072081 28

Danny Lee, Paul Renz, Seungjong Oh, Min-Sig Hwang, Daniel Pavord and Kyung Lim Yun et al.
Online Adaptive MRI-Guided Stereotactic Body Radiotherapy for Pancreatic and Other Intra-Abdominal Cancers
Reprinted from: *Cancers* 2023, *15*, 5272, https://doi.org/10.3390/cancers15215272 54

Hanna Grzbiela, Elzbieta Nowicka, Marzena Gawkowska, Dorota Tarnawska and Rafal Tarnawski
Robotic Stereotactic Radiotherapy for Intracranial Meningiomas—An Opportunity for Radiation Dose De-Escalation
Reprinted from: *Cancers* 2023, *15*, 5436, https://doi.org/10.3390/cancers15225436 68

Felix-Nikolai Oschinka Jegor Habermann, Daniela Schmitt, Thomas Failing, David Alexander Ziegler, Jann Fischer and Laura Anna Fischer et al.
And Yet It Moves: Clinical Outcomes and Motion Management in Stereotactic Body Radiation Therapy (SBRT) of Centrally Located Non-Small Cell Lung Cancer (NSCLC): Shedding Light on the Internal Organ at Risk Volume (IRV) Concept
Reprinted from: *Cancers* 2024, *16*, 231, https://doi.org/10.3390/cancers16010231 81

Michael R. Shurin, Vladimir A. Kirichenko, Galina V. Shurin, Danny Lee, Christopher Crane and Alexander V. Kirichenko
Radiomodulating Properties of Superparamagnetic Iron Oxide Nanoparticle (SPION) Agent Ferumoxytol on Human Monocytes: Implications for MRI-Guided Liver Radiotherapy
Reprinted from: *Cancers* 2024, *16*, 1318, https://doi.org/10.3390/cancers16071318 97

Rachael M. Martin-Paulpeter, P. James Jensen, Luis A. Perles, Gabriel O. Sawakuchi, Prajnan Das and Eugene J. Koay et al.
Daily Diagnostic Quality Computed Tomography-on-Rails (CTOR) Image Guidance for Abdominal Stereotactic Body Radiation Therapy (SBRT)
Reprinted from: *Cancers* 2024, *16*, 3770, https://doi.org/10.3390/cancers16223770 111

Yao Zhao, Adrian Cozma, Yao Ding, Luis Augusto Perles, Reza Reiazi and Xinru Chen et al.
Upper Urinary Tract Stereotactic Body Radiotherapy Using a 1.5 Tesla Magnetic Resonance Imaging-Guided Linear Accelerator: Workflow and Physics Considerations
Reprinted from: *Cancers* 2024, *16*, 3987, https://doi.org/10.3390/cancers16233987 130

Ahmed Hadj Henni, Geoffrey Martinage, Lucie Lebret and Ilias Arhoun
Per-Irradiation Monitoring by kV-2D Acquisitions in Stereotactic Treatment of Spinal and Non-Spinal Bony Metastases Using an On-Board Imager of a Linear Accelerator
Reprinted from: *Cancers* 2024, *16*, 4267, https://doi.org/10.3390/cancers16244267 141

Robert A. Herrera, Eyub Y. Akdemir, Rupesh Kotecha, Kathryn E. Mittauer, Matthew D. Hall and Adeel Kaiser et al.
Evolving Trends and Patterns of Utilization of Magnetic Resonance-Guided Radiotherapy at a Single Institution, 2018–2024
Reprinted from: *Cancers* **2025**, *17*, 208, https://doi.org/10.3390/cancers17020208 . . . . **155**

He Wang, Fahed M. Alsanea, Dong Joo Rhee, Xiaodong Zhang, Wei Liu and Jinzhong Yang et al.
Advanced External Beam Stereotactic Radiotherapy for Skull Base Reirradiation
Reprinted from: *Cancers* **2025**, *17*, 540, https://doi.org/10.3390/cancers17030540 . . . . **168**

About the Editors

Sam Beddar

Sam Beddar is a tenured full professor at the University of Texas MD Anderson Cancer Center, Houston, Texas, in the Division of Radiation Oncology; adjunct professor in the Department of Physics, Physics Engineering and Optics at Laval University, Qubebec City, Quebec, Canada; and adjunct professor in the Department of Medical Physics at The University of Wisconsin School of Medicine, Madison, Wisconsin. He is the Director of Clinical Research in the Department of Radiation Physics within the Division of Radiation Oncology.

He has been the clinical chief of the Gastrointestinal (GI) Service from 2005 to 2020, focusing his clinical attention on developing SPECT, 4D-CT with and without intravenous contrast for the liver, respiratory-gated modalities, and SBRT techniques for GI cancers. He has been the Director of the intraoperative radiation therapy program at MDACC since 2005.

Dr. Beddar has served on many National Institutes of Health study section review panels and has been a PI of numerous NIH/NCI grant awards as well as industrial grants. His laboratory research is actively engaged in the rapidly growing field of scintillation dosimetry and the use of scintillating materials to measure radiation dose. His work ranges from basic research on scintillator properties to detector development, clinical applications, and commercialization. Dr. Beddar's lab is currently using scintillation detectors to perform in vivo dosimetry, external beam radiation therapy, brachytherapy, and proton therapy. His research activities contributed to the EXRADIN W1 and W2 commercial systems from Standard Imaging, Inc. and the HyperScint commercial systems from Medscint, Inc. Recently, his lab has been focusing on the 3D dose imaging of proton beams, prompt gamma imaging, and proton CT and radiography. He has authored more than 200 peer-reviewed publications and 10 patents.

Michael D. Chuong

As an internationally recognized expert in radiation therapy for gastrointestinal (GI) cancers, Michael Chuong, M.D., FACRO, is vice chair and medical director of radiation oncology and leads the GI radiation service at the Miami Cancer Institute. He also serves as the vice chair of education and clinical research and is professor of radiation oncology at the Florida International University Herbert Wertheim College of Medicine.

Dr. Chuong earned his medical degree from the University of South Florida College of Medicine and completed his residency training in radiation oncology at the H. Lee Moffitt Cancer Center, where he served as the chief resident.

Dr. Chuong is frequently invited to speak around the globe about his clinical expertise and research that is impacting the standard of care, especially related to proton therapy and MRI-guided radiation therapy. Dr. Chuong has co-authored over 125 peer-reviewed manuscripts in prestigious journals such as *JAMA Oncology* and the *International Journal of Radiation Oncology, Biology, Physics*, for which he is the GI section editor.

He is a principal investigator for multiple national and international clinical trials that are exploring advanced radiation therapy strategies and unique combinations of radiation therapy with novel therapeutic agents for GI cancers. As an active leader in the medical community, Dr. Chuong is the Protocol Monitoring and Review Committee chair at the Miami Cancer Institute, Disease Site chair of the Proton Collaborative Group, and the Particle Therapy Co-operative Group Gastrointestinal Subcommittee co-chair.

He participates as an active member of the NRG Oncology Non-Colorectal GI subcommittee, NRG Oncology Pancreas working group, and NRG Oncology International Liaison committee.

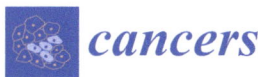

Review

Radiotherapy of the Primary Disease for Synchronous Metastatic Cancer: A Systematic Review

Youssef Ghannam [1,*], Adrien Laville [2], Youlia Kirova [3], Igor Latorzeff [4], Antonin Levy [5,6], Yuedan Zhou [2] and Vincent Bourbonne [7,*]

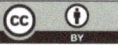

Citation: Ghannam, Y.; Laville, A.; Kirova, Y.; Latorzeff, I.; Levy, A.; Zhou, Y.; Bourbonne, V. Radiotherapy of the Primary Disease for Synchronous Metastatic Cancer: A Systematic Review. *Cancers* **2022**, *14*, 5929. https://doi.org/10.3390/cancers14235929

Academic Editors: Sam Beddar and Michael D. Chuong

Received: 22 October 2022
Accepted: 26 November 2022
Published: 30 November 2022

Publisher's Note: MDPI stays neutral with regard to jurisdictional claims in published maps and institutional affiliations.

Copyright: © 2022 by the authors. Licensee MDPI, Basel, Switzerland. This article is an open access article distributed under the terms and conditions of the Creative Commons Attribution (CC BY) license (https://creativecommons.org/licenses/by/4.0/).

1. Radiation Oncology Department, Centre Paul Papin, Institut de Cancérologie de l'Ouest, 49055 Angers, France
2. Radiation Oncology Department, CHU Amiens-Picardie, 80000 Amiens, France
3. Radiation Oncology Department, Institut Curie Paris, CEDEX 05, 75248 Paris, France
4. Radiation Oncology Department, Bât Atrium Clinique Pasteur, 31300 Toulouse, France
5. Radiation Oncology Department, Gustave Roussy, Université Paris-Saclay, 94805 Villejuif, France
6. Faculté de Médecine, Université Paris-Saclay, 94270 Le Kremlin-Bicêtre, France
7. Radiation Oncology Department, University Hospital, 29200 Brest, France
* Correspondence: idyoussef.ghannam@gmail.com (Y.G.); vincent.bourbonne@chu-brest.fr (V.B.)

Simple Summary: Local radiation treatment of the main tumors in patients with synchronous metastatic illness has traditionally only been used for palliative purposes. The management of patients with de novo metastatic cancer is undergoing a revolution with the advent of new systemic therapies enabling longer overall survival with enhanced quality of life. Numerous studies have looked into the potential survival advantage of treating localized primary tumors at the oligometastatic or oligopersistent stage.

Abstract: In the case of synchronous metastatic disease, the local treatment of primary tumors by radiotherapy has long been reserved for palliative indications. The emergence of the concept of oligometastatic and oligopersistent diseases, the advent of new systemic therapies enabling longer overall survival with an enhanced quality of life, a better understanding of the biologic history of metastatic spread, and technical advances in radiation therapy are revolutionizing the management of patients with de novo metastatic cancer. The prognosis of these patients has been markedly improved and many studies have investigated the survival benefits from the local treatment of various primary tumors in cases of advanced disease at the time of diagnosis or in the case of oligopersistence. This article provides an update on the place of irradiation of the primary tumor in cancer with synchronous metastases, and discusses its interest through published or ongoing trials.

Keywords: primary tumor; locoregional treatment; metastatic cancer; oligometastatic cancer; radiotherapy

1. Introduction

While systemic treatments (chemotherapy, targeted therapies, hormonal therapies, immunotherapies, etc.) are the standard-of-care of synchronous metastatic cancers, local treatment of the primary tumors by surgery or radiotherapy (RT) was mainly used as palliative or symptomatic management (pain, bleeding, etc.). The progress of systemic treatments in recent years has changed the prognosis of these patients, with significantly prolonged survival [1] and sometimes achieved complete remission for several years. This raised the question of treatment of the primary tumors. For some primary diseases, locoregional therapy (LRT) for the intact primary tumor has been hypothesized to improve overall survival (OS), but retrospective series and clinical trials have reported conflicting results. Pooling the data from 4952 patients with various histology subtypes, of whom 1558 received RT and 912 surgery, Ryckman et al. did not find a benefit in progression-free survival (PFS) nor overall survival (OS) [2]. Local treatment of the primary was associated in an OS benefit but only in low metastatic burden patients (HR 0.67, 95% CI 0.52–0.85) while surgery did not improve OS whatever the metastatic burden. When sub-analyzing the results, differential responses may appear depending on the primary and histology. This article thus provides an update on the role of RT on the primary tumors in breast, prostate, and lung cancers with synchronous oligometastatic or oligopersistent disease, and discusses its value through published or ongoing trials.

1.1. Rational

1.1.1. Biological Rational

Stephen Paget formulated the "seed and soil" theory in 1889, whereby metastatic spread is not a random process, but is governed by cooperation between the tumor cells "seeds" and the host organ "soil" [3]. An upstream preparation for metastatic spread requires a suitable microenvironment in the distant organ. A pre-metastatic niche is necessary for metastatic development [4]. This microenvironment consists of a set of immune cells and extracellular matrix proteins forming the metastatic bed. The primary tumor initiates the process of niche formation in distant organs not only by producing growth factors that increase the proliferation of stromal cells, but also by recruiting bone marrow-derived hematopoietic cells to the premetastatic niche [5]. In addition, myeloid precursors are recruited by the primary tumor via cytokines to allow tumor cells to remain undetected by the immune system and thus allowing metastatic development [6]. Primary tumors also secrete exosomes, nanovesicles of 40 to 100 nm in diameter involved in intercellular communication, allowing the exchange of proteins and nucleic acids in particular [7,8].

By secreting a large number of exosomes, primary cancer cells not only influence proximal tumor cells and stromal cells in the local microenvironment, but also have distant systemic effects. They modulate the immune system by stimulating the induction of apoptosis of cytotoxic T cells or the inhibition of natural killer lymphocyte cytotoxicity. These vesicles can also stimulate angiogenesis by interaction with endothelial cells when secreted under hypoxic conditions [9,10]. There is a real molecular communication between the primary tumor and the metastases.

In addition, the primary site may be the source of circulating tumor cells (seeding) which may themselves recolonize the primary tumor (self-seeding) [11,12]. Thus, local irradiation of the primary tumor could suppress this signaling that favors metastatic development. Moreover, lymphocyte activation via DAMPS (damage-associated molecular pattern), a set of pro-inflammatory molecules derived from radiation-induced cell death, could induce an antitumor immune response [13].

A better understanding of the molecular interactions is needed to adapt the therapeutic choices according to the biological profile in order to have a treatment benefit without inducing more toxicity.

1.1.2. Synchronous Metastatic Cancers

The survival of patients with de novo metastatic cancer is very heterogeneous, probably due to the fact that there are several distinct groups of metastatic cancers. Hellman and Weichselbaum named one of the groups: "oligometastatic cancers". It is an intermediate and indolent disease stage with a limited number of metastatic sites (classically fewer than three to five), and is characterized by slow tumor growth (Hellman). Eradicating the metastatic lesions could improve patients' survival [14].

However, a formal demonstration of the benefit of treatment of oligometastases is still lacking. The SABR COMET trial compared stereotactic irradiation of the metastatic sites in addition to systemic treatment with systemic treatment alone in 99 patients with oligo recurrent or metastatic (after initial treatment of primary tumors) [15].

The primary tumor sites included lung (n = 18), breast (n = 18), colon (n = 18), prostate (n = 16), and other localizations (n = 29). Eight-year OS was 27.2% in the SABR arm vs. 13.6% in the control arm (hazard ratio (HR): 0.50; 95% confidence interval (CI): 0.30–0.84; p = 0.008). The heterogeneity of the population makes it impossible to conclude on the value of irradiation of metastatic sites, especially in breast cancer. However, for de novo oligometastatic cancer, the idea of combining maximalist systemic treatments with ablative treatment of the metastases and local treatment of the primary could be an interesting strategy.

2. Irradiation of the Primary Disease for Synchronous Metastatic Breast Cancer

2.1. Retrospective Series

Retrospective studies performed on local treatment of primary tumors examined local treatment options combining surgery with or without postoperative radiotherapy. These studies were mostly performed in a single-center, and presented a variety of methodologies with contradictory findings.

For palliative treatment, local irradiation of the primary tumor seems to control the symptomatology with an acceptable morbidity. In an analysis of the Surveillance, Epidemiology, and End Results (SEER) database of 3660 patients with stage T4M1 breast cancer, 1558 (43%) received surgery (15%), radiation (15%), or both (9%). Symptom improvements were observed in almost 50% of patients, but with an increase in local morbidity (mainly lymphoedema after axillary surgery and neuropathic pain) in 20% of patients who were initially asymptomatic [16].

2.1.1. Impact of Local Treatment on Survival

The first retrospective study to show the benefit of local treatment on the primary tumor was conducted between 1990 and 1993, including 16,023 patients (4.1%) with metastatic breast cancer at the outset. Breast surgery was performed in 9162 patients (57.2%), of which 61.7% were mastectomies. Radiation therapy was performed in 5806 patients, most of whom had undergone surgery [17]. However, the radiation targets (the breast or metastatic lesions) were not specified. The 3-year OS was 17.3% in the no-surgery group, 27.7% in the partial mastectomy group, and 31.8% in the total mastectomy group.

Since then, numerous retrospective studies have shown the benefit of local treatment by surgery with or without complementary irradiation on survival or radical radiotherapy, fueling a debate that is still ongoing (Table 1).

Table 1. Retrospective studies evaluating the impact of local treatment for metastatic breast cancer.

Author	Number of Patients	Local Surgery Number of Patients (%)	Mastectomy Number of Patients or %	Positive Margins	Radiation Therapy	Survival Results with Local Treatment	Survival Results without Local Treatment	p Value	Characteristics Associated with Higher OS Rate in Multivariate Analysis
Khan et al., 2002 [17]	16 023	9162 (57%)	61%	25%	63%	27.7–31.8% (3 years)	17.3% (3 years)	<0.0001	Surgery, systemic treatment, number of metastatic sites
Rapiti et al., 2006 [18]	300	127 (42%)	72%	11%	89%	27% (5 years specific)	12% (5 years)	0.0002	Age < 60 years, no N3 involvement, ER+, no visceral metastasis, no CNS metastasis, hormonal treatment, surgery with negative margins
Babiera et al., 2006 [19]	224	82 (37%)	19	31	0	95% (3 years)	79% (3 years)	0.091	Single metastatic site, HER2 +, Caucasian
Gnerlich et al., 2007 [20]	9734	4578 (47%)	54%	NR	41%	36 months (median)	21 months (median)	<0.001	NR
Fields et al., 2007 [21]	409	187 (46)	54%	33%	0	26.8 months (median)	12.6 months (median)	0.0005	Surgery, exclusive bone metastatic disease
Hazard et al., 2008 [22]	111	47 (42.3%)	67%	29%	67%	43% (3 years)	37% (3 years)	NR	NR
Cady et al., 2008 [23]	622	234 (38%)	NA	NR	NR	44% (3 years)	24% (3 years)	<0.0001	Young patient, HR+, exclusive metastatic bone involvement
Bafford et al., 2008 [24]	147	61 (41%)	65%	NR	NR	42.2 months (median)	28.3 months (median)	0.093	Surgery, no CNS metastasis, HR+, HER 2+++.
Blanchard et al., 2008 [25]	395	242 (61%)	77.7%	NR	99.7%	27.1 months (median)	16.8 months (median)	<0.0001	Surgery, ER+, PR+, number of metastatic sites
Ruiterkamp et al., 2009 [26]	728	288 (39.6%)	66%	NR	34%	24.5% (5 years)	13.1% (5 years)	<0.0001	Surgery, age, no more than one metastatic site, no concurrent disease ($p = 0.06$), systemic therapy
Shien et al., 2009 [27]	344	160 (47)	84%	NR	0	27 months (median)	22 months (median)	0.049	Surgery, age <50 years, soft tissue or bone metastases
Neuman et al., 2010 [28]	186	69 (37%)	40%	41%	13%	NR	NR	NR	ER+, PR+, HER2+++

Table 1. Cont.

Author	Number of Patients	Local Surgery Number of Patients (%)	Mastectomy Number of Patients or %	Positive Margins	Radiation Therapy	Survival Results with Local Treatment	Survival Results without Local Treatment	p Value	Characteristics Associated with Higher OS Rate in Multivariate Analysis
Nguyen et al., 2012 [29]	733	255 (67%)	48.6%	24.3%	RT alone: 22% surgery followed by RT: 11%	21% (5 years)	14% (5 years)	<0.001	Age < 50 years, T1 tumor, RE+, R0 surgery, chemotherapy, hormone therapy, locoregional treatment
Lang et al., 2013 [30]	208	134 (64.4%)	30.6%	NR	32%	56.1 months (median)	37.2 months (median)	0.002	Chemotherapy
Thomas et al., 2016 [31]	21372	13042 (61%)	NR	NR	NA	9.6% (10 years)	2.9% (10 years)	<0.001	NR
Choi et al., 2018 [32]	245	82 (34%)	78%	NR	66%	71% (5 years)	40% (5 years)	<0.001	Endocrine therapy
Le Scodan et al., 2009 [33]	598	320 (55%)	71 (21%)	49 Gy breast/chest wall Boost 22 Gy	RT alone: 78% surgery followed by RT: 13%	43.4% (3 years)	26.7% (3 years)	0.00002	Single metastatic site, young age, locoregional treatment, no visceral metastases, N0
Bourgier et al., 2010 [34]	308	239 (80%)	92 (38%)	50 Gy breast/wall with or without boost	RT alone: 62%	RT alone: 39% (3 years) surgery followed by RT: 57% (3 years)	NR	NR	
Mauro et al., 2016 [35]	125	125	0	50 Gy or hypofractionated 42 Gy: 56% 30 Gy 10 fractions: 40%	RT alone: 100%	23.4 months (median)	NR	NR	Karnofsky, number of metastatic sites, hormone therapy
Pons-Tostivint et al., 2018 [36]	4276	1706 (40%)	55%	NR	RT alone: 31% surgery followed by RT: 43%	63 months (survivors > 1 year)	43.9 months (survivors > 1 an)	0.006	Locoregional treatment; HR+/HER2-; HER2 +++.

Abbreviations: CI confidence interval, CNS central nervous system, HER2 human epidermal growth factor receptor 2, HR+ hormone receptor positive, ER+ estrogen receptor positive, PR+ progesterone receptor positive, RT: radiation therapy, NR: not relevant, NA: not available.

In a more recent retrospective study published by Stahl et al. in 2021, a survival benefit was observed for patients who received either systemic therapy and surgery (HR 0.723; 95% CI 0.671–0.779) or systemic therapy, surgery, and radiation (trimodality: HR 0.640; 95% CI 0.591–0.694) (both $p < 0.0001$) compared with systemic therapy alone [37]. However, once again the LRT seems undistinguishable from distant RT to metastatic sites. Surprisingly, oligometastatic diseases represented 38% of the patients in this series, which is much higher than the usual series, even in academic centers. Furthermore, systemic therapy was used in a small proportion of patients (40% in 2014–2015) which is questionable in stage IV patients.

In addition, the response to systemic treatment seems to be important to consider since some metastatic patients who have effective treatment and stable disease have a better survival than patients with a locally advanced disease without response to systemic treatment [38].

In several retrospective studies, patients with isolated bone metastases appeared to benefit the most from local therapy in terms of overall survival [17,18,39]. Some major prognostic factors of overall survival in favor of local therapy were frequently reported: R0 surgical resection, young age of the operated patients (50–60 years), oligometastatic involvement (one metastasis versus several metastases). Other criteria have been identified: tumor size, hormone receptor status and axillary lymph node involvement. Patients with cancer expressing hormone receptors or HER-2 amplification ($p = 0.004$) would benefit more from local treatment, probably due to the effectiveness of systemic treatment [28].

2.1.2. Impact of Exclusive Irradiation on Survival

Two retrospective French series of studies have examined the impact of exclusive radiotherapy as a local treatment for the primary tumor. In the Curie-Huguenin study reported by Le Scodan et al. of 18,753 patients with breast cancer treated between 1980 and 2004, 598 (3.2%) had metastases at diagnosis [33]. Of the 581 eligible patients, 320 received local treatment, by exclusive radiation in 249 patients (78%), by surgery followed by radiation therapy in 41 patients (13%), or by surgery alone in 30 patients (9%). The average radiation dose was 48 Gy in the breast, with the possibility of a local boost of 22 Gy. With a median follow-up time of 39 months, the probability of survival at 3 years was 43.4% versus 26.7% for the groups with and without local treatment, respectively ($p = 0.00002$).

In the multifactorial analysis, radiotherapy was an independent factor that significantly improved overall survival. The improvement in survival was particularly marked in women with visceral metastases. Authors concluded that radiation therapy could be proposed as an alternative treatment to surgery in patients with metastatic cancer at the time of diagnosis.

The second study by the Gustave Roussy [34] was conducted between 1990 and 2003, among 9138 patients; 308 patients had stage IV disease. The majority of patients (2/3) had a single metastatic site and 49% had non-visceral metastases at diagnosis. LRT was performed in 80% of patients ($n = 239$) either by exclusive radiation ($n = 147$) or by breast and axillary surgery with or without postoperative radiotherapy ($n = 92$). In the operated group, the cancers were of smaller sizes, lower in tumor grade, had less clinical axillary lymph node involvement, and had a lower tumor burden than in the exclusive radiation group. With a median follow-up of 6.5 years, locoregional control was achieved in 85% of patients. The probabilities of metastasis-free survival and overall survival at 3 years were 20% and 39% with exclusive radiation therapy and 39% and 57% with surgery, without significant difference.

Several meta-analyses of these studies, including Gera's work published in 2020, supported LRT to improve survival in these patients with de novo metastatic cancer [40,41].

These results, often from uni- or multifactorial analyses, are sometimes contradictory and should be interpreted with caution because of potential selection bias. The survival advantage of patients undergoing surgery could be explained by selection bias [23]. Published analyses indicate that there is an imbalance between the groups and those patients with lower tumor burden, less dissemination and with a better physiology state (age, comorbidities) are more likely to be candidates for LRT. For example, in the study published by Blanchard et al., it was found that at least 25% of cancers that were operated and 3% of the unoperated tumors were reclassified [25]. This would suggest that their initial presentation was stage I, II or III and only after completion of the extension work-up, they were reclassified as stage IV. This means that for some patients the indication for surgery was based on curative intent and not for palliative purposes [42]. The only way to overcome these selection biases is through prospective randomized trials.

2.2. Prospective Studies

Published prospective studies and ongoing trials on this topic follow two distinct designs (Table 2). The first one was where the patients enrolled received systemic therapy before any LRT. Then, they were registered and if they did not progress after chemotherapy, they were randomized in the LRT group (followed by systemic therapy) or continued systemic therapy alone. The Indian Tata Memorial Center trial included 350 patients under 65 years, with de novo metastatic breast cancer between 2005 and 2013 [43]. Patients were randomized to LRT or no LRT. Among the 350 patients, 336 had unresectable tumors. These received a neoadjuvant chemotherapy and were randomized according to response to receive local or no treatment. One hundred and seventy-three patients underwent surgery (72% mastectomy), and 80% received adjuvant radiotherapy. This trial did not show any benefit in terms of 2-year OS: 41.9% (95% CI 33.9–49.7) in the LRT group versus 43% (35.2–50.8) in the no LRT group. In the multifactorial analysis, global survival was independently associated with hormone receptor expression and a low number of metastatic sites at initial presentation. The site of metastasis at initial presentation was not significantly associated with overall survival. Overall survival in both groups was lower than reported in Western countries, possibly due to the delay in diagnosis. In addition, 107 patients (31%) had HER2-expressing cancers, but due to financial constraints, 98 patients in this subgroup (92%) did not receive anti-HER2 targeted therapy. In this study, LRT resulted in significantly longer locoregional progression-free survival compared with the no-treatment group. This was tempered by the authors, who suggest that initial LRT cannot be justified for local symptom control alone, because only a minority (10%) of patients in the no-local-treatment group still underwent surgery for local palliative reasons.

Table 2. Published randomized trials for metastatic breast cancer.

Trial	Number of Patients	Age (Median)	Local Surgery	Mastectomy	Radiation Therapy	Survival Results with Local Treatment	Survival Results without Local Treatment	p Value	Locoregional Progression with Local Treatment	Locoregional Progression without Local Treatment	Low Metastatic Burden * OS HR (95%CI)
Badwe et al., 2015 [43]	350	48 years	173	72%	80%	Median survival: 19.2 months Survival at 2 years: 41.9%	Median survival: 20.5 months Survival at 2 years: 43%.	HR 1.04, (95% CI 0.81–1.34) p = 0.79	5.3%	10.6%	1.16 (0.69–1.95)
Soran et al., 2018 [44]	274	52 years	138	46%	54%	Survival at 3 years: 60% Survival at 5 years 41.6% (46 months)	Survival at 3 years: 51% Survival at 5 years: 24.4% (37 months)	p = 0.10 p = 0.05	1%	11%	Solitary bone metastases:0.55 (0.36–0.86) Solitary liver/pulmonary metastases: 0.69 (0.37–1.29
Khan et al, 2022 [45]	256	56 years	125	70%	84%	Survival at 3 years: 68.4% (54.9 months)	Survival at 3 years: 67.9% (53.1 months)	HR 1.11, (90% CI 0.82–1.52); p = 0.57	16.3%	39.8%	1.18 (0.38–3.67)

Abbreviations: CI—confidence interval, OS—overall survival. * Low metastatic burden: Badwe et al (Tata Memorial): subgroup of patients with 3 or fewer metastases, Soran et al (MF07-01): oligometastatic subgroups: solitary bone or solitary liver/pulmonary metastasis, Khan et al (E2108): Oligometastasis at registration (exploratory post hoc subgroup analyses).

The recently published North American trial enrolled 390 participants, 256 were randomly assigned: 131 to continued systemic therapy and 125 to early LRT (surgery and radiotherapy) [45]. The 3-year OS was 67.9% without and 68.4% with early LRT (hazard ratio = 1.11; 90% CI, 0.82 to 1.52; $p = 0.57$). Locoregional progression was less frequent in the LRT group (3-year rate: 16.3% v 39.8%; $p < 0.001$). No difference in quality of life was observed between the two arms. Overall survival by tumor subtype for the 20 women with triple-negative breast cancer tended to be worse with the addition of LRT (HR = 3.50).

The Japan Clinical Oncology Group (JCOG) 1017 PRIM-BC is an ongoing trial that was conducted to confirm the superiority, in terms of overall survival, of local treatment of the primary disease with surgery [46]. All patients received a standard systemic treatment after the first registration. After 3 months, patients with non-progressive disease were randomized to surgery with systemic therapy or to systemic therapy alone. The study protocol did not specify whether patients in the surgery group received postoperative radiotherapy.

The second design of the prospective trials was where patients were directly randomized to either to systemic therapy alone or to LRT followed by systemic therapy.

The Turkish randomized trial MF07-01 included 274 patients between 2007 and 2012 [44]. They received local treatment (surgery and radiotherapy in case of conservative surgery) followed by systemic treatment (for 138 patients) or systemic treatment alone (for 136 patients). There was no stratification on baseline characteristics, which explains some of the imbalances between the groups (hormone receptor expression, 85.5% vs. 71.8%, and triple-negative tumors, 7.3% vs. 17.4% in the groups with and without local treatment, respectively). It should be noted that there was a relatively high number of single metastases (30%), while the extension workup included (18 F)-fluorodeoxyglucose PET. Overall survival was significantly prolonged by LRT (at 5 years 41.6% vs. 24.4% $p = 0.005$). An unplanned subgroup analysis showed a significant overall survival advantage with LRT in patients with hormone receptor-positive but non-HER2 cancers, patients with exclusive bone metastases, and patients younger than 55 years. The benefit of local treatment appears particularly clear in the case of single bone metastases.

The Austrian prospective randomized phase III ABCSG-28 POSYTIVE trial attempted to assess median survival by comparing primary surgery followed by systemic therapy to systemic therapy alone in de novo stage IV breast cancer [47]. This trial did not reach full accrual. Ninety-three patients were included against 254 subjects needed. This trial could not demonstrate an overall survival benefit in favor of surgery. Patients randomized to systemic therapy had a median survival rate of 54 months, compared with 34 months in the surgical group. Although the trial was not sufficiently powered, the authors said this trend indicates that caution should be exercised regarding primary surgery in the setting.

Despite several studies on the subject, there is, to date, no clear recommendation or consensus for radiotherapy of the primary disease in synchronous metastatic breast cancer. The negative results of three prospective trials encourage caution regarding LRT, which have to be systematically discussed in multidisciplinary concertation meetings. However, it would appear that LRT by surgery followed by radiation after response to initial systemic therapy would be a good option, particularly in young patients with hormone receptor-expressing, non-HER2, oligometastatic cancer that tends to have bone-only metastases. The systemic treatment remains the standard first-line treatment in the case of metastatic disease and it appears that LRT should not interfere with its implementation, hence the interest in knowing how the new targeted molecules are associated with radiotherapy [48–50].

3. Irradiation of the Primary Tumor for Metastatic Prostate Cancer

Despite implementation of individualized screening, about 10% of patients are diagnosed with initially metastatic prostate cancer [39]. For a long time, metastatic prostate cancers were univocally considered to have a poor prognosis and only systemic treatments were indicated. Many retrospective studies were published suggesting a benefit from local radiotherapy for these patients. Most of them are large population-based studies using propensity-scores [51–58] (Table 3). Two clinical trials and one meta-analysis have suggested the value of local prostate radiotherapy in this context to improve clinical outcomes.

Table 3. Retrospective trials for metastatic prostate cancer.

Author	Number of Patients and Follow Up	Treatment Modalities	Results
Culp et al., 2014 [51]	$n = 8185$	LT = 374	5 years OS
	Median follow-up: 16 months	RP ($n = 245$) BT ($n = 129$) NLT ($n = 7811$)	67.4% 52.6% 22.5% ($p < 0.001$) RP is associated with CSM in MVA: (0.38, CI 0.27–0.53 $p < 0.001$)
Fossati et al., 2015 [52]	$n = 8197$	LT ($n = 628$) (either RP or RT)	Interaction LT and CSM ($p < 0.0001$)
	Median follow-up: 36 months LT, 31 months NLT	NLT ($n = 7569$)	Reduction in CSM for LT with a predicted 3-year mortality < 40% ($p < 0.0001$)
Satkunasivam et al., 2015 [56]	$n = 4069$ Median follow-up: 20 months	LT = 242 RP ($n = 47$)	3-year OS 73%
		IMRT ($n = 88$) CRT ($n = 107$) NLT ($n = 3827$)	72% 37% 34% IMRT was associated with a reduction of CSM (HR 0.38 CI 0.24–0.61 $p < 0.001$)
Rusthoven et al., 2016 [53]	$n = 6382$ Median follow-up: 5.1 years	LT = 538 RP ($n = 69$)	5-year OS 49%
		NLT, ADT alone ($n = 5844$)	25% $p < 0.001$
Löppenberg et al., 2016 [54]	$n = 15501$ Median follow-up: 39 months	LT = 1470 RT ($n = 1131$)	3-year OS 60%
		RP ($n = 294$) BT ($n = 45$) NLT ($n = 14031$)	78% 80% 48% $p < 0.001$ LT was associated with a 39% risk reduction of mortality compared with NLT in MVA adjusted for PSA Gleason score, TNM stage, age
Leyh-Bannurah et al., 2017 [55]	$n = 13692$ Median follow-up: 43.5 months LT, 31 months NLT	LT = 474, NLT = 13218 RT ($n = 161$) RP ($n = 313$)	LT was associated with lower CSM compared with NLT (HR 0.4 IC95% 0.32–0.5)
Parikh et al., 2017 [57]	$n = 6051$	LT = 827	2-year OS 5-year OS
	Median follow-up: 22 months	RP ($n = 622$) IMRT ($n = 52$) CRT ($n = 153$) NLT ($n = 5224$)	72.5% 45.7% LT 80.6% 17.1% NLT ($p < 0.01$) 47.6% 48.9% $p < 0.0001$
Cho et al., 2016 [58]	$n = 140$	LT = 38	3-year OS
	Median follow-up: 34 months	RT ($n = 38$) NLT = 102	69% 43% $p = 0.004$

LT: locally treated, NLT: non locally treated, RP: radical prostatectomy, BT: brachytherapy, OS: overall survival, PFS: progression-free survival, RT: radiotherapy, CSM: cancer-specific mortality, IMRT: intensity-modulated radiotherapy, CRT: conformal radiotherapy, MVA: multivariate analysis.

3.1. HORRAD Trial

HORRAD was the first prospective randomized trial published. This study included 432 metastatic prostate cancer patients, randomized between hormone therapy alone or combined with prostate radiotherapy [59]. The primary endpoint was overall survival, and the secondary endpoint was time to biochemical progression. The median age of the population was 68 years old. The median PSA level was 145 ng/mL. The dose prescribed was 70 Gy in 35 fractions of 2 Gy or 57.76 Gy in 19 fractions of 3.04 Gy. The GTV included the prostate and extensions, the base of the seminal vesicles. Regarding the planning target volume, 1 cm margin in conventional radiotherapy was applied or 8 mm if a position verification protocol with fiducial marker was implanted. Of the patients, 67% had more than five bone metastases at the time of randomization (high volume metastatic burden). With 47 months median follow-up, no difference in overall survival was demonstrated (45 vs. 43 months, HR 0.90; 95% CI [0.70–1.14]. The non-significance could be explained by a lack of statistical power. In the subgroup analysis, patients with fewer than five metastases (n = 160) had a trend towards better overall survival (HR 0.68; 95% CI 0.42–1.10 p = 0.063). Local radiotherapy was associated with 3-month improvement in time without PSA increase (HR = 0.78; 95% CI: [0.63–0.97]; p = 0.02). As suggested by the absence of clear OS benefit despite a benefit in biochemical response, PSA level only should not be used as a surrogate for OS.

A supplementary analysis by Boevé et al. assessed side effects and quality-of-life in this cohort [60]. Apart from local symptoms, there was no significant difference in mean scores on the quality of life items evaluated by QLQ-C30 et QLQ-PR25, with a difference of 10 points from the baseline considered relevant. More frequent urinary and bowel symptoms and diarrhea were found in patients in the prostate radiotherapy group within 3 months after treatment. The bowel symptom score was significantly higher in 22% patients treated with radiotherapy at two years follow-up (HR = 8; CI 95% [4.8–11.1]).

3.2. Stampede Trial

STAMPEDE was a randomized controlled trial who evaluated the benefit of prostate radiotherapy in addition to androgen deprivation therapy in patients with hormone-sensitive metastatic prostate cancer [61]. Totally, 2061 patients were enrolled in this two arms phase III trial randomizing the combination of prostate radiation therapy with androgen suppression or androgen suppression alone. Selected patients were newly diagnosed with metastatic prostate cancer, without prior radical treatment and with metastatic disease confirmed by standard imaging. Radiation could be delivered at a dose of 55 Gy in 20 daily fractions of 2.75 Gy or 36 Gy in 6 weekly fractions of 6 Gy. The planned target volume included the entire prostate +/- seminal vesicles. The primary endpoint was overall survival and failure-free survival (FFS). Secondary endpoints were local symptomatology, progression-free survival (PFS) and metastatic progression free survival. Biological relapse was defined as an increase of at least 50% in PSA level. Patients were divided into subgroups according to their initial metastatic burden based on imaging data (CT, MRI, and scintigraphy). High metastatic burden was defined according to CHAARTED criteria ($\geq$ four bone metastases with $\geq$ one outside the pelvis and vertebrae, or visceral metastases, or both). Patients who did not meet these criteria were classified as low burden. 89% of patients had initially bone metastases. The median PSA level before androgen suppression was 98 ng/mL and 97 ng/mL respectively in each arm. The population median age was 68 years old. Gleason score was $\geq$ 8 in 79% of cases. 40% and 54% of patients had low and high metastatic burden, respectively. It was unknown for 6% of them. In the entire cohort, no significant benefit was found in overall survival with local radiotherapy (HR 0.92; 95% CI [0.8–1.06]; p = 0.27) with a median follow-up of 37 months. Failure-free survival was significantly improved in the radiotherapy arm (HZ= 0.76; 95% CI 0.68–0.84; p = 3.4×10^{-7}). Patients with a low metastatic burden (n = 819) had significantly better overall survival and failure-free survival (HZ= 0.68; 0.52–0.90; p = 0.007). The addition of radiotherapy show a 8% improvement in overall survival in this previously planned subgroup analysis (73% vs. 81% (HR: 0.68; CI 95%: [0.52–0.90]; p = 0.007). The interaction test was significant (p = 0.0098). The hypo fractionated 55 Gy in 20 fractions regimen appeared to be more effective in terms of failure-free survival (HR 0.69, 95% CI 0.59–0.80;

$p < 0.0001$). There was 65% of urinary and 47% of digestive toxicity compared with 71% and 62% in favor of the weekly arm. Prostate radiotherapy appeared to be well tolerated with 4% grade 3–4 toxicity compared to 1% with androgen deprivation alone. For the 533 patients for whom data were available, 15% of patients in the control arm and 13% in the radiotherapy arm had grade $\geq$ three adverse events found at two years of follow-up.

Ali et al. investigated the effect of prostate radiotherapy according to the severity of metastatic spread in the STAMPEDE cohort [39]. More than 2000 patients were randomized, with less than 2% of patients with four or more bone metastases in the spine alone. The survival benefit decreased while increasing number of metastases up to a threshold of three bone metastases. A gain in overall survival was correlated with the number of bone metastases: 8.5%, 6.2% and 5.8% at 3 years follow-up in patients with one, two and three bone metastases respectively. No survival benefit was found in patients with visceral metastases or with strictly more than three bone metastases. For relapse-free survival, nine bone metastases were found as a threshold for benefit. The interaction between the number of bone metastases and treatment adjusted for age, PSA level before androgen suppression, T stage, Gleason score, N stage, metastatic sites, docetaxel use, and RT schedule showed similar results for OS and PFS. In the subgroup analysis, for patients with three or fewer bone metastases with or without non regional lymph node and no visceral metastases, local radiotherapy improved overall survival (3-year survival 85% vs. 75%, HR = 0.64 IC 95% [0.46–0.89]). No survival benefit was associated with four or more bone metastases with or without non-regional lymph node involvement. Classifying low metastatic burden patients as three or fewer bone metastases, regardless of location, with or without non-regional lymph node involvement, with no visceral metastases, the results were significant in overall survival (HR = 0.62 CI 95% [0.46–0.83] $p = 0.01$) and failure-free survival (HR = 0.57 CI 95% [0.47–0.70] $p = 0.001$. The effect of radiotherapy on OS and FFS within patients with low-burden disease did not rely on age, pre-ADT PSA level, World Health Organization performance status, Gleason score, tumor stage, regional nodal stage and schedule. This study supports the value of local radiotherapy in patients with a low number of bone metastases evaluated by conventional imaging.

3.3. STOP-CAP Meta-Analysis

The STOP-CAP meta-analysis pooled the two randomized trials HORRAD and STAMPEDE ($n = 2126$) [62]. No significative improvement in overall survival (HR 0.92, 95% CI 95% [0.81–1.04], $p = 0.195$) or progression-free survival (HR 0.94, CI 95% [0.84–1.05], $p = 0.238$) was found. Biologic progression-free survival (HR 0.74, CI 95% [0.67–0.82], $p = 0.94 \times 10^{-8}$) and failure-free survival (HR 0.76 CI 95% [0.69–0.84] $p= 0.64 \times 10^{-7}$) were improved. The interaction between the number of metastases (<5 vs. >5) and survival was significant (HR = 1.47 CI 95% [1.11–1.94], $p = 0.007$).

Although many patients classified as having a low metastatic burden, as defined by the HORRAD study, are also classified as having a low metastatic burden as defined by the CHAARTED criteria, the definition of tumor volume level remains heterogeneous between these two studies. Modern imaging techniques and molecular signatures would improve the accuracy of patient selection. A number of patients classified as having low metastatic burden would be likely classified as high burden using Choline-PET or PSMA-PET [63]. The benefit of local treatment according to the number of spinal metastases could not be addressed by the analysis of Ali et al. because only 2% of the STAMPEDE cohort had exclusive spinal bone metastatic involvement [39].

3.4. Ongoing Trials

Among the ongoing studies, the PEACE 1 trial is a four-arm multicenter study comparing the combination of androgen suppression, docetaxel chemotherapy +/- prostate radiotherapy (74 Gy in 37 fractions) +/- abiraterone acetate and prednisone. Results regarding the value of local radiotherapy are pending [64]. The NCT03678025 study conducted by the SWOG will evaluate the combination of systemic treatment with local treatment (surgery vs. prostate radiotherapy. Other studies are being conducted to answer the question of a combination of radiotherapy on the primary and oligometastases. PRESTO (prostate-cancer treatment using stereotactic radiotherapy for oligometastases ablation in hormone-sensitive patients) is an ongoing two-arm, multicenter phase III randomized trial. The objective is to evaluate the efficacy of stereotactic radiotherapy applied to all oligometastases in patients with hormone-sensitive oligometastatic prostate cancer, Table 4 [65–73].

Table 4. Ongoing trials for metastatic prostate cancer.

Phase III	Location	Patients Included	Intervention	Outcome	End of Study
PEACE-1 [65]	France	1173	Arm A: ADT + docetaxel Arm B: AA+ADT + docetaxel Arm C: RT+ADT + docetaxel Arm D: AA+RT+ADT + docetaxel	OS PFS	2032
SWOG NCT03678025 [71]	USA	1273	Arm I: Systemic treatment Arm II: Systemic treatment + (RP/RT)	OS	2031
PRESTO [72]	France	350	Arm A: RT + Soc Arm B: Soc	TCR	2027
Phase II					
PLATON [67]	Canada	410	Arm 1: Systemic treatment + prostate directed therapy if low metastatic burden Arm 2: Systemic treatment+ local treatment of all sites	PFS	2025
LoMPII [68]	Belgium	1273	Arm I: RP+/-ADT Arm II: RT+/-ADT	Randomization feasibility	2021
UHSeste NCT02913859 [69]	Croatia	60	Experimental arm: ADT + LHRHa +/- aA + prostate-pelvic RT Standard arm: ADT alone	PFS	2020
IP2 ATLANTA [70]	UK	918	Arm 1: Systemic treatment Arm 2: Systemic treatment + TAMI Arm 3: Systemic treatment + RP/RT +'metastases	pCR Adverse events PFS	2024
MSKCC NCT04262154 [73]	USA	44	Atezolizumab + RT + (aA, prednisone, leuprolide)	2-year FFS	September 2023
MD Anderson NCT01751438 [66]	USA	180	Arm 1: Systemic treatment Arm 2: Systemic treatment + RP/RT	PFS	February 2023

ADT—androgen deprivation therapy, aA—antiandrogen, Soc—standard of care, RP—radical prostatectomy, BT—brachytherapy, OS—overall survival, PFS—progression free survival, RT—radiotherapy, TCR—time to castration resistance (or death from any cause), pCR—complete pathological response.

Local control of the primary matters in selected newly diagnosed hormone-sensitive metastatic prostate cancer. For the majority of patients, prostate radiotherapy could provide a survival benefit with transient and manageable side effects. Although radiotherapy is well tolerated, patients should be informed that radiation is associated with more urinary symptoms and potentially chronic diarrhea. Selection criteria are not consensual and many other questions remain: radiation schedule, technical modalities, association with metastases-directed therapy. The latest recently published international and national guidelines recommend radiation to the primary [74,75]. An ongoing investigation of predictive molecular signatures and advances in nuclear imaging with the use of standardized indices to assess metastatic burden could help with better stratification.

4. Treatment of the Primitive Site in Metastatic Lung Cancer Patients

Lung cancer remains the leading cause of death worldwide with a high percentage being diagnosed as stage IV disease [76]. The arrival of immune checkpoint inhibitors (ICI) in lung cancer patients has completely modified the treatment of those patients, and especially patients with non-small cell lung cancer (NSCLC). At first-line [77,78] and second-line [79,80] treatments, both progression-free survival (PFS) and overall survival (OS) were significantly improved, especially when selecting patients based on the level of PD-L1 expression. Specific biomarkers such as EGFR mutations or ALK rearrangements were identified and could be directly targeted, with prolonged survival when compared to the usual chemotherapy-based regimen [81–85]. Clinicians face new entities of patients, such as long-responders to ICIs or oligometastatic/oligopersistent patients [86], in whom a curative objective could possibly be considered.

With this intent, radiotherapy could be delivered to lower the tumor burden [4,11,12] and possibly increase the PFS/OS. Abscopal responses were also described, yet poorly understood. Several technological advances have been made since the 2000s. Stereotactic radiotherapy allows the delivery of a high dose per fraction in 3–8 fractions, with a high tumor conformation resulting in high local control and a low risk of toxicity [87].

Local treatment has several potential advantages: prevention or treatment of eventual symptoms, prevention of primary/secondary seeding and maintenance with the same treatment and thus differing treatment changes [88].

To this day, several trials have focused on the impact of radiotherapy in metastatic lung cancer. Given the clear differences between NSCLC and small-cell lung cancer (SCLC) but also the lack of data in SCLC patients, this article only focuses on NSCLC patients. Of note, the benefits of a lower dose as thoracic consolidation were assessed in a randomized trial focusing on SCLC patients. The OS benefit was most pronounced when only patients with residual thoracic disease were included. To our knowledge, the CREST trial [89] remains the single published RCT in SCLC patients. Regarding NSCLC patients, local radiotherapy to the primary was investigated more deeply, but with very heterogenous populations.

4.1. Palliative Radiotherapy

According to the NCCN guidelines, local radiotherapy is recommended for palliation or prevention of symptoms such as pain, bleeding or obstruction [90]. In a cohort of 78 patients, palliative thoracic radiotherapy was associated with pain relief in 85.9% in the patients [91]. An improvement of the performance status (PS) was also reported [92], palliative radiotherapy being the possible bridge between palliative care only and systemic treatments [93].

4.2. Oligometastatic NSCLC

The oligometastatic NSCLC stage has been defined with a maximum of five metastases among three or fewer organs, as assessed with ^{18}F-FDG positron emission tomography and brain imaging [94]. Mediastinal lymph nodes are not considered as metastases.

Local radiotherapy to metastatic sites, among which (but not limited to) lung metastases, achieves prolonged survival in selected patients [14,95–98]. These interesting results were first described on retrospective cohorts but later confirmed in several phase II trials. The main concern for patients under systemic treatment is the development of acquired resistance. Locally directed treatment such as radiotherapy could thus increase the PFS and possibly the OS in selected patients with indolent diseases [99]. The benefit of local therapy seems irrespective of the mutational status. Data should, however, be analyzed separately given the different PFS and OS between patients with and without targetable mutations.

4.2.1. NSCLC without Targetable Mutations

One of the largest retrospective cohorts was based on the analysis of 186 patients with oligometastatic NSCLC that were either treated with surgery, local radiotherapy to the primitive (9%), to metastases (17%) and 20% to the primitive and the metastases; the rest did not receive radiotherapy. Radiotherapy was associated with a longer overall survival benefit ($p = 0.04$) but only after propensity score matching [100]. Published meta-analyses are limited by the small number of patients treated with high-dose radiotherapy, as well as a high risk of selection bias. For instance, a meta-analysis reported a 52% decrease in the 1-year death rate when delivering local treatment (74.9% in patients with local treatment and 32.3% in locally untreated patients). The number of metastases was the main prognostic factor [101]. In a meta-analysis aggregating the results of 21 (mainly) retrospective studies, the overall survival reached 20.4 months, with a 1-year survival probability of 70% [102].

Focusing on patients treated with ICIs, robust data remain limited. In a cohort of 148 patients with 38 oligoprogressive patients, switching the therapy group was not superior to continuation of the same ICI with added RT to the progressive lesions [103].

Prospective trials focusing on the benefit of local radiotherapy are very heterogenous regarding their design and treatment modalities. While several phase III trials are ongoing, only phase II results are available. Pre-treatment PET-CT was mandatory in only four out of six trials. The definition of the oligometastatic state varied between fewer than five and fewer than six sites. Among the 209 included patients, 170 patients (81.3%) received either surgery or radiotherapy (normofractionated, moderately hypofractionated or stereotactic) to the primitive and synchronous lesions [14,95–97,104]. In trials in which the overall survival for NSCLC-patients was available, OS ranged from 13.5 to 41.6 months, whereas median PFS ranged from 11.2 to 23.5 months.

For instance, focusing on 49 patients evaluated with a PET-CT ($\leq$ three metastatic sites), the study by Gomez et al. constituted the largest prospective cohort dedicated to oligometastatic NSCLC. OS increased from 17 to 41.2 months ($p = 0.02$) [14,104].

Similar results were found but on smaller or non-NSCLC exclusive cohorts. Bauml et al. included 45 NSCLC patients in which 67% were treated with SBRT and pembrolizumab. In this single arm phase II study, the median OS reached 41.6 months [105]. Of note, patients were included only after the completion of SBRT. With 99 included patients but only 18 patients with NSCLC (18.2%), Palma et al. were able to validate the benefit of local radiotherapy among a variety of oligometastatic cancers, with a median OS of 50 months (vs. 28 in the control arm) [106]. To our knowledge, Palma et al. and Iyengar et al. [107] conducted the two single published prospective studies in which SBRT was mandatory. The main differences between the two were the cancer selection with only NSCLC patients in the Iyengar et al. study and the clinical setting. In the SABR-COMET trial, SBRT was delivered in case of oligorecurrence whereas in the study by Iyengar et al., only synchronous stage IV NSCLC were included.

As presented by Levy et al. [94] and actualized for this review in Table 5, RT modality varied greatly among these prospective trials. Even when SBRT was mandatory, prescriptions differed significantly from one study to the other. Similarly, the rates of patients with brain metastases varied greatly from one study to another.

Table 5. Prospective studies of consolidative radiotherapy in metastatic NSCLC patients, irrespective of the mutational status.

Author	Study Type	Number of Patients	Clinical Stage	Percentage of Patients with Targetable Mutations	Modality of RT	Irradiation of the Primitive and/or Metastases	Control Arm	Percentage of Treated Brain Metastases	Follow-Up	Median PFS	Median OS
Gomez et al. [14]	Randomized phase II	49	Synchronous	12–20%	48% SBRT	Primitive and all residual metastatic sites	Maintenance chemotherapy or watching	25%	38.8 months	14.2 vs. 4.4 months ($p = 0.02$)	41.2 vs. 18.9 months ($p = 0.02$)
Palma et al. [106]	Randomized phase II	18/99	Metachronous Controlled primary	Not defined	100% SBRT	All metastatic sites	Standard	2%	51 months	11.6 vs. 5.4 months ($p = 0.001$)	50.0 vs. 28.0 ($p = 0.006$)
Iyengar et al. [107]	Randomized phase II	29	Synchronous	0%	100% SBRT	Primitive and all metastatic sites	No control arm (concomitant chemotherapy)	0%	9.6 months	9.7 vs. 3.5 months ($p = 0.1$)	Not reached vs. 17 months
Bauml et al. [105]	Single arm phase II	45	Synchronous or Metachronous	Not defined	67% SBRT	Primitive and all metastatic sites	No control arm (concomitant pembrolizumab)	36%	25 months	18.7 months	41.6 months
De Ruysscher et al. [95]	Single arm phase II	39	Synchronous	7.7%	0% SBRT to the primitive	Primitive and all metastatic sites	No control arm	43.6%	27.7 months	12.1 months	13.5 months
Collen et al. [96]	Single arm phase II	26	Synchronous or Metachronous	7.7%	100% SBRT	Primitive and all metastatic sites	No control arm	13%	16.4 months	11.2 months	23 months
Petty et al. [97]	Single arm phase II	27	Synchronous	Not defined	Not defined	All sites of residual disease	No control arm	41%	24.2 months	11.2 months	28.4 months
Arrieta et al. [98]	Single arm phase II	37	Synchronous	43.2%	18.9% SBRT	Primitive and all metastatic sites	No control arm	43.2%	32.5 months	23.5 months	Not reached
Wang et al. [108]	Randomized phase II	127	Synchronous	100% mEGFR	100% SBRT	Primitive and all metastatic sites	Standard: first-line TKI	0%	23.6 months	20.2 vs. 12.5 months ($p < 0.001$)	25.5 vs. 17.4 months ($p < 0.001$)

Abbreviations: RT—radiotherapy, PFS—progression-free survival, OS—overall survival, SBRT—stereotactic body radiotherapy, mEGFR—mutated epidermal growth factor receptor, TKI—tyrosine kinase inhibitor.

Of note, patients with EGFR mutations could be included in some trials, with the rates reaching 12–20% [14,104] or even 43.2% [98]. In contrast, in a study in which patients with oncodrivers were excluded, local therapy increased the median PFS by only 6.2 months [107]. A separate focus on mutated-NSCLC seems necessary.

4.2.2. NSCLC with Targetable Mutations: EGFR, ALK, ROS1

Interesting results were also obtained in patients with EGFR mutations [109]. Approximately half of recurrences after EGFR-targeted therapy occur first in the primary or pre-existing metastatic sites [88]. The primary lung tumor size appears as the strongest risk factor for failure in the original sites. In some reports, the local recurrence rate even reaches 60% as the site of first failure and the only site of failure for 30% [110]. Given the indolent pattern of certain NSCLCs under tyrosine-kinase inhibitors (TKIs), the evidence for benefit from RT seems more robust, with the lack of phase III trials.

Radiotherapy was evaluated as a consolidation treatment in 145 patients under TKIs, with 35.2% having received radiotherapy on the primitive and the metastases, 37.9% on either the primitive or the metastases and 26.9% having received no radiotherapy. Median PFS and OS of 20.6 months and 40.9 months were obtained [111]. Using a propensity-matching and a cohort of 308 patients among which only 46 patients received TKI and SBRT, a significant PFS benefit was obtained in comparison with patients treated with TKIs only ($p = 0.03$). No significant OS benefit was shown [108]. These retrospective results were further confirmed in a phase III randomized trial [112]. Among the 631 screened patients, 136 patients were enrolled and randomly assigned to either first-generation TKI (gefitinib, erlotinib or icotinib) alone or upfront RT prior to TKI. With a median follow-up of 23.6 months, 133 patients were analyzable. The majority of patients had one to four metastases (> 85% in both arms). Upfront RT followed by TKI significantly prolonged PFS from 12.5 months (CI 95% 11.6–13.4) to 20.2 months (CI 95% 17.9–22.5) and OS from 17.6 (CI 95% 15.4–19.8) to 25.5 months (23.2–27.8) ($p < 0.001$). A currently ongoing phase II trial (NCT02314364) focuses on the benefit of consolidative SBRT on residual disease in the lung, liver, adrenal glands, and/or spine within 6 months of initiating TKI treatment in patients with oncogene-driven NSCLC (with alterations in EGFR, ALK, ROS1). A phase II study (ATOM) assessed the efficacy of SBRT delivered to residual oligometastases (after 3 months TKI) in 16 patients. When compared to screen-failed patients (unfit for SBRT), patients that benefited from SBRT had a higher PFS (HR 0.41, $p = 0.01$) [113]. This PFS benefit was confirmed by OS in a previously presented multi-institutional phase II trial including 12–20% patients with oncogene-driven NSCLC (41.2 vs. 17.0 months) [14,104].

In case of oligoprogression, RT is considered as a way to overcome treatment resistance and especially resistance to EGFR TKIs. In a phase II trial comparing erlotinib vs. erlotinib + RT in patients experiencing progression after an EGFR TKI [114], RT was associated with a modest PFS of 5.8 months (95% CI 2.5–11.3) and OS of 2.9 years (95% CI 1.1–2.9). The benefit of adding RT to first and second generation TKI must be further explored given the positive results of third generation EGFR TKIs [115]. Several studies in which both PFS and OS benefits were retrospectively [116,117] and prospectively [118] reported, suggesting that local SBRT should be further evaluated in large scale RCTs. SBRT has seen a growing interest for oligoprogressive patients under TKIs [119,120]. Available data remain scarce in this situation [121]. The results of several trials are, however, awaited (NCT01573702; NCT02450591).

4.3. Ongoing Trials for Oligometastatic NSCLC Patients

The SARON trial [122] (NCT02417662) is a randomized phase III trial focusing on patients with oligometastatic EGFR, ALK and ROS1 mutation negative NSCLC; the oligometastatic state being defined by the presence of one to three sites of synchronous metastatic disease, among which one must be extracranial. While the control arm is a standard platinum-doublet chemotherapy, the investigational arm will evaluate the benefit of delivering RT to the primary and then the metastatic sites. With 340 awaited patients, the main drawback will be a comparison with a chemotherapy-only based treatment and not a chemo-immunotherapy one. Focusing on a similar clinical setting, the TRAILOCLORI trial (NCT05111197) will evaluate the benefit of stereotactic radiotherapy to oligopersistent sites in NSCLC patients, the disease controlled with long-term immunotherapy. With a more aggressive approach, the CHESS trial (NCT03965468) will evaluate the benefits of a multidisciplinary approach combining PD-L1 inhibitor and chemotherapy as well as SBRT to all metastatic lesions. If there is no disease progression at 3 months, normofractionated radiotherapy will be delivered to the primary tumor while continuing the PD-L1 inhibitor.

With a similar approach but focusing on the primary, the PRIME-LUNG (NCT05222087) will evaluate the benefits of upfront SBRT to the primary in combination with chemo-immunotherapy, compared to chemo-immunotherapy alone as a first-line treatment for de novo stage IV NSCLC patients.

The NIRVANA trial (NCT03774732) is a phase III trial evaluating the benefits of localized radiotherapy (conformational or stereotactic radiotherapy) to the primitive or metastatic lesions in patients treated with a PD-1 inhibitor and concomitant chemotherapy for a stage IV NSCLC.

The LONESTAR trial (NCT03391869) is an ongoing phase III randomized trial evaluating the benefit of local consolidative treatment (LCT) in EGFR/ALK negative NSCLC patients treated with nivolumab + ipilimumab. Of note, the LCT could either be radiotherapy or surgery.

Similar studies are also being conducted in EGFR/ALK/ROS1-mutated patients. In the NORTHSTAR trial (NCT03410043), patients treated with frontline osimertinib are randomized between osimertinib alone vs. osimertinib + consolidation treatment to as many sites as feasible; the primary endpoint being the PFS.

Irrespective of the histology or the mutational status, the SABR-COMET 3 (NCT03862911 and SABR-COMET 10 (NCT03721341) trials are phase III comparing standard of care vs. standard of care + SBRT in patients with, respectively, up to 3 or 10 metastases. These trials and several other trials are further detailed in Table 6 giving an overview of ongoing prospective trials.

Table 6. Overview of currently ongoing prospective trials in metastatic NSCLC patients, irrespective of the mutational status.

NCT	Clinical Setting	Definition of the Oligometastatic Stage	Study Type	Interventional Arm	Control Arm	Primary Endpoint
NCT03965468	Synchronous oligometastatic and not-mutated NSCLC	≤3 distant metastases One metastasis must be extra-cerebral	Phase II single arm	First phase: PD-L1 inhibitor (durvalumab)Carboplatin + paclitaxelSBRT to all oligometastatic lesions Restaging at 3 months: if no progression, normofractionated to the primary	No control arm	12 months PFS
NCT05278052	Synchronous oligometastatic and not-mutated NSCLC	1–5 metastatic sites ≤3 metastases per organ	Phase III	Standard maintenance therapy + Local RT to all oligometastatic sites including the primary loco-regional disease	Standard maintenance therapy	OS
NCT03391869	Metastatic and not-mutated NSCLC	Not restricted to oligometastatic NSCLC	Phase III	Nivolumab + ipilimumab + local treatment of the primary (surgery of RT) after 2 cycles of immunotherapy	Nivolumab + Ipilimumab	OS
NCT05222087	Metastatic and not-mutated NSCLC	Not restricted to oligometastatic NSCLC	Phase II/III	First-line chemo-immunotherapy +/- SBRT to the primary	Chemo-immunotherapy	OS
NCT02417662	Synchronous oligometastatic and not-mutated NSCLC	1–5 metastatic sites ≤3 metastases per organ	Phase III	Platinum-doublet chemotherapy + RT to the primary and the metastatic sites	Platinum-doublet chemotherapy	OS
NCT03774732	Advanced and not-mutated NSCLC	Not restricted to oligometastatic NSCLC	Phase III	Pembrolizumab + chemotherapy + RT to the primary and the metastatic sites	Pembrolizumab + chemotherapy	OS
NCT04908956	Synchronous oligometastatic and EGFR mutated NSCLC	1–5 metastatic sites	Phase II single arm	Osimertinib + SBRT to the primary tumor and all metastatic sites	No control arm	Safety
NCT05277844	Synchronous oligometastatic and EGFR mutated NSCLC	1–5 metastatic sites ≤3 metastases per organ	Randomized phase II	TKI + SBRT to the primary tumor and all metastatic sites	TKI alone	PFS
NCT03410043	Advanced and EGFR mutated NSCLC	Not restricted to oligometastatic NSCLC	Randomized phase II	Osimertinib + Local treatment (Surgery or RT) to the primary and/or metastatic sites	Osimertinib	PFS

Table 6. Cont.

NCT	Clinical Setting	Definition of the Oligometastatic Stage	Study Type	Interventional Arm	Control Arm	Primary Endpoint
NCT03705403	Oligometastatic NSCLC	1–5 metastatic sites ≤2 brain metastases	Randomized phase II	RT to all metastatic sites + immunocytokine L19-IL2 (darleukin)	Standard of care: systemic treatment or local treatment (RT or surgery) or wait and see	PFS
NCT05111197	Oligopersistent and not-mutated EGFR	1–5 metastatic sites ≤3 brain metastases	Randomized phase III	PD-1 or PD-L1 inhibitor + SBRT to metastatic and persistent sites	PD-1 or PD-L1 inhibitor	OS
NCT03822577	Oligopersistent or oligorecurrent with controlled primary	1–3 metastatic sites	Randomized phase III	Standard medical treatment + LAT (SBRT, RFA or surgery)	Standard medical treatment	OS
NCT03862911	Oligopersistent or oligorecurrent with controlled primary	1–3 metastatic sites	Randomized phase III	Standard medical treatment + SBRT to metastatic and persistent sites	Standard medical treatment	OS
NCT03721341	Oligopersistent or oligorecurrent with controlled primary	4–10 metastatic sites	Randomized phase III	Standard medical treatment + SBRT to metastatic and persistent sites	Standard medical treatment	OS
NCT03137771	Metastatic NSCLC stable under standard medical treatment	Not restricted to oligometastatic NSCLC	Randomized phase II/III	Maintenance therapy + SBRT/RT to a single extracranial site	Maintenance therapy	Phase II: PFS Phase III: OS
NCT03256981	Oligoprogressive mutated EGFR	1–3 oligoprogressive sites	Randomized II	Continued TKI therapy + SBRT	Continued TKI therapy	PFS
NCT04405401	Oligoprogression on ICI or TKI	1–5 metastatic sites	Randomized II	Continued therapy + SBRT	Standard medical treatment	PFS/OS
NCT02756793	Oligoprogressive NSCLC	1–5 metastatic sites	Randomized II	Continued therapy + SBRT	Standard medical treatment	PFS

Abbreviations: NCT—National Clinical Trial number, NSCLC—non-small cell lung cancer, PD-L1—programmed death ligand 1, SBRT—stereotactic body radiotherapy, PFS—progression-free survival, RT—radiotherapy, OS—overall survival, TKI—tyrosine kinase inhibitor, LAT—local ablative therapy, RFA—radiofrequency ablation, ICI—immune checkpoint inhibitor.

Prospective and phase III data supporting the OS benefit of local consolidative radiotherapy in the NSCLC setting remain scarce but tend to favor RT with a low and acceptable toxicity profile. This therapeutic approach remains currently evaluated in several ongoing phase II/III trials and should be offered to patients within clinical trials.

5. Conclusions

Despite many retrospective and prospective studies, the local treatment of synchronous metastatic cancer by irradiation of the primary disease for breast or non-small cell lung cancer has not yet been validated as a standard of care. Trials are underway to justify the survival benefit. The challenge will be to determine the group of patients who can benefit from it. In the meantime, the indications must be discussed on a case-by-case basis in a multidisciplinary consultation meeting. In the case of metastatic oligometastatic prostate cancer, the indication for radiotherapy of the primary site has demonstrated a significant increase in overall survival and progression-free survival and is now considered as a standard of care. This indication will be reinforced by ongoing trials. The combination of local treatment of the primary tumor and all metastatic lesions by stereotactic irradiation, particularly in the case of oligometastatic cancer, seems to be an interesting strategy while awaiting the results of the many ongoing trials on this subject.

Author Contributions: Conceptualization, Y.G., A.L. (Adrien Laville) and V.B.; methodology, Y.G., A.L. (Adrien Laville) and V.B.; validation, Y.G., A.L. (Adrien Laville) and V.B.; formal analysis, Y.G., A.L. (Adrien Laville) and V.B.; data curation, Y.G., A.L. (Adrien Laville) and V.B.; writing—original draft preparation, Y.G., A.L., (Adrien Laville) V.B. and Y.Z.; writing—review and editing, Y.G., A.L. (Adrien Laville), V.B., Y.Z., Y.K., A.L. (Antonin Levy) and I.L.; visualization, V.B.; supervision, Y.K., A.L. (Antonin Levy) and I.L.; project administration, Y.G. and V.B. All authors have read and agreed to the published version of the manuscript.

Funding: This research received no external funding.

Conflicts of Interest: The authors declare no conflict of interest.

References

1. Hölzel, D.; Eckel, R.; Bauerfeind, I.; Baier, B.; Beck, T.; Braun, M.; Ettl, J.; Hamann, U.; Kiechle, M.; Mahner, S.; et al. Improved Systemic Treatment for Early Breast Cancer Improves Cure Rates, Modifies Metastatic Pattern and Shortens Post-Metastatic Survival: 35-Year Results from the Munich Cancer Registry. *J. Cancer Res. Clin. Oncol.* **2017**, *143*, 1701–1712. [CrossRef] [PubMed]
2. Ryckman, J.M.; Thomas, T.V.; Wang, M.; Wu, X.; Siva, S.; Spratt, D.E.; Slotman, B.; Pal, S.; Chapin, B.F.; Fitzal, F.; et al. Local Treatment of the Primary Tumor for Patients With Metastatic Cancer (PRIME-TX): A Meta-Analysis. *Int. J. Radiat. Oncol. Biol. Phys.* **2022**, *114*, 919–935. [CrossRef] [PubMed]
3. Paget, S. The Distribution of Secondary Growths in Cancer of the Breast. *Cancer Metastasis Rev.* **1989**, *8*, 98–101. [CrossRef] [PubMed]
4. Kaplan, R.N.; Rafii, S.; Lyden, D. Preparing the "Soil": The Premetastatic Niche: Figure 1. *Cancer Res.* **2006**, *66*, 11089–11093. [CrossRef] [PubMed]
5. Kaplan, R.N.; Psaila, B.; Lyden, D. Bone Marrow Cells in the "Pre-Metastatic Niche": Within Bone and Beyond. *Cancer Metastasis Rev.* **2006**, *25*, 521–529. [CrossRef] [PubMed]
6. Akhtar, M.; Haider, A.; Rashid, S.; Al-Nabet, A.D.M.H. Paget's "Seed and Soil" Theory of Cancer Metastasis: An Idea Whose Time Has Come. *Adv. Anat. Pathol.* **2019**, *26*, 69–74. [CrossRef]
7. Weidle, U.H.; Birzele, F.; Kollmorgen, G.; Rüger, R. The Multiple Roles of Exosomes in Metastasis. *Cancer Genomics Proteomics* **2017**, *14*, 1–16. [CrossRef]
8. Théry, C.; Zitvogel, L.; Amigorena, S. Exosomes: Composition, Biogenesis and Function. *Nat. Rev. Immunol.* **2002**, *2*, 569–579. [CrossRef]
9. Rashed, M.H.; Bayraktar, E.; Helal, G.K.; Abd-Ellah, M.; Amero, P.; Chavez-Reyes, A.; Rodriguez-Aguayo, C. Exosomes: From Garbage Bins to Promising Therapeutic Targets. *Int. J. Mol. Sci.* **2017**, *18*, 538. [CrossRef]
10. Soung, Y.H.; Nguyen, T.; Cao, H.; Lee, J.; Chung, J. Emerging Roles of Exosomes in Cancer Invasion and Metastasis. *BMB Rep.* **2016**, *49*, 18–25. [CrossRef]
11. Kim, M.-Y.; Oskarsson, T.; Acharyya, S.; Nguyen, D.X.; Zhang, X.H.-F.; Norton, L.; Massagué, J. Tumor Self-Seeding by Circulating Cancer Cells. *Cell* **2009**, *139*, 1315–1326. [CrossRef] [PubMed]
12. Comen, E.; Norton, L.; Massagué, J. Clinical Implications of Cancer Self-Seeding. *Nat. Rev. Clin. Oncol.* **2011**, *8*, 369–377. [CrossRef]

13. Bockel, S.; Antoni, D.; Deutsch, É.; Mornex, F. Immunothérapie et radiothérapie. *Cancer/Radiothérapie* **2017**, *21*, 244–255. [CrossRef] [PubMed]
14. Gomez, D.R.; Tang, C.; Zhang, J.; Blumenschein, G.R.; Hernandez, M.; Lee, J.J.; Ye, R.; Palma, D.A.; Louie, A.V.; Camidge, D.R.; et al. Local Consolidative Therapy Vs. Maintenance Therapy or Observation for Patients With Oligometastatic Non-Small-Cell Lung Cancer: Long-Term Results of a Multi-Institutional, Phase II, Randomized Study. *J. Clin. Oncol. Off. J. Am. Soc. Clin. Oncol.* **2019**, *37*, 1558–1565. [CrossRef] [PubMed]
15. Harrow, S.; Palma, D.A.; Olson, R.; Gaede, S.; Louie, A.V.; Haasbeek, C.; Mulroy, L.; Lock, M.; Rodrigues, G.B.; Yaremko, B.P.; et al. Stereotactic Radiation for the Comprehensive Treatment of Oligometastases (SABR-COMET)–Extended Long-Term Outcomes. *Int. J. Radiat. Oncol.* **2022**, *114*, 611–616. [CrossRef]
16. Fairweather, M.; Jiang, W.; Keating, N.L.; Freedman, R.A.; King, T.A.; Nakhlis, F. Morbidity of Local Therapy for Locally Advanced Metastatic Breast Cancer: An Analysis of the Surveillance, Epidemiology, and End Results (SEER)–Medicare Registry. *Breast Cancer Res. Treat.* **2018**, *169*, 287–293. [CrossRef]
17. Khan, S.A.; Stewart, A.K.; Morrow, M. Does Aggressive Local Therapy Improve Survival in Metastatic Breast Cancer? *Surgery* **2002**, *132*, 620–627. [CrossRef]
18. Rapiti, E.; Verkooijen, H.M.; Vlastos, G.; Fioretta, G.; Neyroud-Caspar, I.; Sappino, A.P.; Chappuis, P.O.; Bouchardy, C. Complete Excision of Primary Breast Tumor Improves Survival of Patients With Metastatic Breast Cancer at Diagnosis. *J. Clin. Oncol.* **2006**, *24*, 2743–2749. [CrossRef]
19. Babiera, G.V.; Rao, R.; Feng, L.; Meric-Bernstam, F.; Kuerer, H.M.; Singletary, S.E.; Hunt, K.K.; Ross, M.I.; Gwyn, K.M.; Feig, B.W.; et al. Effect of Primary Tumor Extirpation in Breast Cancer Patients Who Present with Stage IV Disease and an Intact Primary Tumor. *Ann. Surg. Oncol.* **2006**, *13*, 776–782. [CrossRef]
20. Gnerlich, J.; Jeffe, D.B.; Deshpande, A.D.; Beers, C.; Zander, C.; Margenthaler, J.A. Surgical Removal of the Primary Tumor Increases Overall Survival in Patients with Metastatic Breast Cancer: Analysis of the 1988-2003 SEER Data. *Ann. Surg. Oncol.* **2007**, *14*, 2187–2194. [CrossRef]
21. Fields, R.C.; Jeffe, D.B.; Trinkaus, K.; Zhang, Q.; Arthur, C.; Aft, R.; Dietz, J.R.; Eberlein, T.J.; Gillanders, W.E.; Margenthaler, J.A. Surgical Resection of the Primary Tumor Is Associated with Increased Long-Term Survival in Patients with Stage IV Breast Cancer after Controlling for Site of Metastasis. *Ann. Surg. Oncol.* **2007**, *14*, 3345–3351. [CrossRef] [PubMed]
22. Hazard, H.W.; Gorla, S.R.; Scholtens, D.; Kiel, K.; Gradishar, W.J.; Khan, S.A. Surgical Resection of the Primary Tumor, Chest Wall Control, and Survival in Women with Metastatic Breast Cancer. *Cancer* **2008**, *113*, 2011–2019. [CrossRef] [PubMed]
23. Cady, B.; Nathan, N.R.; Michaelson, J.S.; Golshan, M.; Smith, B.L. Matched Pair Analyses of Stage IV Breast Cancer with or Without Resection of Primary Breast Site. *Ann. Surg. Oncol.* **2008**, *15*, 3384–3395. [CrossRef] [PubMed]
24. Bafford, A.C.; Burstein, H.J.; Barkley, C.R.; Smith, B.L.; Lipsitz, S.; Iglehart, J.D.; Winer, E.P.; Golshan, M. Breast Surgery in Stage IV Breast Cancer: Impact of Staging and Patient Selection on Overall Survival. *Breast Cancer Res. Treat.* **2009**, *115*, 7–12. [CrossRef] [PubMed]
25. Blanchard, D.K.; Shetty, P.B.; Hilsenbeck, S.G.; Elledge, R.M. Association of Surgery With Improved Survival in Stage IV Breast Cancer Patients. *Ann. Surg.* **2008**, *247*, 732–738. [CrossRef]
26. Ruiterkamp, J.; Ernst, M.F.; van de Poll-Franse, L.V.; Bosscha, K.; Tjan-Heijnen, V.C.G.; Voogd, A.C. Surgical Resection of the Primary Tumour Is Associated with Improved Survival in Patients with Distant Metastatic Breast Cancer at Diagnosis. *Eur. J. Surg. Oncol. J. Eur. Soc. Surg. Oncol. Br. Assoc. Surg. Oncol.* **2009**, *35*, 1146–1151. [CrossRef] [PubMed]
27. Shien, T.; Kinoshita, T.; Shimizu, C.; Hojo, T.; Taira, N.; Doihara, H.; Akashi-Tanaka, S. Primary Tumor Resection Improves the Survival of Younger Patients with Metastatic Breast Cancer. *Oncol. Rep.* **2009**, *21*, 827–832. [CrossRef]
28. Neuman, H.B.; Morrogh, M.; Gonen, M.; Van Zee, K.J.; Morrow, M.; King, T.A. Stage IV Breast Cancer in the Era of Targeted Therapy: Does Surgery of the Primary Tumor Matter? *Cancer* **2010**, *116*, 1226–1233. [CrossRef]
29. Nguyen, D.H.A.; Truong, P.T.; Alexander, C.; Walter, C.V.; Hayashi, E.; Christie, J.; Lesperance, M. Can Locoregional Treatment of the Primary Tumor Improve Outcomes for Women with Stage IV Breast Cancer at Diagnosis? *Int. J. Radiat. Oncol. Biol. Phys.* **2012**, *84*, 39–45. [CrossRef]
30. Lang, J.E.; Tereffe, W.; Mitchell, M.P.; Rao, R.; Feng, L.; Meric-Bernstam, F.; Bedrosian, I.; Kuerer, H.M.; Hunt, K.K.; Hortobagyi, G.N.; et al. Primary Tumor Extirpation in Breast Cancer Patients Who Present with Stage IV Disease Is Associated with Improved Survival. *Ann. Surg. Oncol.* **2013**, *20*, 1893–1899. [CrossRef]
31. Thomas, A.; Khan, S.A.; Chrischilles, E.A.; Schroeder, M.C. Initial Surgery and Survival in Stage IV Breast Cancer in the United States, 1988-2011. *JAMA Surg.* **2016**, *151*, 424–431. [CrossRef]
32. Choi, S.H.; Kim, J.W.; Choi, J.; Sohn, J.; Kim, S.I.; Park, S.; Park, H.S.; Jeong, J.; Suh, C.-O.; Keum, K.C.; et al. Locoregional Treatment of the Primary Tumor in Patients With De Novo Stage IV Breast Cancer: A Radiation Oncologist's Perspective. *Clin. Breast Cancer* **2018**, *18*, e167–e178. [CrossRef] [PubMed]
33. Le Scodan, R.; Stevens, D.; Brain, E.; Floiras, J.L.; Cohen-Solal, C.; De La Lande, B.; Tubiana-Hulin, M.; Yacoub, S.; Gutierrez, M.; Ali, D.; et al. Breast Cancer With Synchronous Metastases: Survival Impact of Exclusive Locoregional Radiotherapy. *J. Clin. Oncol.* **2009**, *27*, 1375–1381. [CrossRef]
34. Bourgier, C.; Khodari, W.; Vataire, A.-L.; Pessoa, E.L.; Dunant, A.; Delaloge, S.; Uzan, C.; Balleyguier, C.; Mathieu, M.-C.; Marsiglia, H.; et al. Breast Radiotherapy as Part of Loco-Regional Treatments in Stage IV Breast Cancer Patients with Oligometastatic Disease. *Radiother. Oncol.* **2010**, *96*, 199–203. [CrossRef] [PubMed]

35. Mauro, G.P.; de Andrade Carvalho, H.; Stuart, S.R.; Mano, M.S.; Marta, G.N. Effects of Locoregional Radiotherapy in Patients with Metastatic Breast Cancer. *Breast Edinb. Scotl.* **2016**, *28*, 73–78. [CrossRef] [PubMed]
36. Pons-Tostivint, E.; Kirova, Y.; Lusque, A.; Campone, M.; Geffrelot, J.; Rivera, S.; Mailliez, A.; Pasquier, D.; Madranges, N.; Firmin, N.; et al. Radiation Therapy to the Primary Tumor for de Novo Metastatic Breast Cancer and Overall Survival in a Retrospective Multicenter Cohort Analysis. *Radiother. Oncol. J. Eur. Soc. Ther. Radiol. Oncol.* **2020**, *145*, 109–116. [CrossRef]
37. Stahl, K.; Wong, W.; Dodge, D.; Brooks, A.; McLaughlin, C.; Olecki, E.; Lewcun, J.; Newport, K.; Vasekar, M.; Shen, C. Benefits of Surgical Treatment of Stage IV Breast Cancer for Patients With Known Hormone Receptor and HER2 Status. *Ann. Surg. Oncol.* **2021**, *28*, 2646–2658. [CrossRef]
38. Thery, L.; Arsene-Henry, A.; Carroll, S.; Peurien, D.; Bazire, L.; Robilliard, M.; Fourquet, A.; Kirova, Y.M. Use of Helical Tomotherapy in Locally Advanced and/or Metastatic Breast Cancer for Locoregional Treatment. *Br. J. Radiol.* **2018**, *91*, 20170822. [CrossRef]
39. Ali, A.; Hoyle, A.; Haran, Á.M.; Brawley, C.D.; Cook, A.; Amos, C.; Calvert, J.; Douis, H.; Mason, M.D.; Dearnaley, D.; et al. Association of Bone Metastatic Burden with Survival Benefit from Prostate Radiotherapy in Patients with Newly Diagnosed Metastatic Prostate Cancer: A Secondary Analysis of a Randomized Clinical Trial. *JAMA Oncol.* **2021**, *7*, 555–563. [CrossRef]
40. Xiao, W.; Zou, Y.; Zheng, S.; Hu, X.; Liu, P.; Xie, X.; Yu, P.; Tang, H.; Xie, X. Primary Tumor Resection in Stage IV Breast Cancer: A Systematic Review and Meta-Analysis. *Eur. J. Surg. Oncol.* **2018**, *44*, 1504–1512. [CrossRef]
41. Gera, R.; Chehade, H.E.L.H.; Wazir, U.; Tayeh, S.; Kasem, A.; Mokbel, K. Locoregional Therapy of the Primary Tumour in de Novo Stage IV Breast Cancer in 216 066 Patients: A Meta-Analysis. *Sci. Rep.* **2020**, *10*, 2952. [CrossRef]
42. Khodari, W.; Sedrati, A.; Naisse, I.; Bosc, R.; Belkacemi, Y. Impact of Loco-Regional Treatment on Metastatic Breast Cancer Outcome: A Review. *Crit. Rev. Oncol. Hematol.* **2013**, *87*, 69–79. [CrossRef] [PubMed]
43. Badwe, R.; Hawaldar, R.; Nair, N.; Kaushik, S.; Parmar, V.; Siddique, S.; Budrukkar, A.; Mittra, I.; Gupta, S. Locoregional Treatment versus No Treatment of the Primary Tumour in Metastatic Breast Cancer: An Open-Label Randomised Controlled Trial. *Lancet Oncol.* **2015**, *16*, 1380–1388. [CrossRef] [PubMed]
44. Soran, A.; Ozmen, V.; Ozbas, S.; Karanlik, H.; Muslumanoglu, M.; Igci, A.; Canturk, Z.; Utkan, Z.; Ozaslan, C.; Evrensel, T.; et al. Randomized Trial Comparing Resection of Primary Tumor with No Surgery in Stage IV Breast Cancer at Presentation: Protocol MF07-01. *Ann. Surg. Oncol.* **2018**, *25*, 3141–3149. [CrossRef] [PubMed]
45. Khan, S.A.; Zhao, F.; Goldstein, L.J.; Cella, D.; Basik, M.; Golshan, M.; Julian, T.B.; Pockaj, B.A.; Lee, C.A.; Razaq, W.; et al. Early Local Therapy for the Primary Site in De Novo Stage IV Breast Cancer: Results of a Randomized Clinical Trial (E2108). *J. Clin. Oncol.* **2022**, *40*, 978–987. [CrossRef]
46. Shien, T.; Mizutani, T.; Tanaka, K.; Kinoshita, T.; Hara, F.; Fujisawa, N.; Masuda, N.; Tamura, K.; Hojo, T.; Kanbayashi, C.; et al. A Randomized Controlled Trial Comparing Primary Tumor Resection plus Systemic Therapy with Systemic Therapy Alone in Metastatic Breast Cancer (JCOG1017 PRIM-BC). *J. Clin. Oncol.* **2017**, *35*, TPS588. [CrossRef]
47. Fitzal, F.; Bjelic-Radisic, V.; Knauer, M.; Steger, G.; Hubalek, M.; Balic, M.; Singer, C.; Bartsch, R.; Schrenk, P.; Soelkner, L.; et al. Impact of Breast Surgery in Primary Metastasized Breast Cancer: Outcomes of the Prospective Randomized Phase III ABCSG-28 POSYTIVE Trial. *Ann. Surg.* **2019**, *269*, 1163–1169. [CrossRef]
48. Beddok, A.; Xu, H.P.; Henry, A.A.; Porte, B.; Fourquet, A.; Cottu, P.; Kirova, Y. Concurrent Use of Palbociclib and Radiation Therapy: Single-Centre Experience and Review of the Literature. *Br. J. Cancer* **2020**, *123*, 905–908. [CrossRef]
49. Loap, P.; Loirat, D.; Berger, F.; Cao, K.; Ricci, F.; Jochem, A.; Raizonville, L.; Mosseri, V.; Fourquet, A.; Kirova, Y. Combination of Olaparib with Radiotherapy for Triple-negative Breast Cancers: One-year Toxicity Report of the RADIOPARP Phase I Trial. *Int. J. Cancer* **2021**, *149*, 1828–1832. [CrossRef]
50. Zolcsák, Z.; Loirat, D.; Fourquet, A.; Kirova, Y.M. Adjuvant Trastuzumab Emtansine (T-DM1) and Concurrent Radiotherapy for Residual Invasive HER2-Positive Breast Cancer: Single-Center Preliminary Results. *Am. J. Clin. Oncol.* **2020**, *43*, 895–901. [CrossRef]
51. Culp, S.H.; Schellhammer, P.F.; Williams, M.B. Might Men Diagnosed with Metastatic Prostate Cancer Benefit from Definitive Treatment of the Primary Tumor? A SEER-Based Study. *Eur. Urol.* **2014**, *65*, 1058–1066. [CrossRef]
52. Fossati, N.; Trinh, Q.-D.; Sammon, J.; Sood, A.; Larcher, A.; Sun, M.; Karakiewicz, P.; Guazzoni, G.; Montorsi, F.; Briganti, A.; et al. Identifying Optimal Candidates for Local Treatment of the Primary Tumor among Patients Diagnosed with Metastatic Prostate Cancer: A SEER-Based Study. *Eur. Urol.* **2015**, *67*, 3–6. [CrossRef]
53. Rusthoven, C.G.; Jones, B.L.; Flaig, T.W.; Crawford, E.D.; Koshy, M.; Sher, D.J.; Mahmood, U.; Chen, R.C.; Chapin, B.F.; Kavanagh, B.D.; et al. Improved Survival With Prostate Radiation in Addition to Androgen Deprivation Therapy for Men With Newly Diagnosed Metastatic Prostate Cancer. *J. Clin. Oncol. Off. J. Am. Soc. Clin. Oncol.* **2016**, *34*, 2835–2842. [CrossRef] [PubMed]
54. Löppenberg, B.; Dalela, D.; Karabon, P.; Sood, A.; Sammon, J.D.; Meyer, C.P.; Sun, M.; Noldus, J.; Peabody, J.O.; Trinh, Q.-D.; et al. The Impact of Local Treatment on Overall Survival in Patients with Metastatic Prostate Cancer on Diagnosis: A National Cancer Data Base Analysis. *Eur. Urol.* **2017**, *72*, 14–19. [CrossRef] [PubMed]
55. Leyh-Bannurah, S.-R.; Gazdovich, S.; Budäus, L.; Zaffuto, E.; Briganti, A.; Abdollah, F.; Montorsi, F.; Schiffmann, J.; Menon, M.; Shariat, S.F.; et al. Local Therapy Improves Survival in Metastatic Prostate Cancer. *Eur. Urol.* **2017**, *72*, 118–124. [CrossRef] [PubMed]

56. Satkunasivam, R.; Kim, A.E.; Desai, M.; Nguyen, M.M.; Quinn, D.I.; Ballas, L.; Lewinger, J.P.; Stern, M.C.; Hamilton, A.S.; Aron, M.; et al. Radical Prostatectomy or External Beam Radiation Therapy vs No Local Therapy for Survival Benefit in Metastatic Prostate Cancer: A SEER-Medicare Analysis. *J. Urol.* **2015**, *194*, 378–385. [CrossRef]
57. Parikh, R.R.; Byun, J.; Goyal, S.; Kim, I.Y. Local Therapy Improves Overall Survival in Patients With Newly Diagnosed Metastatic Prostate Cancer. *Prostate* **2017**, *77*, 559–572. [CrossRef]
58. Cho, Y.; Chang, J.S.; Rha, K.H.; Hong, S.J.; Choi, Y.D.; Ham, W.S.; Kim, J.W.; Cho, J. Does Radiotherapy for the Primary Tumor Benefit Prostate Cancer Patients with Distant Metastasis at Initial Diagnosis? *PLoS ONE* **2016**, *11*, e0147191. [CrossRef]
59. Boevé, L.M.S.; Hulshof, M.C.C.M.; Vis, A.N.; Zwinderman, A.H.; Twisk, J.W.R.; Witjes, W.P.J.; Delaere, K.P.J.; van Moorselaar, R.J.A.; Verhagen, P.C.M.S.; van Andel, G. Effect on Survival of Androgen Deprivation Therapy Alone Compared to Androgen Deprivation Therapy Combined with Concurrent Radiation Therapy to the Prostate in Patients with Primary Bone Metastatic Prostate Cancer in a Prospective Randomised Clinical Trial: Data from the HORRAD Trial. *Eur. Urol.* **2019**, *75*, 410–418. [CrossRef]
60. Boevé, L.; Hulshof, M.C.C.M.; Verhagen, P.C.M.S.; Twisk, J.W.R.; Witjes, W.P.J.; de Vries, P.; van Moorselaar, R.J.A.; van Andel, G.; Vis, A.N. Patient-Reported Quality of Life in Patients with Primary Metastatic Prostate Cancer Treated with Androgen Deprivation Therapy with and Without Concurrent Radiation Therapy to the Prostate in a Prospective Randomised Clinical Trial; Data from the HORRAD Trial. *Eur. Urol.* **2021**, *79*, 188–197. [CrossRef]
61. Parker, C.C.; James, N.D.; Brawley, C.D.; Clarke, N.W.; Hoyle, A.P.; Ali, A.; Ritchie, A.W.S.; Attard, G.; Chowdhury, S.; Cross, W.; et al. Radiotherapy to the Primary Tumour for Newly Diagnosed, Metastatic Prostate Cancer (STAMPEDE): A Randomised Controlled Phase 3 Trial. *Lancet* **2018**, *392*, 2353–2366. [CrossRef] [PubMed]
62. Burdett, S.; Boevé, L.M.; Ingleby, F.C.; Fisher, D.J.; Rydzewska, L.H.; Vale, C.L.; van Andel, G.; Clarke, N.W.; Hulshof, M.C.; James, N.D.; et al. Prostate Radiotherapy for Metastatic Hormone-Sensitive Prostate Cancer: A STOPCAP Systematic Review and Meta-Analysis. *Eur. Urol.* **2019**, *76*, 115–124. [CrossRef] [PubMed]
63. Barbato, F.; Fendler, W.P.; Rauscher, I.; Herrmann, K.; Wetter, A.; Ferdinandus, J.; Seifert, R.; Nader, M.; Rahbar, K.; Hadaschik, B.; et al. PSMA-PET for the Assessment of Metastatic Hormone-Sensitive Prostate Cancer Volume of Disease. *J. Nucl. Med. Off. Publ. Soc. Nucl. Med.* **2021**, *62*, 1747–1750. [CrossRef] [PubMed]
64. Fizazi, K.; Foulon, S.; Carles, J.; Roubaud, G.; McDermott, R.; Fléchon, A.; Tombal, B.; Supiot, S.; Berthold, D.; Ronchin, P.; et al. Abiraterone plus Prednisone Added to Androgen Deprivation Therapy and Docetaxel in de Novo Metastatic Castration-Sensitive Prostate Cancer (PEACE-1): A Multicentre, Open-Label, Randomised, Phase 3 Study with a 2 × 2 Factorial Design. *Lancet* **2022**, *399*, 1695–1707. [CrossRef] [PubMed]
65. UNICANCER. *A Prospective Randomised Phase III Study Of Androgen Deprivation Therapy with or without Docetaxel with or without Local Radiotherapy with or Without Abiraterone Acetate and Prednisone in Patients with Metastatic Hormone-Naïve Prostate Cancer*; Clinicaltrials.gov: Bethesda, MD, USA, 2021.
66. MD Anderson Cancer Center. *A Prospective, Multi-Institutional, Randomized, Phase II Trial of Best Systemic Therapy or Best Systemic Therapy (BST) Plus Definitive Treatment (Radiation or Surgery) of the Primary Tumor in Metastatic (M1) Prostate Cancer (PC)*; Clinicaltrials.gov: Bethesda, MD, USA, 2022.
67. Canadian Cancer Trials Group. *A Randomized Phase III Trial of Local Ablative Therapy for Hormone Sensitive Oligometastatic Prostate Cancer [PLATON]*; Clinicaltrials.gov: Bethesda, MD, USA, 2022.
68. University Hospital, Ghent. *Cytoreductive Prostatectomy versus Cytoreductive Prostate Irradiation as a Local Treatment Option for Metastatic Prostate Cancer: A Multicentric Feasibility Trial*; Clinicaltrials.gov: Bethesda, MD, USA, 2018.
69. Frobe, A. *Hormone Therapy with or without Definitive Radiotherapy in Metastatic Prostate Cancer*; Clinicaltrials.gov: Bethesda, MD, USA, 2018.
70. Imperial College London. *Local Cytoreductive Treatments for Men with Newly Diagnosed Metastatic Prostate Cancer in Addition to Standard of Care Treatment*; Clinicaltrials.gov: Bethesda, MD, USA, 2021.
71. Southwest Oncology Group. *Phase III Randomized Trial of Standard Systemic Therapy (SST) versus Standard Systemic Therapy Plus Definitive Treatment (Surgery or Radiation) of the Primary Tumor in Metastatic Prostate Cancer*; Clinicaltrials.gov: Bethesda, MD, USA, 2021.
72. UNICANCER. *Prostate-Cancer Treatment Using Stereotactic Radiotherapy for Oligometastases Ablation in Hormone-Sensitive Patients—A GETUG-AFU Phase III Randomized Controlled Trial*; Clinicaltrials.gov: Bethesda, MD, USA, 2022.
73. Memorial Sloan Kettering Cancer Center. *SAABR: Single Arm Phase II Study of Abiraterone + Atezolizumab + GnRH Analog and Stereotactic Body Radiotherapy (SBRT) to the Prostate in Men with Newly Diagnosed Hormone-Sensitive Metastatic Prostate Cancer*; Clinicaltrials.gov: Bethesda, MD, USA, 2022.
74. Mottet, N.; van den Bergh, R.C.N.; Briers, E.; Van den Broeck, T.; Cumberbatch, M.G.; De Santis, M.; Fanti, S.; Fossati, N.; Gandaglia, G.; Gillessen, S.; et al. EAU-EANM-ESTRO-ESUR-SIOG Guidelines on Prostate Cancer—2020 Update. Part 1: Screening, Diagnosis, and Local Treatment with Curative Intent. *Eur. Urol.* **2021**, *79*, 243–262. [CrossRef]
75. De Crevoisier, R.; Supiot, S.; Créhange, G.; Pommier, P.; Latorzeff, I.; Chapet, O.; Pasquier, D.; Blanchard, P.; Schick, U.; Marchesi, V.; et al. External Radiotherapy for Prostatic Cancers. *Cancer/Radiothérapie* **2022**, *26*, 329–343. [CrossRef] [PubMed]
76. Goldstraw, P.; Chansky, K.; Crowley, J.; Rami-Porta, R.; Asamura, H.; Eberhardt, W.E.E.; Nicholson, A.G.; Groome, P.; Mitchell, A.; Bolejack, V.; et al. The IASLC Lung Cancer Staging Project: Proposals for Revision of the TNM Stage Groupings in the Forthcoming (Eighth) Edition of the TNM Classification for Lung Cancer. *J. Thorac. Oncol. Off. Publ. Int. Assoc. Study Lung Cancer* **2016**, *11*, 39–51. [CrossRef]

77. Borghaei, H.; Langer, C.J.; Paz-Ares, L.; Rodríguez-Abreu, D.; Halmos, B.; Garassino, M.C.; Houghton, B.; Kurata, T.; Cheng, Y.; Lin, J.; et al. Pembrolizumab plus Chemotherapy versus Chemotherapy Alone in Patients with Advanced Non–Small Cell Lung Cancer without Tumor PD-L1 Expression: A Pooled Analysis of 3 Randomized Controlled Trials. *Cancer* **2020**, *126*, 4867–4877. [CrossRef] [PubMed]
78. Gandhi, L.; Rodríguez-Abreu, D.; Gadgeel, S.; Esteban, E.; Felip, E.; De Angelis, F.; Domine, M.; Clingan, P.; Hochmair, M.J.; Powell, S.F.; et al. Pembrolizumab plus Chemotherapy in Metastatic Non–Small-Cell Lung Cancer. *N. Engl. J. Med.* **2018**, *378*, 2078–2092. [CrossRef]
79. Borghaei, H.; Paz-Ares, L.; Horn, L.; Spigel, D.R.; Steins, M.; Ready, N.E.; Chow, L.Q.; Vokes, E.E.; Felip, E.; Holgado, E.; et al. Nivolumab versus Docetaxel in Advanced Nonsquamous Non–Small-Cell Lung Cancer. *N. Engl. J. Med.* **2015**, *373*, 1627–1639. [CrossRef] [PubMed]
80. Herbst, R.S.; Baas, P.; Kim, D.-W.; Felip, E.; Pérez-Gracia, J.L.; Han, J.-Y.; Molina, J.; Kim, J.-H.; Arvis, C.D.; Ahn, M.-J.; et al. Pembrolizumab versus Docetaxel for Previously Treated, PD-L1-Positive, Advanced Non-Small-Cell Lung Cancer (KEYNOTE-010): A Randomised Controlled Trial. *Lancet* **2016**, *387*, 1540–1550. [CrossRef] [PubMed]
81. Remon, J.; Steuer, C.E.; Ramalingam, S.S.; Felip, E. Osimertinib and Other Third-Generation EGFR TKI in EGFR-Mutant NSCLC Patients. *Ann. Oncol. Off. J. Eur. Soc. Med. Oncol.* **2018**, *29*, i20–i27. [CrossRef]
82. Wu, Y.-L.; Zhou, C.; Liam, C.-K.; Wu, G.; Liu, X.; Zhong, Z.; Lu, S.; Cheng, Y.; Han, B.; Chen, L.; et al. First-Line Erlotinib versus Gemcitabine/Cisplatin in Patients with Advanced EGFR Mutation-Positive Non-Small-Cell Lung Cancer: Analyses from the Phase III, Randomized, Open-Label, ENSURE Study. *Ann. Oncol. Off. J. Eur. Soc. Med. Oncol.* **2015**, *26*, 1883–1889. [CrossRef] [PubMed]
83. Yang, Z.; Hackshaw, A.; Feng, Q.; Fu, X.; Zhang, Y.; Mao, C.; Tang, J. Comparison of Gefitinib, Erlotinib and Afatinib in Non-Small Cell Lung Cancer: A Meta-Analysis. *Int. J. Cancer* **2017**, *140*, 2805–2819. [CrossRef] [PubMed]
84. Shaw, A.T.; Bauer, T.M.; de Marinis, F.; Felip, E.; Goto, Y.; Liu, G.; Mazieres, J.; Kim, D.-W.; Mok, T.; Polli, A.; et al. First-Line Lorlatinib or Crizotinib in Advanced ALK-Positive Lung Cancer. *N. Engl. J. Med.* **2020**, *383*, 2018–2029. [CrossRef]
85. Camidge, D.R.; Kim, H.R.; Ahn, M.-J.; Yang, J.C.-H.; Han, J.-Y.; Lee, J.-S.; Hochmair, M.J.; Li, J.Y.-C.; Chang, G.-C.; Lee, K.H.; et al. Brigatinib versus Crizotinib in ALK-Positive Non-Small-Cell Lung Cancer. *N. Engl. J. Med.* **2018**, *379*, 2027–2039. [CrossRef]
86. Guckenberger, M.; Lievens, Y.; Bouma, A.B.; Collette, L.; Dekker, A.; deSouza, N.M.; Dingemans, A.-M.C.; Fournier, B.; Hurkmans, C.; Lecouvet, F.E.; et al. Characterisation and Classification of Oligometastatic Disease: A European Society for Radiotherapy and Oncology and European Organisation for Research and Treatment of Cancer Consensus Recommendation. *Lancet Oncol.* **2020**, *21*, e18–e28. [CrossRef]
87. Giraud, N.; Abdiche, S.; Trouette, R. Stereotactic Radiotherapy in Targeted Therapy Treated Oligo-Metastatic Oncogene-Addicted (Non-Small-Cell) Lung Cancer. *Cancer Radiother. J. Soc. Francaise Radiother. Oncol.* **2019**, *23*, 346–354. [CrossRef]
88. Al-Halabi, H.; Sayegh, K.; Digamurthy, S.R.; Niemierko, A.; Piotrowska, Z.; Willers, H.; Sequist, L.V. Pattern of Failure Analysis in Metastatic EGFR-Mutant Lung Cancer Treated with Tyrosine Kinase Inhibitors to Identify Candidates for Consolidation Stereotactic Body Radiation Therapy. *J. Thorac. Oncol. Off. Publ. Int. Assoc. Study Lung Cancer* **2015**, *10*, 1601–1607. [CrossRef]
89. Slotman, B.J.; van Tinteren, H.; Praag, J.O.; Knegjens, J.L.; El Sharouni, S.Y.; Hatton, M.; Keijser, A.; Faivre-Finn, C.; Senan, S. Use of Thoracic Radiotherapy for Extensive Stage Small-Cell Lung Cancer: A Phase 3 Randomised Controlled Trial. *Lancet Lond. Engl.* **2015**, *385*, 36–42. [CrossRef]
90. Ettinger, D.S.; Wood, D.E.; Aisner, D.L.; Akerley, W.; Bauman, J.R.; Bharat, A.; Bruno, D.S.; Chang, J.Y.; Chirieac, L.R.; D'Amico, T.A.; et al. NCCN Guidelines Insights: Non-Small Cell Lung Cancer, Version 2.2021. *J. Natl. Compr. Cancer Netw. JNCCN* **2021**, *19*, 254–266. [CrossRef]
91. Topkan, E.; Yildirim, B.A.; Guler, O.C.; Parlak, C.; Pehlivan, B.; Selek, U. Safety and Palliative Efficacy of Single-Dose 8-Gy Reirradiation for Painful Local Failure in Patients with Stage IV Non-Small Cell Lung Cancer Previously Treated with Radical Chemoradiation Therapy. *Int. J. Radiat. Oncol. Biol. Phys.* **2015**, *91*, 774–780. [CrossRef]
92. Lupattelli, M.; Maranzano, E.; Bellavita, R.; Chionne, F.; Darwish, S.; Piro, F.; Latini, P. Short-Course Palliative Radiotherapy in Non-Small-Cell Lung Cancer: Results of a Prospective Study. *Am. J. Clin. Oncol.* **2000**, *23*, 89–93. [CrossRef] [PubMed]
93. Zhou, Y.; Yu, F.; Zhao, Y.; Zeng, Y.; Yang, X.; Chu, L.; Chu, X.; Li, Y.; Zou, L.; Guo, T.; et al. A Narrative Review of Evolving Roles of Radiotherapy in Advanced Non-Small Cell Lung Cancer: From Palliative Care to Active Player. *Transl. Lung Cancer Res.* **2020**, *9*, 2479–2493. [CrossRef] [PubMed]
94. Levy, A.; Roux, C.; Mercier, O.; Issard, J.; Botticella, A.; Barlesi, F.; Le Péchoux, C. Radiotherapy for oligometastatic non-small cell lung cancer patients. *Cancer/Radiothérapie* **2021**, *25*, 517–522. [CrossRef] [PubMed]
95. De Ruysscher, D.; Wanders, R.; van Baardwijk, A.; Dingemans, A.-M.C.; Reymen, B.; Houben, R.; Bootsma, G.; Pitz, C.; van Eijsden, L.; Geraedts, W.; et al. Radical Treatment of Non-Small-Cell Lung Cancer Patients with Synchronous Oligometastases: Long-Term Results of a Prospective Phase II Trial (Nct01282450). *J. Thorac. Oncol. Off. Publ. Int. Assoc. Study Lung Cancer* **2012**, *7*, 1547–1555. [CrossRef]
96. Collen, C.; Christian, N.; Schallier, D.; Meysman, M.; Duchateau, M.; Storme, G.; De Ridder, M. Phase II Study of Stereotactic Body Radiotherapy to Primary Tumor and Metastatic Locations in Oligometastatic Nonsmall-Cell Lung Cancer Patients. *Ann. Oncol. Off. J. Eur. Soc. Med. Oncol.* **2014**, *25*, 1954–1959. [CrossRef] [PubMed]

97. Petty, W.J.; Urbanic, J.J.; Ahmed, T.; Hughes, R.; Levine, B.; Rusthoven, K.; Papagikos, M.; Ruiz, J.R.; Lally, B.E.; Chan, M.; et al. Long-Term Outcomes of a Phase 2 Trial of Chemotherapy With Consolidative Radiation Therapy for Oligometastatic Non-Small Cell Lung Cancer. *Int. J. Radiat. Oncol. Biol. Phys.* **2018**, *102*, 527–535. [CrossRef] [PubMed]
98. Arrieta, O.; Barrón, F.; Maldonado, F.; Cabrera, L.; Corona-Cruz, J.F.; Blake, M.; Ramírez-Tirado, L.A.; Zatarain-Barrón, Z.L.; Cardona, A.F.; García, O.; et al. Radical Consolidative Treatment Provides a Clinical Benefit and Long-Term Survival in Patients with Synchronous Oligometastatic Non-Small Cell Lung Cancer: A Phase II Study. *Lung Cancer Amst. Neth.* **2019**, *130*, 67–75. [CrossRef]
99. Park, K.; Ahn, M.; Yu, C.; Kim, S.; Lin, M.; Sriuranpong, V.; Tsai, C.; Lee, J.; Kang, J.; Perez-Moreno, P.; et al. Aspiration: First-Line Erlotinib (E) Until and Beyond Recist Progression (Pd) in Asian Patients (Pts) with Egfr Mutation-Positive (Mut+) Nsclc. *Ann. Oncol.* **2014**, *25*, iv426. [CrossRef]
100. Parikh, R.B.; Cronin, A.M.; Kozono, D.E.; Oxnard, G.R.; Mak, R.H.; Jackman, D.M.; Lo, P.C.; Baldini, E.H.; Johnson, B.E.; Chen, A.B. Definitive Primary Therapy in Patients Presenting with Oligometastatic Non-Small Cell Lung Cancer. *Int. J. Radiat. Oncol. Biol. Phys.* **2014**, *89*, 880–887. [CrossRef]
101. Li, D.; Zhu, X.; Wang, H.; Qiu, M.; Li, N. Should Aggressive Thoracic Therapy Be Performed in Patients with Synchronous Oligometastatic Non-Small Cell Lung Cancer? A Meta-Analysis. *J. Thorac. Dis.* **2017**, *9*, 310–317. [CrossRef]
102. Petrelli, F.; Ghidini, A.; Cabiddu, M.; Tomasello, G.; De Stefani, A.; Bruschieri, L.; Vitali, E.; Ghilardi, M.; Borgonovo, K.; Barni, S.; et al. Addition of Radiotherapy to the Primary Tumour in Oligometastatic NSCLC: A Systematic Review and Meta-Analysis. *Lung Cancer Amst. Neth.* **2018**, *126*, 194–200. [CrossRef]
103. Kagawa, Y.; Furuta, H.; Uemura, T.; Watanabe, N.; Shimizu, J.; Horio, Y.; Kuroda, H.; Inaba, Y.; Kodaira, T.; Masago, K.; et al. Efficacy of Local Therapy for Oligoprogressive Disease after Programmed Cell Death 1 Blockade in Advanced Non-Small Cell Lung Cancer. *Cancer Sci.* **2020**, *111*, 4442–4452. [CrossRef] [PubMed]
104. Gomez, D.R.; Blumenschein, G.R.; Lee, J.J.; Hernandez, M.; Ye, R.; Camidge, D.R.; Doebele, R.C.; Skoulidis, F.; Gaspar, L.E.; Gibbons, D.L.; et al. Local Consolidative Therapy versus Maintenance Therapy or Observation for Patients with Oligometastatic Non-Small-Cell Lung Cancer without Progression after First-Line Systemic Therapy: A Multicentre, Randomised, Controlled, Phase 2 Study. *Lancet Oncol.* **2016**, *17*, 1672–1682. [CrossRef] [PubMed]
105. Bauml, J.M.; Mick, R.; Ciunci, C.; Aggarwal, C.; Davis, C.; Evans, T.; Deshpande, C.; Miller, L.; Patel, P.; Alley, E.; et al. Pembrolizumab After Completion of Locally Ablative Therapy for Oligometastatic Non-Small Cell Lung Cancer: A Phase 2 Trial. *JAMA Oncol.* **2019**, *5*, 1283–1290. [CrossRef] [PubMed]
106. Palma, D.A.; Olson, R.; Harrow, S.; Gaede, S.; Louie, A.V.; Haasbeek, C.; Mulroy, L.; Lock, M.; Rodrigues, G.B.; Yaremko, B.P.; et al. Stereotactic Ablative Radiotherapy for the Comprehensive Treatment of Oligometastatic Cancers: Long-Term Results of the SABR-COMET Phase II Randomized Trial. *J. Clin. Oncol.* **2020**, *38*, 2830–2838. [CrossRef]
107. Iyengar, P.; Wardak, Z.; Gerber, D.E.; Tumati, V.; Ahn, C.; Hughes, R.S.; Dowell, J.E.; Cheedella, N.; Nedzi, L.; Westover, K.D.; et al. Consolidative Radiotherapy for Limited Metastatic Non-Small-Cell Lung Cancer: A Phase 2 Randomized Clinical Trial. *JAMA Oncol.* **2018**, *4*, e173501. [CrossRef]
108. Wang, X.; Zeng, Z.; Cai, J.; Xu, P.; Liang, P.; Luo, Y.; Liu, A. Efficacy and Acquired Resistance for EGFR-TKI plus Thoracic SBRT in Patients with Advanced EGFR-Mutant Non-Small-Cell Lung Cancer: A Propensity-Matched Retrospective Study. *BMC Cancer* **2021**, *21*, 482. [CrossRef]
109. Campo, M.; Al-Halabi, H.; Khandekar, M.; Shaw, A.T.; Sequist, L.V.; Willers, H. Integration of Stereotactic Body Radiation Therapy With Tyrosine Kinase Inhibitors in Stage IV Oncogene-Driven Lung Cancer. *The Oncologist* **2016**, *21*, 964–973. [CrossRef]
110. Patel, S.; Rimner, A.; Foster, A.; Zhang, Z.-F.; Woo, K.; Yu, H.A.; Riely, G.; Wu, A. Pattern of Failure in Metastatic EGFR-Mutant NSCLC Treated With Erlotinib: A Role for Upfront Radiation Therapy? *Int. J. Radiat. Oncol. Biol. Phys.* **2014**, *90*, S643. [CrossRef]
111. Xu, Q.; Zhou, F.; Liu, H.; Jiang, T.; Li, X.; Xu, Y.; Zhou, C. Consolidative Local Ablative Therapy Improves the Survival of Patients With Synchronous Oligometastatic NSCLC Harboring EGFR Activating Mutation Treated With First-Line EGFR-TKIs. *J. Thorac. Oncol. Off. Publ. Int. Assoc. Study Lung Cancer* **2018**, *13*, 1383–1392. [CrossRef] [PubMed]
112. Wang, X.-S.; Bai, Y.-F.; Verma, V.; Yu, R.-L.; Tian, W.; Ao, R.; Deng, Y.; Xia, J.-L.; Zhu, X.-Q.; Liu, H.; et al. Randomized Trial of First-Line Tyrosine Kinase Inhibitor With or Without Radiotherapy for Synchronous Oligometastatic EGFR-Mutated Non-Small Cell Lung Cancer. *JNCI J. Natl. Cancer Inst.* **2022**, *114*, djac015. [CrossRef]
113. Chan, O.S.H.; Lam, K.C.; Li, J.Y.C.; Choi, F.P.T.; Wong, C.Y.H.; Chang, A.T.Y.; Mo, F.K.F.; Wang, K.; Yeung, R.M.W.; Mok, T.S.K. ATOM: A Phase II Study to Assess Efficacy of Preemptive Local Ablative Therapy to Residual Oligometastases of NSCLC after EGFR TKI. *Lung Cancer Amst. Neth.* **2020**, *142*, 41–46. [CrossRef] [PubMed]
114. Weiss, J.; Kavanagh, B.D.; Deal, A.M.; Zagar, T.; Marks, L.B.; Stinchcombe, T.; Borghaei, H.; West, H.J.; Morris, D.E.; Villaruz, L.C.; et al. Phase II Study of Stereotactic Radiosurgery or Other Local Ablation Followed by Erlotinib for Patients with EGFR Mutation Who Have Previously Progressed on an EGFR Tyrosine Kinase Inhibitor (TKI). *J. Clin. Oncol.* **2017**, *35*, e20623. [CrossRef]
115. Andrews Wright, N.M.; Goss, G.D. Third-Generation Epidermal Growth Factor Receptor Tyrosine Kinase Inhibitors for the Treatment of Non-Small Cell Lung Cancer. *Transl. Lung Cancer Res.* **2019**, *8*, S247–S264. [CrossRef] [PubMed]
116. Jiang, T.; Chu, Q.; Wang, H.; Zhou, F.; Gao, G.; Chen, X.; Li, X.; Zhao, C.; Xu, Q.; Li, W.; et al. EGFR-TKIs plus Local Therapy Demonstrated Survival Benefit than EGFR-TKIs Alone in EGFR-Mutant NSCLC Patients with Oligometastatic or Oligoprogressive Liver Metastases. *Int. J. Cancer* **2019**, *144*, 2605–2612. [CrossRef] [PubMed]

117. Borghetti, P.; Bonù, M.L.; Giubbolini, R.; Levra, N.G.; Mazzola, R.; Perna, M.; Visani, L.; Meacci, F.; Taraborrelli, M.; Triggiani, L.; et al. Concomitant Radiotherapy and TKI in Metastatic EGFR- or ALK-Mutated Non-Small Cell Lung Cancer: A Multicentric Analysis on Behalf of AIRO Lung Cancer Study Group. *Radiol. Med.* **2019**, *124*, 662–670. [CrossRef]
118. Wang, X.; Zeng, M. First-Line Tyrosine Kinase Inhibitor with or without Aggressive Upfront Local Radiation Therapy in Patients with EGFRm Oligometastatic Non-Small Cell Lung Cancer: Interim Results of a Randomized Phase III, Open-Label Clinical Trial (SINDAS) (NCT02893332). *J. Clin. Oncol.* **2020**, *38*, 9508. [CrossRef]
119. Yu, H.A.; Sima, C.S.; Huang, J.; Solomon, S.B.; Rimner, A.; Paik, P.; Pietanza, M.C.; Azzoli, C.G.; Rizvi, N.A.; Krug, L.M.; et al. Local Therapy with Continued EGFR Tyrosine Kinase Inhibitor Therapy as a Treatment Strategy in EGFR-Mutant Advanced Lung Cancers That Have Developed Acquired Resistance to EGFR Tyrosine Kinase Inhibitors. *J. Thorac. Oncol. Off. Publ. Int. Assoc. Study Lung Cancer* **2013**, *8*, 346–351. [CrossRef]
120. Yoshida, T.; Yoh, K.; Niho, S.; Umemura, S.; Matsumoto, S.; Ohmatsu, H.; Ohe, Y.; Goto, K. RECIST Progression Patterns during EGFR Tyrosine Kinase Inhibitor Treatment of Advanced Non-Small Cell Lung Cancer Patients Harboring an EGFR Mutation. *Lung Cancer Amst. Neth.* **2015**, *90*, 477–483. [CrossRef] [PubMed]
121. Doebele, R.C.; Pilling, A.B.; Aisner, D.L.; Kutateladze, T.G.; Le, A.T.; Weickhardt, A.J.; Kondo, K.L.; Linderman, D.J.; Heasley, L.E.; Franklin, W.A.; et al. Mechanisms of Resistance to Crizotinib in Patients with ALK Gene Rearranged Non-Small Cell Lung Cancer. *Clin. Cancer Res. Off. J. Am. Assoc. Cancer Res.* **2012**, *18*, 1472–1482. [CrossRef] [PubMed]
122. Conibear, J.; Chia, B.; Ngai, Y.; Bates, A.T.; Counsell, N.; Patel, R.; Eaton, D.; Faivre-Finn, C.; Fenwick, J.; Forster, M.; et al. Study Protocol for the SARON Trial: A Multicentre, Randomised Controlled Phase III Trial Comparing the Addition of Stereotactic Ablative Radiotherapy and Radical Radiotherapy with Standard Chemotherapy Alone for Oligometastatic Non-Small Cell Lung Cancer. *BMJ Open* **2018**, *8*, e020690. [CrossRef] [PubMed]

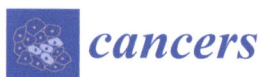 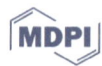

Review

Stereotactic Magnetic Resonance-Guided Adaptive and Non-Adaptive Radiotherapy on Combination MR-Linear Accelerators: Current Practice and Future Directions

John Michael Bryant, Joseph Weygand, Emily Keit, Ruben Cruz-Chamorro, Maria L. Sandoval, Ibrahim M. Oraiqat, Jacqueline Andreozzi, Gage Redler, Kujtim Latifi, Vladimir Feygelman and Stephen A. Rosenberg *

Department of Radiation Oncology, H. Lee Moffitt Cancer Center and Research Institute, Tampa, FL 33612, USA; john.bryant@moffitt.org (J.M.B.)
* Correspondence: stephen.rosenberg@moffitt.org

Simple Summary: Stereotactic body radiotherapy (SBRT) is an effective radiation therapy technique that heavily relies upon daily image guidance to achieve the necessary precision. Magnetic resonance imaging (MRI) offers significant advantages over computed tomography (CT), which has traditionally been used for daily image guidance for SBRT. Hybrid MRI and linear accelerators (MRLs) allow for the delivery of stereotactic MR-guided adaptive radiotherapy (SMART) and improve patient outcomes for many types of tumors. In this review, we summarized the evidence for SMART as it related to ablative treatments and explored how multi-parametric MRIs could continue to improve patient outcomes.

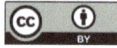

Citation: Bryant, J.M.; Weygand, J.; Keit, E.; Cruz-Chamorro, R.; Sandoval, M.L.; Oraiqat, I.M.; Andreozzi, J.; Redler, G.; Latifi, K.; Feygelman, V.; et al. Stereotactic Magnetic Resonance-Guided Adaptive and Non-Adaptive Radiotherapy on Combination MR-Linear Accelerators: Current Practice and Future Directions. *Cancers* **2023**, *15*, 2081. https://doi.org/10.3390/cancers15072081

Academic Editors: Sam Beddar and Michael D. Chuong

Received: 13 March 2023
Revised: 27 March 2023
Accepted: 29 March 2023
Published: 30 March 2023

Copyright: © 2023 by the authors. Licensee MDPI, Basel, Switzerland. This article is an open access article distributed under the terms and conditions of the Creative Commons Attribution (CC BY) license (https://creativecommons.org/licenses/by/4.0/).

Abstract: Stereotactic body radiotherapy (SBRT) is an effective radiation therapy technique that has allowed for shorter treatment courses, as compared to conventionally dosed radiation therapy. As its name implies, SBRT relies on daily image guidance to ensure that each fraction targets a tumor, instead of healthy tissue. Magnetic resonance imaging (MRI) offers improved soft-tissue visualization, allowing for better tumor and normal tissue delineation. MR-guided RT (MRgRT) has traditionally been defined by the use of offline MRI to aid in defining the RT volumes during the initial planning stages in order to ensure accurate tumor targeting while sparing critical normal tissues. However, the ViewRay MRIdian and Elekta Unity have improved upon and revolutionized the MRgRT by creating a combined MRI and linear accelerator (MRL), allowing MRgRT to incorporate online MRI in RT. MRL-based MR-guided SBRT (MRgSBRT) represents a novel solution to deliver higher doses to larger volumes of gross disease, regardless of the proximity of at-risk organs due to the (1) superior soft-tissue visualization for patient positioning, (2) real-time continuous intrafraction assessment of internal structures, and (3) daily online adaptive replanning. Stereotactic MR-guided adaptive radiation therapy (SMART) has enabled the safe delivery of ablative doses to tumors adjacent to radiosensitive tissues throughout the body. Although it is still a relatively new RT technique, SMART has demonstrated significant opportunities to improve disease control and reduce toxicity. In this review, we included the current clinical applications and the active prospective trials related to SMART. We highlighted the most impactful clinical studies at various tumor sites. In addition, we explored how MRL-based multiparametric MRI could potentially synergize with SMART to significantly change the current treatment paradigm and to improve personalized cancer care.

Keywords: radiation therapy; RT; ultra-hypofractionated radiation therapy; ablative radiation therapy; adaptive radiation therapy; image guided radiotherapy; magnetic resonance imaging; MRI; MR-guided radiation therapy; MRgRT; stereotactic body radiotherapy; SBRT; stereotactic ablative radiotherapy; SABR; stereotactic magnetic resonance-guided adaptive radiotherapy; SMART; plan optimization; tumor motion management; multiparametric MRI; mpMRI

1. Introduction

Cancer continues to be a major global health concern and a leading cause of death. There were an estimated 19.3 million new cancer diagnoses and 10.0 million cancer-related deaths worldwide in 2020 [1]. By 2040, it is estimated that there will be 29.5 million new cases and 16.3 million deaths annually worldwide [2]. Radiotherapy (RT) remains a fundamental component of an effective cancer treatment program [2]. An estimated 50% of all cancer patients receive RT as part of their care [3]. Therefore, advances within the field of radiation oncology are paramount to the improvement of cancer outcomes. Stereotactic body radiotherapy (SBRT) has emerged as a highly effective RT modality that allows for radiotherapeutic-dose escalation that can be delivered in fewer fractions, as compared to conventionally dosed RT [4]. However, this new modality requires more exact targeting to ensure that these high doses are delivered to the tumor, not the healthy, tissue. SBRT has traditionally relied on planar or volumetric (e.g., cone-beam computed tomography (CBCT)) X-ray imaging techniques to ensure proper treatment planning each day to improve accuracy [5]. However, X-ray imaging techniques are insensitive to morphological changes, relative to the tumor, in the surrounding soft tissue [6], which are often the most radiosensitive and at risk of significant treatment-related toxicity [7–9]. CBCT has lacked the ability to accurately delineate the interface between tumor and normal soft tissue, which has limited the dose that could be safely planned for delivery [10]. Additionally, intrafraction motion management with X-ray-based imaging has often relied on a surrogate, such as an external patient surface and internal fiducial markers [11]. A recent development within the field of radiation oncology is the magnetic resonance imaging-guided linear accelerators (MRLs) that can overcome some of the challenges associated with X-ray/CT-based systems.

Magnetic resonance imaging (MRI) offers improved soft-tissue delineation, allowing for the better visualization and discrimination of normal tissues and tumor targets, while being able to detect subtle physiological changes within the tissues, as well [12,13]. MR-guided RT (MRgRT) has traditionally used offline MRI to assist in defining volumes during the initial planning stages [14,15]. This contrasts with online MRgRT, which allows for daily on-table MRI and for the direct monitoring of targets and critical organs at risk (OARs) during treatment. Online MRI is the defining feature of MRL that provides all its unique capabilities and online adaptive workflow, as shown in Figure 1. MRL can acquire MR images for both treatment planning and daily set-up verification with the patient in the treatment position. Prior to treatment, each MRI acquired can be used for adjusting the plan to account for the exact positions of the targets and the normal tissue when fused with a treatment-planning CT [16,17]. When combined with dedicated software and efficient workflows, this daily MR-based adaptive planning allows for improved target coverage, opportunities for isotoxic dose delivery, and reduced normal tissue toxicity. This is called online adaptive radiotherapy and may increase the therapeutic window of RT. In addition, the MRL is capable of real-time (cine) MRI while the treatment is being delivered according to a rapid and balanced steady-state free-precession MRI acquisition technique [18], allowing for treatment-gating based on the patient anatomy directly (e.g., the tumor target) for motion control. These capabilities reduce the uncertainties in external beam radiation therapy delivery. Traditionally, larger planning target volume (PTV) margins have been used to account for these uncertainties and ensure that we treat the target appropriately. However, the unique capabilities of MRL allow for margin reduction. This, in turn, allows for higher tumor doses while conserving the normal tissue and, Therefore, widening the therapeutic window for the safe and effective delivery of MRI-guided SBRT (MRgSBRT).

This increased therapeutic window allows for safer isotoxic dose escalation. Online adaptive SBRT in an MRL is commonly referred to as stereotactic magnetic resonance-guided adaptive radiotherapy (SMART). SMART is an advanced SBRT modality that is currently being utilized for many tumor types in clinics around the globe to improve therapeutic efficacy and safety [17,19]. The global adoption of this novel MRL technology for SMART continues to accelerate. This has led to a multitude of innovative trials and registries [19,20] that explore and expand the impact of this new treatment modality. Table 1 lists all currently active trials exploring either nonadaptive MRL-based SBRT (MRL-SBRT) and SMART registered on ClinicalTrials.gov, accessed on 12 March 2023.

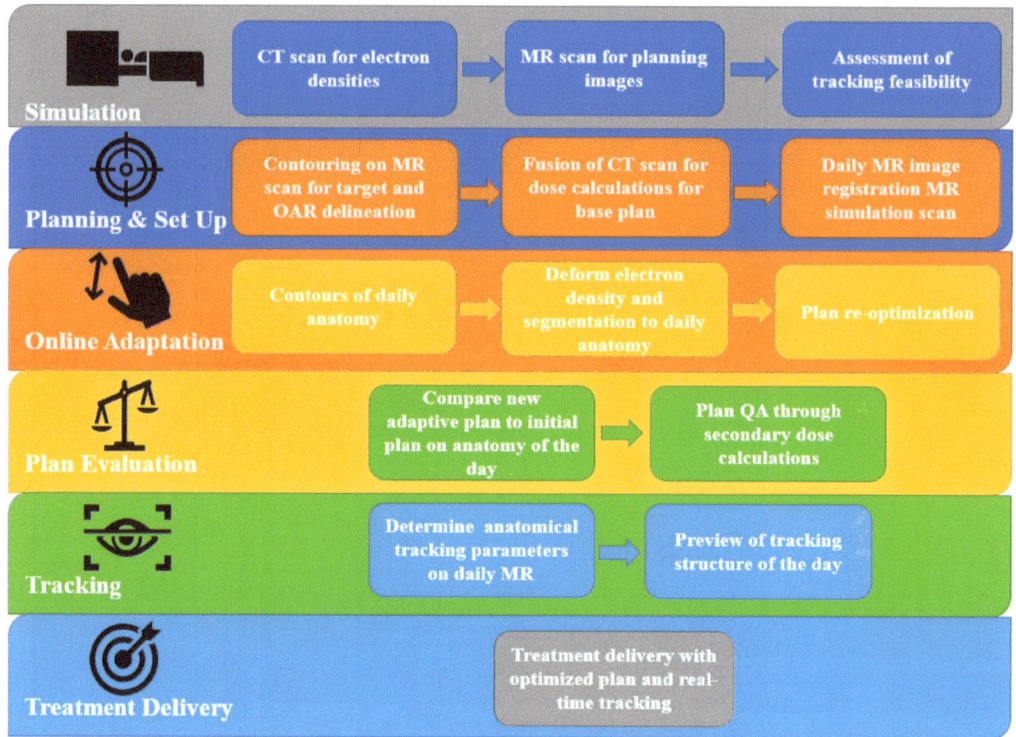

Figure 1. MRL workflow. CT: Computed tomography; MR: magnetic resonance; MRL: MR linear accelerator; OAR: organ at risk; QA: quality assurance.

Table 1. Active SMART and nonadaptive MRL-SBRT clinical trials registered on ClinicTrials.gov. Both actively recruiting and active but not-yet-recruiting trials were included.

Study Title	Sponsor	Site	Condition/Disease	Estimated Enrollment	ClinicalTrials.gov Identifier
A Master Protocol of Stereotactic Magnetic Resonance Guided Adaptive Radiation Therapy (SMART)	Dana–Farber Cancer Institute	All/Multiple sites	N/A	1000	NCT04115254
The MR-Linac Technical Feasibility Protocol (UMBRELLA-II)	The Netherlands Cancer Institute	All/Multiple sites	N/A	140	NCT04351204
The Multiple Outcome Evaluation of Radiation Therapy Using the MR-Linac Study (MOMENTUM)	UMC Utrecht	All/Multiple sites	N/A	6000	NCT04075305
Magnetic Resonance Guided Radiation Therapy (CONFIRM)	Dana–Farber Cancer Institute	All/Multiple sites	Gastric Cancer, Invasive Breast Cancer, in Situ Breast Cancer, Mantle Cell Lymphoma, Larynx Cancer, Bladder Cancer	70	NCT04368702

Table 1. Cont.

Study Title	Sponsor	Site	Condition/Disease	Estimated Enrollment	ClinicalTrials.gov Identifier
Immune Checkpoint Inhibitor and MR-guided SBRT for Limited Progressive Metastatic Carcinoma	Baptist Health South Florida	All/Multiple sites	Metastatic tumors	52	NCT04376502
Stereotactic MRI-guided Adaptive Radiation Therapy (SMART) in One Fraction (SMART-ONE)	Baptist Health South Florida	All/Multiple sites	Oligometastatic cancer, up to 10 sites of disease	30	NCT04939246
Real-Time MRI-Guided 3-Fraction Accelerated Partial Breast Irradiation in Early Breast Cancer (MAPBI)	University of Wisconsin, Madison	Breast	Breast Cancer, DCIS	30	NCT03936478
MR-Linac Guided Adaptive FSRT for Brain Metastases From Non-small Cell Lung Cancer	Sun Yat-Sen University	Central Nervous System	Brain Metastases from Non-Small Cell Lung Cancer	55	NCT04946019
Pilot Study of Same-session MR-only Simulation and Treatment With Stereotactic MRI-guided Adaptive Radiotherapy (SMART) for Oligometastases of the Spine	Washington University School of Medicine	Central Nervous System	Oligometastases of the Spine	10	NCT03878485
Locally Advanced Pancreatic Cancer Treated With ABLAtivE Stereotactic MRI-guided Adaptive Radiation Therapy (LAP-ABLATE)	ViewRay Inc.	Gastrointestinal	Pancreatic Cancer	267	NCT05585554
Sequential Treatment With GEMBRAX and Then FOLFIRINOX Followed by Stereotactic MRI-guided Radiotherapy in Patients With Locally Advanced Pancreatic Cancer (GABRINOX-ART)	Institut du Cancer de Montpellier—Val d'Aurelle	Gastrointestinal	Pancreatic Cancer	103	NCT04570943
MR-Guided Adaptive SBRT of Primary Tumor for Pain Control in Metastatic PDAC (MASPAC)	Ludwig-Maximilians—University of Munich	Gastrointestinal	Pancreatic Cancer	92	NCT05114213
Stereotactic Radiotherapy vs. Best Supportive Care in Unfit Pancreatic Cancer Patients (PANCOSAR)	Amsterdam UMC	Gastrointestinal	Pancreatic Cancer	98	NCT05265663
Precision Radiotherapy Using MR-linac for Pancreatic Neuroendocrine Tumours in MEN1 Patients (PRIME)	J.M. de Laat	Gastrointestinal	Pancreatic Neuroendocrine Tumors	20	NCT05037461
MR-guided Pre-operative RT in Gastric Cancer	Washington University School of Medicine	Gastrointestinal	Gastric cancer	36	NCT04162665
Magnetic Resonance-guided Adaptive Stereotactic Body Radiotherapy for Hepatic Metastases (MAESTRO)	University Hospital Heidelberg	Gastrointestinal	Liver Metastases	90	NCT05027711
OAR-Based, Dose Escalated SBRT With Real-time Adaptive MRI Guidance for Liver Metastases	University of Wisconsin, Madison	Gastrointestinal	Liver Metastases	48	NCT04020276

Table 1. *Cont.*

Study Title	Sponsor	Site	Condition/Disease	Estimated Enrollment	ClinicalTrials.gov Identifier
Adaptative MR-Guided Stereotactic Body Radiotherapy of Liver Tumors (RASTAF)	Centre Georges Francois Leclerc	Gastrointestinal	Liver Metastases	46	NCT04242342
Radiotherapy With Iron Oxide Nanoparticles (SPION) on MR-Linac for Primary & Metastatic Hepatic Cancers	Allegheny Singer Research Institute	Gastrointestinal	Liver tumors	25	NCT04682847
Stereotactic MRI-guided Radiation Therapy for Localized Prostate Cancer (SMILE)	University Hospital Heidelberg	Genitourinary	Prostate Cancer	68	NCT04845503
Randomized Trial of Five or Two MRI-Guided Adaptive Radiotherapy Treatments for Prostate Cancer (FORT)	Weill Medical College of Cornell University	Genitourinary	Prostate Cancer	136	NCT04984343
MR-linac Guided Ultra-hypofractionated RT for Prostate Cancer	Chinese Academy of Medical Sciences	Genitourinary	Prostate Cancer	50	NCT05183074
Randomized Phase-II Trial of Salvage Radiotherapy for Prostate Cancer In 4 Weeks vs. 2 Weeks	Weill Medical College of Cornell University	Genitourinary	Prostate Cancer	134	NCT04422132
MR-Linac for Head and Neck SBRT	Sunnybrook Health Sciences Centre	Head and Neck	Head and Neck Cancer	30	NCT04809792
Nano-SMART: Nanoparticles with MR Guided SBRT in Centrally Located Lung Tumors and Pancreatic Cancer	Dana–Farber Cancer Institute	Thorax	Non-small Cell Lung Cancer, Pancreatic Cancer	100	NCT04789486
Magnetic Resonance Guided Adaptive Stereotactic Body Radiotherapy for Lung Tumors in Ultra-central Location (MAGELLAN)	University Hospital Heidelberg	Thorax	Non-small Cell Lung Cancer, Metastatic tumors	38	NCT04925583
Study of LUNG Stereotactic Adaptive Ablative Radiotherapy (LUNG STAAR)	Baptist Health South Florida	Thorax	Non-small Cell Lung Cancer	60	NCT04917224
A Multicenter Phase-II Study of Stereotactic Radiotherapy for Centrally Located Lung Tumors (STRICT-LUNG STUDY) and Ultra-centrally Located Lung Tumors (STAR-LUNG STUDY)	Rigshospitalet, Denmark	Thorax	Primary Lung Cancer, Metastatic tumors	138	NCT05354596

The two most common commercially available MRLs are the ViewRay MRIdian (ViewRay Technologies Inc., Oakwood Village, OH, USA) and Elekta Unity (Elekta AB, Stockholm, Sweden). The global adoption of MRL technology has been driven by these 2 systems, with 112 (56 of each) ViewRay MRIdian and Elekta Unity systems having been installed as of 31 December 2022 (Figure 2). Since 2019, these systems have combined to perform an estimated 37,500 treatments (Figure 3). The MRIdian system combines a 0.345 T-field strength split-bore magnet MRI with a 28 cm gap that contains the 6 MV flattening filter-free (FFF) linear accelerator components [21]. ViewRay originally produced a tri-^{60}Co unit; however, these have all been upgraded (except for one) to MRL [22]. The Elekta Unity combines a 1.5 T MRI (Philips, Amsterdam, The Netherlands) and a 7 MV FFF linear accelerator irradiating through a cryostat [16]. Although both ViewRay MRIdian and Elekta Unity are MRLs and can be utilized for the purposes of SMART, there are important distinctions between the two machines regarding their capabilities. The most obvious difference is the conventional (i.e., 1.5 T) static magnetic field (B_0) strength of Elekta Unity, as compared to the low-field (i.e., 0.345 T) MRIdian system. Higher B_0 improves the signal-to-noise ratio and generally improves overall image quality. However, the relationship between the field strength and contrast-to-noise ratio, which is important for target-tracking, is not straightforward [23]. The higher B_0 also makes multiparametric imaging easier to perform as well as provides the general capability to immediately utilize pulse sequences developed for diagnostic MRI purposes at the same field strength. However, since both system-specific and patient-induced (e.g., chemical shift and magnetic susceptibility effects) geometric distortion also scales with B_0, it is easier to manage in the low-field machine [13,24]. Lastly, the MRIdian system has had real-time tumor-tracking with automatic beam-gating since its launch, whereas the Unity system achieved FDA approval for tracking on 28 February 2023.

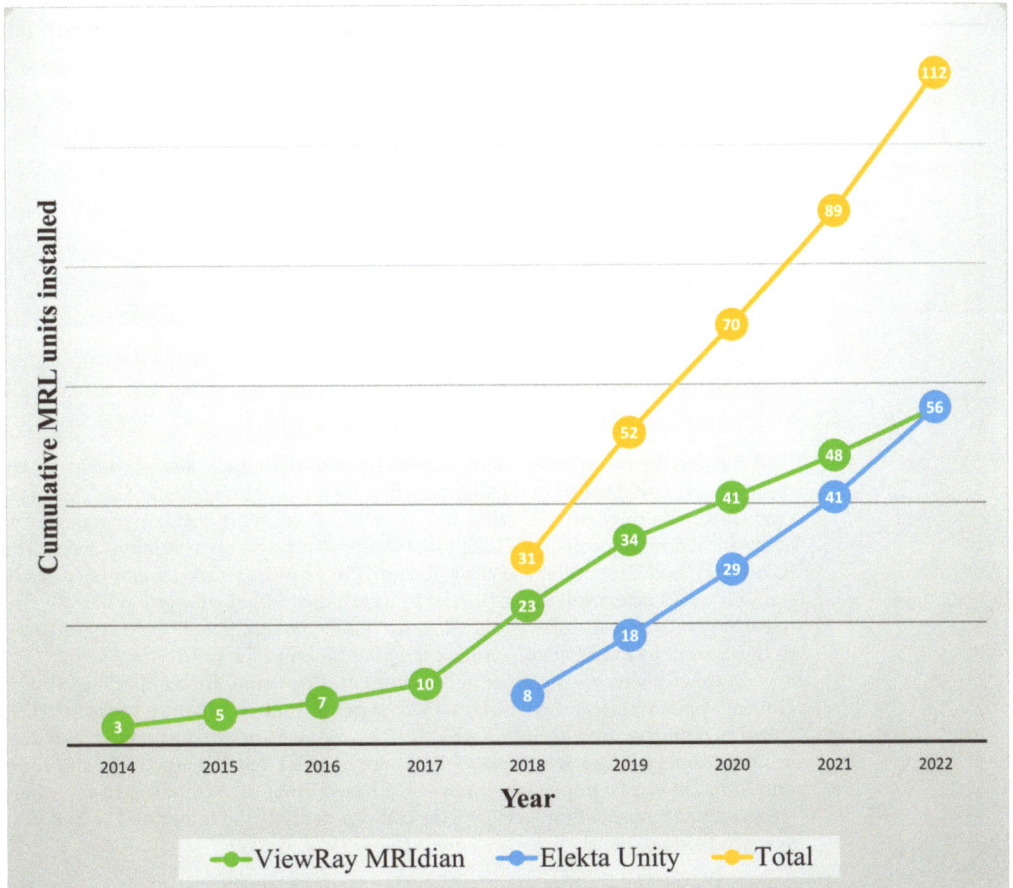

Figure 2. Cumulative installations of ViewRay MRIdian and Elekta Unity MRLs over time. ViewRay MRIdian was initially a tri-^{60}Co system, with MRL installations beginning in 2017. All existing ViewRay MRIdian systems, except for one, have been upgraded to MRLs. Elekta Unity systems were initially pre-clinical until late 2019. All existing Elekta Unity systems have been upgraded to fully clinical systems. Data used for the creation of Figure 2 were directly provided by Elekta and ViewRay team members.

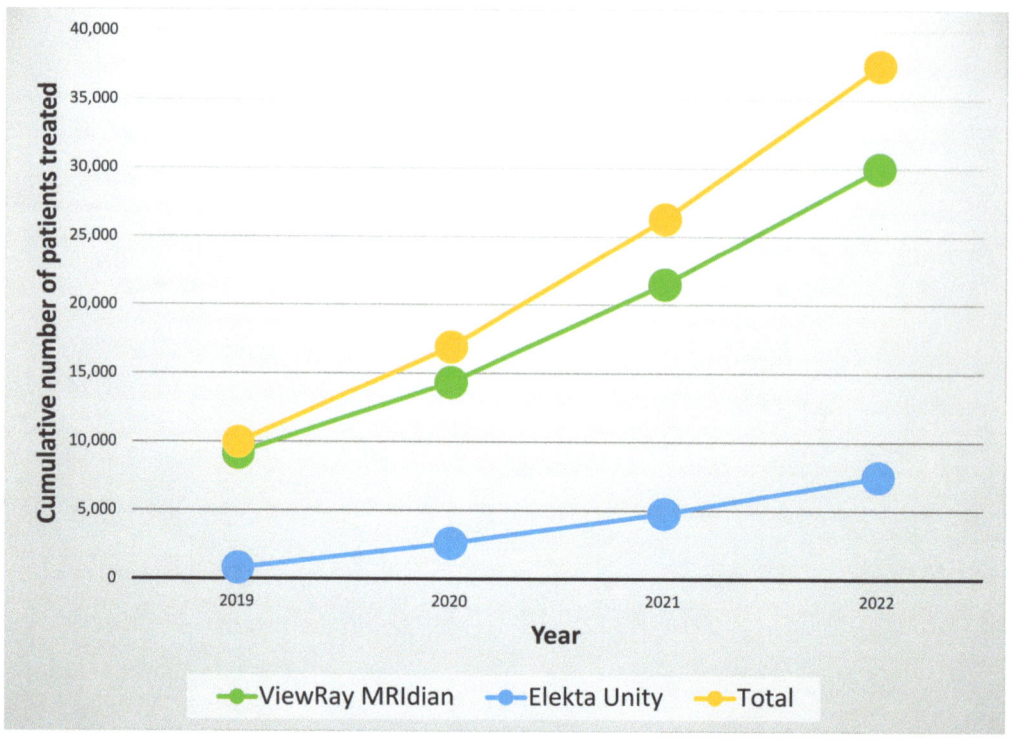

Figure 3. Cumulative treatments of ViewRay MRIdian and Elekta Unity MRLs per year since 2019. Data used for the creation of Figure 3 were directly provided by ViewRay and from data presented at the 9th annual MR in RT symposium [25].

Despite the improvements in personalized radiotherapy already achieved by MRLs, their full potential is not yet realized. MRLs could enable significant strides in personalized cancer therapy by analyzing the daily MR images for subtle intra- and peri-tumor anatomical and physiological/functional changes in response to ablative doses. The ability to identify and determine the clinical significance of the tumoral response during each fraction could be exploited for further individualized plan adaptation [26–28]; Therefore, these MRI radiomic features could allow for online biological and physiological, in addition to the current morphological, online plan adaptation in the future.

In this review, we summarized current and potential future directions for SMART clinical applications and trials, by cancer type. Although we only focused on sites that could benefit the most from SMART, this review was not comprehensive in scope. We focused on as many sites as possible where SMART has been actively improving care and has evidence of improvement over CT-based SBRT. In addition, in a separate section, we explored how existing technologies could potentially be integrated with current MRL systems to significantly improve personalized radiotherapy.

2. SMART Clinical Applications

2.1. Head and Neck Cancer

MRI plays an important role in the diagnosis and treatment of head and neck cancers (HNCs) due to the improved visualization of the muscle invasion, the perineural invasion, and the extracapsular extension [29,30]. Therefore, MRI could improve target delineation and expand the role of adaptive RT in these cancers [31]. Early data has suggested that an offline adaptation with MRL could be efficacious [32]. The limited evidence on the treatment of HNC utilizing the tri-^{60}Co system demonstrated effective tumor control with low toxicity rates [33,34]. The early evidence on the treatment of HNC using an MRL demonstrated similar feasibility and safety [19,35,36]. An early report from the MOMENTUM study (NCT04075305) demonstrated the feasibility of MRgRT with a 1.5 T MRL in 13 patients with HNC [19]. These initial data have helped establish the feasibility of conventionally fractionated HNC radiotherapy using MRLs. SBRT has become an important tool for radiation oncologists in the treatment of many types of de novo and recurrent HNCs, although concerns remain regarding toxicity and appropriate tumor selection [37,38]. The advantages of SMART over conventional SBRT modalities could expand the therapeutic window of HNC SBRT. Currently, there is a prospective early-phase trial exploring SMART feasibility and safety for HNC utilizing the 1.5 T MRL (NCT04809792) that is expected to complete enrollment in late 2023.

2.2. Central and Ultra-Central Lung Tumors

SBRT is part of the standard of care for early-stage, non-operable non-small-cell lung cancer (NSCLC) [39] and has been commonly used to treat metastatic lesions in the lungs [40,41]. Lung SBRT has been demonstrated to have excellent local control and minimal toxicity rates [42–44]. However, concerns remain for using SBRT on more centrally located lung lesions due to high rates of toxicity [45]. These central lesions, defined as being within two cm of the proximal bronchial tree (PBT) by the Radiation Therapy Oncology Group (RTOG) [46], and ultra-central (UC) lesions, defined as being within one cm of the PBT, have had significantly higher rates of SBRT-related grade-3–5 toxicity, as compared to more peripherally located tumors [45–49]. Up to one-third of patients with UC lung tumors have experienced grade-3 or higher SBRT-related toxicity, and 15% died as a result of the treatment [49]. These high rates of toxicity were likely related to the uncertainty of the large internal target volume (ITV) and soft-tissue organs at risk (OARs) in the positional planning with CT-based SBRT, leading to unintentionally high doses delivered to the PBT.

SMART has overcome these limitations with the use of MR-guided online plan adaptation to push unacceptably high doses away from OARs and real-time tumor-tracking to control for respiratory motion during treatment [50–55]. SMART for central and UC lesions has been associated with local control rates approaching 96% for both primary and metastatic cancers [53]. In addition, the toxicity rates were comparable to those in peripheral lesions [53,54]. Importantly, recent evidence did not correlate the risk of late intrapulmonary hemorrhage with SMART [56], which was a primary cause of treatment-related death [49] with CT-based SBRT. These initial experiences led to the development of multiple prospective studies exploring SMART for central and ultra-central lesions. Trials such as LUNG Stereotactic Adaptive Ablative Radiotherapy (LUNG STAAR; NCT04917224) Stereotactic Radiotherapy for Centrally Located Lung Tumors (STRICT-LUNG STUDY; NCT04917224); and Ultra-Centrally Located Lung Tumors (STAR-LUNG STUDY; NCT05354596) are exploring the clinical outcomes of SMART for primary early-stage NSCLC and metastatic lesions.

2.3. Cardiac Metastases

The heart and pericardial tissues are rare sites of malignancy, with the most generous estimates of the incidence of primary and metastatic lesions being $\leq 0.03\%$ and $\leq 3\%$, respectively [57,58]. As survival continues to improve in the metastatic setting, particularly in melanoma, the incidence of cardiac metastases has increased [59,60]. The surgical resection of these lesions has traditionally been the only means of definitive therapy [61], with RT playing a purely palliative role [62]. Advances in the field of radiation oncology have indicated the feasible effective treatment of these lesions with SBRT [63]. SMART has the potential to improve the delivery of SBRT to these highly mobile lesions that have been difficult to identify with CT imaging. Currently, SMART data are very limited for these rare tumors. A single institutional experiment in five patients with cardiac lesions that were treated with SMART reported excellent tumor coverage and minimal toxicity [64]. Larger series are required to optimize the dosage for various histologies and to better explore the role of MRgRT in cardiac tumors.

2.4. Pancreatic Cancer

The role of SBRT in borderline resectable (BRPC) and locally advanced pancreatic cancer (LAPC) has been controversial [65–70]. Although SBRT appeared to significantly improve local control, the concerns regarding the lack of improvement in overall survival and toxicity have persisted [65–72]. Data suggested that the dose escalation could have been associated with the improvements in both local control and overall survival [73–78]. Dose-escalated SBRT has historically been limited in practice due to the radiosensitive gastrointestinal organs that surround the pancreas. However, SBRT via SMART could overcome these toxicity-related challenges in pancreatic cancer due to the excellent soft-tissue visualization and online plan adaptation and gating [79–81].

Ablative SMART (A-SMART) demonstrated an excellent safety profile [82,83] and even appeared to be an effective option for elderly patients with unresectable pancreatic cancer who were at increased risk for treatment-related toxicities [84]. Initial studies exploring A-SMART for BRPC and LAPC demonstrated limited toxicity and improved clinical outcomes, with local control and overall survival rates approaching 90% and 70%, respectively [80,81,83,85–87]. In addition, pre-operative A-SMART for BRPC patients was associated with excellent negative resection rates and did not appear to increase the intra- or post-operative mortality [88]. The results of the multicenter phase-II trial, SMART for Locally Advanced Pancreatic Cancer (NCT03621644), were recently presented and demonstrated a median overall survival of 22.5 months and a 1-year overall survival of 94% [89]. The incidence of grade-3 or higher toxicity related to A-SMART was 2.2%. Due to these positive results, a phase-III trial has been announced, the Locally Advanced Pancreatic Cancer Treated with Ablative Stereotactic MRI-guided Adaptive Radiation Therapy (LAP-ABLATE) trial (NCT05585554), which will compare the standard chemotherapy to sequential chemotherapy, followed by A-SMART. Additional phase-II clinical trials exploring SMART for pancreatic pain control in metastatic disease (NCT05114213), SMART in frail and elderly patients (NCT05265663), a combination of intensified sequential chemotherapy with A-SMART (NCT04570943), and SMART for neuroendocrine pancreatic tumors (NCT05037461) are ongoing.

2.5. Liver Tumors

Surgical resection is the standard of care for primary hepatocellular carcinoma (HCC) [90] and hepatic oligometastases [91,92]; however, only one-fifth of patients are deemed eligible for surgery [93]. For unresectable hepatic tumors, SBRT could be a potential treatment option that has the advantage of not being an invasive procedure [94–96]. Over three years, SBRT achieved local control rates of over 90% for metastatic lesions, if treated with ablative doses [97]. Due to the parallel architecture of the liver, it can withstand high doses of radiation in small areas but is at high risk of radiation-induced liver disease (RILD) with larger targets [98]. In addition, the local radiosensitive gastrointestinal organs are at high risk of toxicity during liver irradiation. SBRT, in particular, has been associated with a risk of grade-3 or higher toxicity in up to one-third of patients [99], thus limiting patient selection and dose escalation. However, MR-guided SBRT can overcome many of the challenges faced by CT-based SBRT.

SMART has reduced irradiated liver volumes without an ITV (on some MRL systems that provide patient anatomy tracking/gating) and tighter PTV margins and ensured tolerances for nearby radiosensitive structures were safely and reliably respected while achieving the requisite ablative doses [50,87,100–102]. Patients have also forgone the need for invasive fiducial markers for gating and tracking with SMART. SMART for primary and metastatic liver lesions has been demonstrated to have local control rates between 75% and 100% at 21 months with a grade-3 toxicity rate of only 8% and no grade-4 toxicity or treatment-related deaths [101]. These initial reports of SMART in hepatic lesions are promising but limited due to their retrospective nature and short follow-up periods. Multiple trials exploring liver-focused SMART have been initiated to better define its role. The phase-II Magnetic Resonance-Guided Adaptive Stereotactic Body Radiotherapy for Hepatic Metastases (MAESTRO) randomized trial is currently recruiting patients to compare ITV-based SBRT and SMART. The Adaptive MR-Guided Stereotactic Body Radiotherapy of Liver Tumors (RASTAF) phase-II trial (NCT04242342) is exploring dose escalation of up to 60 Gy in 5 fractions with SMART in all types of liver tumors. The OAR-Based, Dose-Escalated SBRT With Real-time Adaptive MRI Guidance for Liver Metastases trial (NCT04020276) is a 2-staged phase-I study that is exploring dose escalation of up to 80 Gy in a 4-plus-4 with a confirmatory expansion cohort design.

2.6. Adrenal Metastases

The adrenal gland is a common site of metastases from many malignancies [103] and the indications have been increasing for a definitive treatment in metastatic adrenal lesions [104,105]. There was insufficient evidence to determine the best local treatment modality for isolated and limited adrenal metastases [106]. While surgery is a curative modality option for isolated adrenal metastasis, it has often been contraindicated in the presence of more extensive disease, in elderly patients, and in those with other significant co-morbidities [103,107,108]. Additionally, the recovery time of these procedures usually requires lengthy hospital stays [103]. SBRT is a valid alternative when surgery is not feasible [106,109–111]. However, patients have historically presented significantly worse tumor control, as compared to adrenalectomy [108]. This has likely been due to dose limitations in conventional CT-based SBRT because of the interfractional movement of OARs [112,113], which can be up to 3 cm for local radiosensitive gastrointestinal organs, as well as intrafractional respiratory-induced movement [114]. However, a BED_{10} of >100 Gy was associated with tumor control approaching that of a resection [111,115]. SMART was capable of respiratory-motion management and online plan adaptation for positional changes in local OARs, making it feasible for the delivery of ablative doses. The early data supported the feasibility and the efficacy of SMART in these tumors [86,116]. The recent data has supported this approach by demonstrating 1-year local control rates of 100% in a limited series [117]. The MRL Dana–Farber master trial (NCT04115254) and the SMART-ONE trial (NCT03878485) will help define the feasibility and the role of SMART for adrenal SBRT.

2.7. Kidney Cancer

The role of radiotherapy and SBRT has been limited in the treatment of primary kidney cancer [118]. SBRT could offer a benefit in large tumors (>4 cm) that are not suitable for surgical resection [119]. SBRT appeared to demonstrate exponential cell death in renal cell carcinoma, as compared to conventional fractionation [120]. However, CT-based SBRT often must use large margins [121] to account for movements during therapy [122]. MRL-based SBRT had an advantage over CT-based SBRT by eliminating the need for ITVs, one of the reasons for large margins [123]. The early data has suggested that SMART could be well tolerated with clinically meaningful disease control [124,125]. Therefore, if currently active trials establish a larger role of SBRT [126,127], SMART could play an important part in kidney cancer radiotherapy in the future.

2.8. Breast Cancer

Breast conservation is important to many people with breast cancer, and treatment strategies to avoid mastectomies have been developed that are effective and widely adopted for early-stage breast cancer. RT played an integral role in this treatment design to ensure the clinical outcomes were similar to that of mastectomy [128]. Due to concerns of normal tissue exposure and the inconvenience of 5–6 weeks of daily RT in traditional post-partial mastectomy whole-breast RT, accelerated partial-breast irradiation (APBI) was explored as a potential alternative in specially selected patients with favorable patient and tumor characteristics [129,130]. APBI focuses solely on the areas surrounding the surgical bed and is typically delivered within 1–2 weeks. Both brachytherapy and external beam techniques were explored to determine their unique advantages and drawbacks [131,132]. Brachytherapy offers excellent conformality but is a more invasive procedure. External beam radiotherapy (EBRT) is non-invasive but requires larger margins due to the uncertainties in the daily design and the intrafractional motion management. The high dose per fraction for EBRT ABPI could have contributed to late cosmetic toxicity, although evidence for this has been mixed [131,133,134], with a larger percentage of treated breast volume being a predictor for adverse cosmetic outcomes [135]. SMART could be an excellent external beam APBI modality to improve clinical outcomes. SMART could improve upon existing external beam ABPI due to its superior soft-tissue visualization of the resected cavity and online plan adaptation for the daily design that could allow for a smaller PTV, or even a zero-margin PTV, without sacrificing coverage.

A single institution prospective trial of a 10-fraction with zero-margin PTV APBI on a 0.35 T MRL in 30 patients reduced treatment volumes by 52%, as compared to conventional APBI [136]. These data supported the exploration of APBI delivered with SMART. An early dosimetric analysis demonstrated that 88.5% of the possible dosimetric objectives were fulfilled during planning [137]. The early evidence of APBI delivered with MRLs demonstrated dosimetric advantages over traditional CT-based strategies. If long-term clinical and cosmetic outcome data for APBI delivered with SMART are favorable, this could become an important modality for elderly people with early-stage breast cancer, as approximately 40% of these patients are unable to complete their 5-year hormone therapy, which significantly increases the risk of disease recurrence [138]. However, the clinical benefit of SMART APBI remains unclear, as long-term outcomes for CT-based APBI are excellent. Therefore, whether the dosimetric advantages translate into clinically meaningful improvements over existing APBI techniques is not yet known. The phase-II trial, Real-Time MRI-Guided Three-Fraction Accelerated Partial-Breast Irradiation in Early Breast Cancer (MAPBI) (NCT03936478), is exploring cosmetic and clinical outcomes with SMART APBI.

2.9. Prostate Cancer

There has been an increased utilization of SBRT to reduce the length of treatment and take advantage of the low α/β ratio in prostate cancer [139,140]. The early studies demonstrated significant gastrointestinal and genitourinary toxicity [141,142]. Recent large phase-III trials have had conflicting evidence regarding toxicity [143,144]. MR-guided SBRT (Non-MRL based) is one strategy that has been employed to reduce toxicity. MRI is regularly used in the diagnosis, staging, and management of prostate cancer [145,146] due to its excellent visualization of lesions in both the prostate and the normal surrounding tissue [147]. MRI has been used during treatment planning to better visualize the critical OARs [148], to aid in contouring, and more recently, to help guide boosters to high-risk foci [149]. Therefore, nonadaptive MRL-SBRT and SMART appear to be a logical evolution in prostate SBRT [150,151].

SMART and nonadaptive MRL-SBRT offer multiple advantages over CT-based prostate SBRT, which includes include inter- and intra-fractional rectal motion management and proper daily alignment for urethral-sparing techniques. In addition, SMART and nonadaptive MRL-SBRT do not require the invasive implantation of fiducial markers for daily alignment, which is often a transrectal procedure that has been associated with complications that impacted the quality of life in up to one-third of patients [152,153]. SMART feasibility for prostate cancer is well established [154–156]. Urethral-sparing techniques demonstrated significantly low rates of acute genitourinary toxicity [157]. The results from the SCIMITAR trial, a phase-II, dual-center, single-arm trial that treated post-operative prostate cancer at high-risk for recurrence, with SBRT, demonstrated worse gastrointestinal toxicity of up to 6 months in patients treated with CT-based SBRT, as compared to MRL-SBRT [158].

The MIRAGE trial (NCT04384770) was the first phase-III trial to compare SMART with CT-based SBRT [159]. MIRAGE sought to evaluate if the aggressive margin reduction that had been made feasible with MRL-based treatment would significantly reduce acute grade-2 or higher genitourinary toxicity, as compared to CT-guided treatment [159]. MRL-based MRgSBRT demonstrated a significant reduction in grade-2 or higher acute genitourinary (24.4% (95% CI, 15.4–35.4%) vs. 43.4% (95% CI, 32.1–55.3%); $p = 0.01$) and gastrointestinal (0.0% (95% CI, 0–4.6%) vs. 10.5% (95% CI, 4.7–19.7%); $p = 0.003$) toxicity [159]. This first prospective head-to-head study of CT-based SBRT and MRL-based MRgSBRT clearly demonstrated how MRL capabilities could translate into improved clinical outcomes.

There are multiple current phase-II trials exploring SMART in prostate cancer. The European Stereotactic MRI-Guided Radiation Therapy for Localized Prostate Cancer (SMILE) trial (NCT04845503) is exploring SMART feasibility within an estimated cohort of 68 males. In addition, a phase-II trial (NCT05183074) is exploring the utilization of an MRL to deliver SMART with simultaneously integrated boosters for MR-prominent tumor foci. Another phase-II trial (NCT04984343) is exploring SMART hypofractionation, reducing the standard 5 fractions to 2, to continue reducing treatment time in this very common cancer.

2.10. Spinal Metastases

Spine RT is an important part of metastatic disease management to improve pain, prevent pathological fractures, and prevent neurological morbidity. SBRT had improved efficacy, as compared to conventional forms of radiotherapy [160]. MRIs have been used in spine SBRT to accurately delineate the spinal cord and create a 1–2 mm planning OAR volume (PRV) to decrease disease coverage [160]. Bony structures act as surrogates for the daily design in conventional CBCT image guidance, but CBCTs are not reliable for the accurate visualization of the spinal cord. Therefore, a spinal cord PRV is created during treatment planning to account for daily motion management. MRLs could provide a benefit due to their superior demarcation of the spinal cord and other soft-tissue OAR positions with daily MRIs, as compared to CBCTs [10]. Dosimetric feasibility studies suggested that design improvements with MRI could reduce the dose to the spinal cord [161]. Daily MRIs allow for direct plan registration of the spinal cord, thereby eliminating the need for cord PRVs and allowing for greater tumor coverage. Additionally, the comparatively low fields of the MRLs, as compared to many diagnostic MRIs, have also decreased the artifact and geometric distortions caused by metal hardware [162]. Utilizing an MRL for spine SBRT also improved the integration of the CT treatment planning scan because the radiation oncologist was able to ensure the same patient position [163,164]. These advantages could allow for reduced margins and safe dose escalation. However, it remains unclear if these dosimetric advantages will be clinically meaningful, as compared to CBCT-based spine SBRT. The results of a current phase-I/II trial treating all sites of disease with SMART, including the spine (NCT04115254), and the Pilot Study of Same-Session MR-Only Simulation and Treatment with SMART for Oligometastases of the Spine (NCT03878485) could help determine the feasibility of this technique.

2.11. Oligometastatic Cancer

The increasing data have demonstrated that patients with limited metastases who were treated in a definitive manner at all sites of disease had increased overall survival [165]. This limited metastatic state is termed oligometastatic, and it blurs the line between localized and incurable systemic disease. Recent clinical trials have demonstrated the benefit of SBRT for patients with oligometastatic cancer, typically defined as between one and five metastatic lesions. Randomized phase-II studies of oligometastatic NSCLC [166] and prostate cancer [167] showed improved outcomes with SBRT at all metastatic sites. The phase-II SABR-COMET trial demonstrated that SBRT had improved overall and progression-free survival for various histologies, as compared to standard palliative therapy [168]. However, multi-site SBRT has a significant risk of increased toxicity. The NRG BR-001 trial that delivered SBRT to all sites of metastatic disease demonstrated a rate of late grade-3 or higher toxicity to be 20% at 2 years [169]. Similarly, SABR-COMET reported a 29% rate of grade-2 or higher toxicity, including 3 treatment-related deaths, in the SBRT group, as compared to only 9% in the control group. SMART was uniquely suited for delivering high-dose SBRT to multiple sites concurrently due to its excellent therapeutic window [170]. In addition, SMART has also enabled safe isotoxic dose escalation [82,86], with increased local control and overall survival rates.

Data have been limited concerning the use of SMART in an oligometastatic setting, but SMART has been well tolerated [86,102,171]. Several ongoing clinical trials are evaluating the use of MRgRT in the management of oligometastatic disease. Notably, the SMART-ONE trial is a single-arm trial that is investigating the feasibility of delivering single-fraction MR-guided SBRT to up to 10 sites of disease (NCT04939246). The Washington University School of Medicine is exploring the use of SMART in oligometastatic disease of the spine (NCT03878485). We eagerly await the results of these trials to establish the feasibility, efficacy, and safety of MRgRT in an oligometastatic setting.

2.12. Ablative Dose Re-Irradiation

Re-irradiation (reRT) has historically been limited due to the increased risk of severe toxicity due to cumulatively high OAR doses; however, it also could provide a significant benefit in carefully selected patients with locally recurrent or progressive cancer [172,173]. Therefore, dose selection in reRT is a delicate balance between prioritizing tumor control and patient safety that usually results in modest dose delivery. Historically, these doses did not offer robust local control, especially in patients who did not proceed to surgery [174]. However, dose escalation could improve long-term local control and overall survival in reRT [174–176]. The improved therapeutic ratio of SMART could allow for the safe delivery of dose-escalated reRT.

SMART reRT data have been limited, but the treatment has been well tolerated. SMART reRT in the abdomen and pelvis demonstrated a 1-year local control rate approaching 90% [177]. With a median follow-up of 14 months, there was no acute or late grade-3 or higher toxicity, demonstrating the safety of this modality. Another recent report focused only on prostate reRT and demonstrated a 1-year disease progression-free survival rate that also approached 90%, while maintaining minimal toxicity [178]. SMART reRT appears to be associated with strong local disease control and minimal toxicity, which could warrant further investigation in clinical trials.

3. Future Directions

SMART has enabled the delivery of greater doses to tumors surrounded by some of the most radiosensitive normal tissue within the body, and this has indicated potential dose-escalated treatments that were previously thought to be infeasible, as discussed. Although this has been primarily achieved with MR-guided anatomic adaptation, we believe that the future of SMART may lie in advanced adaptation techniques. This requires the immense data stored in daily MRIs to better understand the tumoral response to treatment throughout the course of radiotherapy, and then these daily insights must be used to adjust both the dosage and fractions throughout the treatment. This would represent major a paradigm shift in the field of radiation oncology. Traditionally, dosage and fractionations were determined prior to and during treatment planning. Even with the current advances in SMART, we continue to use this approach and merely adapt to improve the delivery of a predetermined dose and fractionation. However, studying the tumor changes in response to treatment via daily MRI could provide deeper insights into the nature of a specific tumor and how it will ultimately respond to the current dose and fractionation plan.

Two novel studies, Adaptive Radiation for Locally Advanced Rectal Adenocarcinoma (NCT05108428) and Theragnostic Utilities for Neoplastic Diseases of the Rectum by MRI-Guided Radiotherapy (THUNDER2; NCT04815694), are already utilizing MRL to explore plan adaptation based on tumoral response. They are relying on the tumoral volumetric changes to identify which rectal tumors would benefit the most from sequential booster-dose escalation. Guiding treatment planning based upon volumetric response for certain cancers is clinically feasible when using MRL in longer treatment courses of conventional and minimally hypofractionated radiotherapy. However, utilizing this same technique with SMART is far more difficult due to the significantly shorter treatment course that often does not allow enough time for tumors to demonstrate a clinically obvious volumetric response. Therefore, the more subtle and less well-understood peri- and intra-tumoral changes during therapy should be utilized to guide physiologically and biologically adaptive radiotherapy. The multiparametric MRI (mpMRI) allows for a wider breadth of imaging data to better investigate these often-imperceptible changes.

MRL-Based Multiparametric MRI

MRL adaptation has traditionally been employed for the management of interfractional tumoral and OAR changes in shape and position. However, MRI has also been used for assessing biological and physiological information [179–181], as well as for MRI techniques termed mpMRI [182]. One such technique is diffusion-weighted imaging [183] which enabled the detection of changes in water mobility [184]. These changes were correlated with tumor growth [185] and necrosis [186]. This was facilitated by mapping a parameter known as the apparent diffusion coefficient (ADC), which was then used to track the response to radiation therapy [187]. ADC mapping is particularly attractive in adaptive radiotherapy since the changes in ADC could be noted before morphological changes in the tumor [188], and these changes in diffusion could be used to guide dose-escalation strategies and biologically guided radiation plan adaptation [189,190]. Diffusion-weighted imaging has been applied using a 1.5 T linear accelerator [191–193]. Although technical challenges have been reported [194], DWI was included as an option in this simulation [35]. DWI was initially applied using the 0.35 T tri-^{60}Co system [195,196] and was shown to be predictive of tumor histology [197] and, in combination with deep learning, therapeutic response [198]. Technical challenges were reported [199] when the 0.35 T MRgRT system had transitioned from the tri-^{60}Co system to MRL, but recent applications using DWI with a 0.35 T MRL have appeared promising [200].

A potential application of MRL-based adaptive radiotherapy is the use of metabolic changes to guide RT, as this has been utilized in the recently developed PET/CT-guided radiotherapy delivery systems [201]. Cancer metabolism is severely dysregulated [202], and this dysregulation is reflected downstream, as the concentrations of many metabolites are modulated in cancer cells [203]. While positron-emission tomography (PET) [204–206] has traditionally been applied to observe the metabolic accumulation in tumor cells, MR-based techniques, such as magnetic resonance spectroscopic imaging (MRSI) [207], chemical exchange saturation transfer (CEST) [208,209], and hyperpolarized dynamic magnetic resonance spectroscopy [210], were able to interrogate metabolic processes further downstream [211]. MRSI allowed for the noninvasive mapping of a number of metabolite concentrations by simultaneously acquiring MR data in the spatial frequency and temporal domains [212]. It was applied to produce high-resolution metabolite maps in gliomas [213], and lactate mapping of glioblastoma has been performed using deuterium [214]. Additionally, using phosphorus-based MRSI, the mapping of intra- and extra-cellular pH in tumors was demonstrated [215]. The technical limitations concerning the online incorporation of MRSI with MRL as a work flow have persisted due to the relatively long scan times [216] and low sensitivity in conventional magnetic-field-strength systems [217]. Sensitivity could be counteracted by hyperpolarizing the nucleus, which has resulted in a large increase in sensitivity for a short period of time [218]. The main application has been to observe the dynamic conversion of pyruvate into lactate in tumors [219]. Lastly, CEST allowed for the indirect detection of low concentration solutes via their effect on the water MR signal [220]. CEST has been shown to predict the chemo-radiotherapeutic response of tumors [221,222].

While these MR-based metabolic-imaging techniques have yet to be incorporated into online MRgRT due to the technical challenges, they have significant potential for assessing biological behavior in adaptive RT. The additional incorporation of artificial intelligence into the interpretation of mpMRI data could facilitate biologically driven RT plan adaptation [223,224].

4. Barriers and Limitations

Although MRLs represent one of the most exciting advancements within the field of radiation oncology, these combined linear accelerators have limitations. This novel technology is resource intensive, requiring considerable financial and time investments for operation. The commissioning of MRL requires the development of departmental MR-safety protocols similar to those for diagnostic MRIs, which include MRI safety questionnaires for all patients and thorough MRI safety training for all users with an emphasis on ferrous-material awareness [225]. MRL uses a different workflow, as compared to other linear accelerators; thus, all members of the treatment team, including the physician, physicists, and therapists, must learn to properly operate MRLs [226]. Furthermore, the daily time requirement for online adaptive radiotherapy can be substantial, from 30 to 60 min per treatment, to allow for adequate plan evaluation, adaptation, and treatment delivery, even with an experienced team. This limits total patient throughput and can often require considerable time-at-machine for physicians and physicists.

MRLs also have physical limitations due to the special physics of concurrent MRI with external beam radiotherapy. Lorentz forces have resulted in overdosing hollow organs and required an advanced treatment planning system [227]. MRI geometric distortion, the uncertainty associated with MRI regarding radiation isocenter distance, the multi-leaf collimator position error, and the uncertainties in voxel size and tracking have presented additional physical limitations [101]. Therefore, the familiarity and expertise of physicians, dosimetrists, and physicists regarding these special physics were required for optimal treatment planning and establishing more robust quality assurance methods [86]. MRIs lack electron density and attenuation coefficient information. Therefore, CT images are still required for treatment planning. Additionally, there is a lack of a six-degree couch for adjustments due to the confined space of the MRLinac system.

Patient selection is critical for a successful MRL program. Special attention is required for patients with claustrophobia, large body habitus, and MRI-incompatible implanted devices. Patients with claustrophobia may require pre-treatment anxiolytic therapy or may not be able to tolerate it at all. Patients with large body habitus may not be able to fit within the geometric dimensions of the machine. Even if the patient physically fits into the machine, they may exceed the maximal field-of-view, which can result in aliasing artifacts. This is especially important when using special devices, such as coils, depending on the treatment site.

Diligent screening for all potentially implanted ferromagnetic devices is required for all patients, and alternative treatment options should be considered in these cases.

MRL has many advantages over CT-based linear accelerators. However, MRL was not designed to be a replacement for CT-based linear accelerators. We found that MRL was best suited in cases where its unique advantages were required to deliver a treatment that would be too dangerous in a CT-based linear accelerator.

5. Conclusions

MRL is rapidly becoming an integral instrument for personalized radiotherapy. SMART represents the next generation of SBRT by expanding the therapeutic window due to its vastly improved precision through enhanced soft-tissue resolution and daily MR-guided online adaptation, along with real-time gating in MRIdian. Safe dose escalation using isotoxic approaches with SMART appears to be improving disease outcomes across multiple tumor sites. There are a multitude of cutting-edge clinical trials currently in progress to establish this new modality's role in many types of cancer. Looking forward, MRL and mpMRI appear to have significant synergistic potential, in conjunction with SMART, in personalized cancer therapy.

Author Contributions: Conceptualization, J.M.B. and S.A.R.; methodology, J.M.B.; writing—original draft preparation, J.M.B. and J.W.; writing—review and editing, J.M.B., J.W., E.K., R.C.-C., M.L.S., I.M.O., J.A., G.R., K.L.; visualization, J.M.B.; supervision, S.A.R. and V.F.; project administration, J.M.B. and S.A.R.; funding acquisition, S.A.R. All authors have read and agreed to the published version of the manuscript.

Funding: Submission fees were paid by ViewRay, Inc., Oakwood, OH, USA.

Data Availability Statement: The data presented in this study are available in this article.

Acknowledgments: We thank the ViewRay and Elekta team members who provided us with an MRL installation and treatment data.

Conflicts of Interest: Stephen Rosenberg has received research grants from ViewRay, Inc. He also received an honorarium and has served on the Lung Research Consortium Advisory Board for ViewRay, Inc. Vladimir Feygelman and Kujtim Latifi have received consulting fees from ViewRay, Inc. No other authors have any conflict of interest to declare.

References

1. Sung, H.; Ferlay, J.; Siegel, R.L.; Laversanne, M.; Soerjomataram, I.; Jemal, A.; Bray, F. Global Cancer Statistics 2020: GLOBOCAN Estimates of Incidence and Mortality Worldwide for 36 Cancers in 185 Countries. *CA Cancer J. Clin.* **2021**, *71*, 209–249. [CrossRef] [PubMed]
2. Abdel-Wahab, M.; Gondhowiardjo, S.S.; Rosa, A.A.; Lievens, Y.; El-Haj, N.; Polo Rubio, J.A.; Prajogi, G.B.; Helgadottir, H.; Zubizarreta, E.; Meghzifene, A.; et al. Global Radiotherapy: Current Status and Future Directions-White Paper. *JCO Glob. Oncol.* **2021**, *7*, 827–842. [CrossRef] [PubMed]
3. Atun, R.; Jaffray, D.A.; Barton, M.B.; Bray, F.; Baumann, M.; Vikram, B.; Hanna, T.P.; Knaul, F.M.; Lievens, Y.; Lui, T.Y.; et al. Expanding global access to radiotherapy. *Lancet Oncol.* **2015**, *16*, 1153–1186. [CrossRef]
4. Onishi, H.; Shirato, H.; Nagata, Y.; Hiraoka, M.; Fujino, M.; Gomi, K.; Niibe, Y.; Karasawa, K.; Hayakawa, K.; Takai, Y.; et al. Hypofractionated stereotactic radiotherapy (HypoFXSRT) for stage I non-small cell lung cancer: Updated results of 257 patients in a Japanese multi-institutional study. *J. Thorac. Oncol.* **2007**, *2*, S94–S100. [CrossRef]
5. Jaffray, D.A. Image-guided radiotherapy: From current concept to future perspectives. *Nat. Rev. Clin. Oncol.* **2012**, *9*, 688–699. [CrossRef]
6. Letourneau, D.; Martinez, A.A.; Lockman, D.; Yan, D.; Vargas, C.; Ivaldi, G.; Wong, J. Assessment of residual error for online cone-beam CT-guided treatment of prostate cancer patients. *Int. J. Radiat. Oncol. Biol. Phys.* **2005**, *62*, 1239–1246. [CrossRef]
7. Thomas, D.H.; Santhanam, A.; Kishan, A.U.; Cao, M.; Lamb, J.; Min, Y.; O'Connell, D.; Yang, Y.; Agazaryan, N.; Lee, P.; et al. Initial clinical observations of intra- and interfractional motion variation in MR-guided lung SBRT. *Br. J. Radiol.* **2018**, *91*, 20170522. [CrossRef] [PubMed]
8. Byun, D.J.; Gorovets, D.J.; Jacobs, L.M.; Happersett, L.; Zhang, P.; Pei, X.; Burleson, S.; Zhang, Z.; Hunt, M.; McBride, S.; et al. Strict bladder filling and rectal emptying during prostate SBRT: Does it make a dosimetric or clinical difference? *Radiat. Oncol.* **2020**, *15*, 239. [CrossRef] [PubMed]
9. Loi, M.; Magallon-Baro, A.; Suker, M.; van Eijck, C.; Sharma, A.; Hoogeman, M.; Nuyttens, J. Pancreatic cancer treated with SBRT: Effect of anatomical interfraction variations on dose to organs at risk. *Radiother. Oncol.* **2019**, *134*, 67–73. [CrossRef]
10. Noel, C.E.; Parikh, P.J.; Spencer, C.R.; Green, O.L.; Hu, Y.; Mutic, S.; Olsen, J.R. Comparison of onboard low-field magnetic resonance imaging versus onboard computed tomography for anatomy visualization in radiotherapy. *Acta Oncol.* **2015**, *54*, 1474–1482. [CrossRef]
11. Casamassima, F.; Cavedon, C.; Francescon, P.; Stancanello, J.; Avanzo, M.; Cora, S.; Scalchi, P. Use of motion tracking in stereotactic body radiotherapy: Evaluation of uncertainty in off-target dose distribution and optimization strategies. *Acta Oncol.* **2006**, *45*, 943–947. [CrossRef] [PubMed]
12. Yousaf, T.; Dervenoulas, G.; Politis, M. Advances in MRI Methodology. *Int. Rev. Neurobiol.* **2018**, *141*, 31–76. [CrossRef]
13. Weygand, J.; Fuller, C.D.; Ibbott, G.S.; Mohamed, A.S.; Ding, Y.; Yang, J.; Hwang, K.P.; Wang, J. Spatial Precision in Magnetic Resonance Imaging-Guided Radiation Therapy: The Role of Geometric Distortion. *Int. J. Radiat. Oncol. Biol. Phys.* **2016**, *95*, 1304–1316. [CrossRef] [PubMed]
14. Chang, J.H.; Lim Joon, D.; Nguyen, B.T.; Hiew, C.Y.; Esler, S.; Angus, D.; Chao, M.; Wada, M.; Quong, G.; Khoo, V. MRI scans significantly change target coverage decisions in radical radiotherapy for prostate cancer. *J. Med. Imaging Radiat. Oncol.* **2014**, *58*, 237–243. [CrossRef] [PubMed]
15. Dhermain, F. Radiotherapy of high-grade gliomas: Current standards and new concepts, innovations in imaging and radiotherapy, and new therapeutic approaches. *Chin. J. Cancer* **2014**, *33*, 16–24. [CrossRef]
16. Lagendijk, J.J.; Raaymakers, B.W.; van Vulpen, M. The magnetic resonance imaging-linac system. *Semin. Radiat. Oncol.* **2014**, *24*, 207–209. [CrossRef]

17. Acharya, S.; Fischer-Valuck, B.W.; Kashani, R.; Parikh, P.; Yang, D.; Zhao, T.; Green, O.; Wooten, O.; Li, H.H.; Hu, Y.; et al. Online Magnetic Resonance Image Guided Adaptive Radiation Therapy: First Clinical Applications. *Int. J. Radiat. Oncol. Biol. Phys.* **2016**, *94*, 394–403. [CrossRef] [PubMed]
18. Carr, H.Y. Steady-State Free Precession in Nuclear Magnetic Resonance. *Phys. Rev.* **1958**, *112*, 1693–1701. [CrossRef]
19. De Mol van Otterloo, S.R.; Christodouleas, J.P.; Blezer, E.L.A.; Akhiat, H.; Brown, K.; Choudhury, A.; Eggert, D.; Erickson, B.A.; Daamen, L.A.; Faivre-Finn, C.; et al. Patterns of Care, Tolerability, and Safety of the First Cohort of Patients Treated on a Novel High-Field MR-Linac within the MOMENTUM Study: Initial Results from a Prospective Multi-Institutional Registry. *Int. J. Radiat. Oncol. Biol. Phys.* **2021**, *111*, 867–875. [CrossRef] [PubMed]
20. De Leon, J.; Woods, A.; Twentyman, T.; Meade, M.; Sproule, V.; Chandran, S.; Christiansen, J.; Kennedy, N.; Marney, M.; Barooshian, K.; et al. Analysis of data to Advance Personalised Therapy with MR-Linac (ADAPT-MRL). *Clin. Transl. Radiat. Oncol.* **2021**, *31*, 64–70. [CrossRef]
21. Menard, C.; van der Heide, U.A. Introduction: Magnetic resonance imaging comes of age in radiation oncology. *Semin. Radiat. Oncol.* **2014**, *24*, 149–150. [CrossRef] [PubMed]
22. Mutic, S.; Dempsey, J.F. The ViewRay system: Magnetic resonance-guided and controlled radiotherapy. *Semin. Radiat. Oncol.* **2014**, *24*, 196–199. [CrossRef] [PubMed]
23. Wachowicz, K.; De Zanche, N.; Yip, E.; Volotovskyy, V.; Fallone, B.G. CNR considerations for rapid real-time MRI tumor tracking in radiotherapy hybrid devices: Effects of B0 field strength. *Med. Phys.* **2016**, *43*, 4903. [CrossRef]
24. Hori, M.; Hagiwara, A.; Goto, M.; Wada, A.; Aoki, S. Low-Field Magnetic Resonance Imaging: Its History and Renaissance. *Investig. Radiol.* **2021**, *56*, 669–679. [CrossRef] [PubMed]
25. Shultz, D.C. High Field MR Guided Using the Unity Platform. In Proceedings of the 9th MR in RT Symposium, Los Angeles, CA, USA, 7 February 2023.
26. Gillies, R.J.; Bhujwalla, Z.M.; Evelhoch, J.; Garwood, M.; Neeman, M.; Robinson, S.P.; Sotak, C.H.; Van Der Sanden, B. Applications of magnetic resonance in model systems: Tumor biology and physiology. *Neoplasia* **2000**, *2*, 139–151. [CrossRef] [PubMed]
27. Tomaszewski, M.R.; Gillies, R.J. The Biological Meaning of Radiomic Features. *Radiology* **2021**, *299*, E256. [CrossRef]
28. Tomaszewski, M.R.; Latifi, K.; Boyer, E.; Palm, R.F.; El Naqa, I.; Moros, E.G.; Hoffe, S.E.; Rosenberg, S.A.; Frakes, J.M.; Gillies, R.J. Delta radiomics analysis of Magnetic Resonance guided radiotherapy imaging data can enable treatment response prediction in pancreatic cancer. *Radiat. Oncol.* **2021**, *16*, 237. [CrossRef]
29. Park, S.I.; Guenette, J.P.; Suh, C.H.; Hanna, G.J.; Chung, S.R.; Baek, J.H.; Lee, J.H.; Choi, Y.J. The diagnostic performance of CT and MRI for detecting extranodal extension in patients with head and neck squamous cell carcinoma: A systematic review and diagnostic meta-analysis. *Eur. Radiol.* **2021**, *31*, 2048–2061. [CrossRef] [PubMed]
30. Sumi, M.; Nakamura, T. Extranodal spread in the neck: MRI detection on the basis of pixel-based time-signal intensity curve analysis. *J. Magn. Reson. Imaging* **2011**, *33*, 830–838. [CrossRef] [PubMed]
31. Boeke, S.; Monnich, D.; van Timmeren, J.E.; Balermpas, P. MR-Guided Radiotherapy for Head and Neck Cancer: Current Developments, Perspectives, and Challenges. *Front. Oncol.* **2021**, *11*, 616156. [CrossRef] [PubMed]
32. Chuter, R.W.; Pollitt, A.; Whitehurst, P.; MacKay, R.I.; van Herk, M.; McWilliam, A. Assessing MR-linac radiotherapy robustness for anatomical changes in head and neck cancer. *Phys. Med. Biol.* **2018**, *63*, 125020. [CrossRef]
33. Fischer-Valuck, B.W.; Henke, L.; Green, O.; Kashani, R.; Acharya, S.; Bradley, J.D.; Robinson, C.G.; Thomas, M.; Zoberi, I.; Thorstad, W.; et al. Two-and-a-half-year clinical experience with the world's first magnetic resonance image guided radiation therapy system. *Adv. Radiat. Oncol.* **2017**, *2*, 485–493. [CrossRef]
34. Chen, A.M.; Cao, M.; Hsu, S.; Lamb, J.; Mikaeilian, A.; Yang, Y.; Agazaryan, N.; Low, D.A.; Steinberg, M.L. Magnetic resonance imaging guided reirradiation of recurrent and second primary head and neck cancer. *Adv. Radiat. Oncol.* **2017**, *2*, 167–175. [CrossRef]
35. McDonald, B.A.; Vedam, S.; Yang, J.; Wang, J.; Castillo, P.; Lee, B.; Sobremonte, A.; Ahmed, S.; Ding, Y.; Mohamed, A.S.R.; et al. Initial Feasibility and Clinical Implementation of Daily MR-Guided Adaptive Head and Neck Cancer Radiation Therapy on a 1.5T MR-Linac System: Prospective R-IDEAL 2a/2b Systematic Clinical Evaluation of Technical Innovation. *Int. J. Radiat. Oncol. Biol. Phys.* **2021**, *109*, 1606–1618. [CrossRef] [PubMed]
36. Chen, A.M.; Hsu, S.; Lamb, J.; Yang, Y.; Agazaryan, N.; Steinberg, M.L.; Low, D.A.; Cao, M. MRI-guided radiotherapy for head and neck cancer: Initial clinical experience. *Clin. Transl. Oncol.* **2018**, *20*, 160–168. [CrossRef] [PubMed]
37. Malik, N.H.; Kim, M.S.; Chen, H.; Poon, I.; Husain, Z.; Eskander, A.; Boldt, G.; Louie, A.V.; Karam, I. Stereotactic Radiation Therapy for De Novo Head and Neck Cancers: A Systematic Review and Meta-Analysis. *Adv. Radiat. Oncol.* **2021**, *6*, 100628. [CrossRef]
38. Strom, T.; Wishka, C.; Caudell, J.J. Stereotactic Body Radiotherapy for Recurrent Unresectable Head and Neck Cancers. *Cancer Control* **2016**, *23*, 6–11. [CrossRef] [PubMed]
39. Sebastian, N.T.; Xu-Welliver, M.; Williams, T.M. Stereotactic body radiation therapy (SBRT) for early stage non-small cell lung cancer (NSCLC): Contemporary insights and advances. *J. Thorac. Dis.* **2018**, *10*, S2451–S2464. [CrossRef]
40. Wulf, J.; Hädinger, U.; Oppitz, U.; Thiele, W.; Ness-Dourdoumas, R.; Flentje, M. Stereotactic radiotherapy of targets in the lung and liver. *Strahlenther. Onkol.* **2001**, *177*, 645–655. [CrossRef]

41. Palma, D.A.; Olson, R.; Harrow, S.; Gaede, S.; Louie, A.V.; Haasbeek, C.; Mulroy, L.; Lock, M.; Rodrigues, G.B.; Yaremko, B.P.; et al. Stereotactic ablative radiotherapy versus standard of care palliative treatment in patients with oligometastatic cancers (SABR-COMET): A randomised, phase 2, open-label trial. *Lancet* **2019**, *393*, 2051–2058. [CrossRef] [PubMed]
42. Videtic, G.M.M.; Donington, J.; Giuliani, M.; Heinzerling, J.; Karas, T.Z.; Kelsey, C.R.; Lally, B.E.; Latzka, K.; Lo, S.S.; Moghanaki, D.; et al. Stereotactic body radiation therapy for early-stage non-small cell lung cancer: Executive Summary of an ASTRO Evidence-Based Guideline. *Pract. Radiat. Oncol.* **2017**, *7*, 295–301. [CrossRef] [PubMed]
43. Timmerman, R.; Paulus, R.; Galvin, J.; Michalski, J.; Straube, W.; Bradley, J.; Fakiris, A.; Bezjak, A.; Videtic, G.; Johnstone, D.; et al. Stereotactic Body Radiation Therapy for Inoperable Early Stage Lung Cancer. *JAMA* **2010**, *303*, 1070–1076. [CrossRef] [PubMed]
44. Timmerman, R.D.; Hu, C.; Michalski, J.M.; Bradley, J.C.; Galvin, J.; Johnstone, D.W.; Choy, H. Long-term Results of Stereotactic Body Radiation Therapy in Medically Inoperable Stage I Non–Small Cell Lung Cancer. *JAMA Oncol.* **2018**, *4*, 1287–1288. [CrossRef] [PubMed]
45. Timmerman, R.; McGarry, R.; Yiannoutsos, C.; Papiez, L.; Tudor, K.; DeLuca, J.; Ewing, M.; Abdulrahman, R.; DesRosiers, C.; Williams, M.; et al. Excessive toxicity when treating central tumors in a phase II study of stereotactic body radiation therapy for medically inoperable early-stage lung cancer. *J. Clin. Oncol.* **2006**, *24*, 4833–4839. [CrossRef] [PubMed]
46. Bezjak, A.; Paulus, R.; Gaspar, L.E.; Timmerman, R.D.; Straube, W.L.; Ryan, W.F.; Garces, Y.I.; Pu, A.T.; Singh, A.K.; Videtic, G.M.; et al. Safety and Efficacy of a Five-Fraction Stereotactic Body Radiotherapy Schedule for Centrally Located Non-Small-Cell Lung Cancer: NRG Oncology/RTOG 0813 Trial. *J. Clin. Oncol.* **2019**, *37*, 1316–1325. [CrossRef]
47. Fakiris, A.J.; McGarry, R.C.; Yiannoutsos, C.T.; Papiez, L.; Williams, M.; Henderson, M.A.; Timmerman, R. Stereotactic body radiation therapy for early-stage non-small-cell lung carcinoma: Four-year results of a prospective phase II study. *Int. J. Radiat. Oncol. Biol. Phys.* **2009**, *75*, 677–682. [CrossRef] [PubMed]
48. Chaudhuri, A.A.; Tang, C.; Binkley, M.S.; Jin, M.; Wynne, J.F.; von Eyben, R.; Hara, W.Y.; Trakul, N.; Loo, B.W., Jr.; Diehn, M. Stereotactic ablative radiotherapy (SABR) for treatment of central and ultra-central lung tumors. *Lung Cancer* **2015**, *89*, 50–56. [CrossRef]
49. Lindberg, K.; Grozman, V.; Karlsson, K.; Lindberg, S.; Lax, I.; Wersall, P.; Persson, G.F.; Josipovic, M.; Khalil, A.A.; Moeller, D.S.; et al. The HILUS-Trial-a Prospective Nordic Multicenter Phase 2 Study of Ultracentral Lung Tumors Treated With Stereotactic Body Radiotherapy. *J. Thorac. Oncol.* **2021**, *16*, 1200–1210. [CrossRef]
50. Henke, L.; Kashani, R.; Yang, D.; Zhao, T.; Green, O.; Olsen, L.; Rodriguez, V.; Wooten, H.O.; Li, H.H.; Hu, Y.; et al. Simulated Online Adaptive Magnetic Resonance-Guided Stereotactic Body Radiation Therapy for the Treatment of Oligometastatic Disease of the Abdomen and Central Thorax: Characterization of Potential Advantages. *Int. J. Radiat. Oncol. Biol. Phys.* **2016**, *96*, 1078–1086. [CrossRef]
51. Regnery, S.; Buchele, C.; Weykamp, F.; Pohl, M.; Hoegen, P.; Eichkorn, T.; Held, T.; Ristau, J.; Rippke, C.; Konig, L.; et al. Adaptive MR-Guided Stereotactic Radiotherapy is Beneficial for Ablative Treatment of Lung Tumors in High-Risk Locations. *Front. Oncol.* **2021**, *11*, 757031. [CrossRef] [PubMed]
52. Ligtenberg, H.; Hackett, S.L.; Merckel, L.G.; Snoeren, L.; Kontaxis, C.; Zachiu, C.; Bol, G.H.; Verhoeff, J.J.C.; Fast, M.F. Towards mid-position based Stereotactic Body Radiation Therapy using online magnetic resonance imaging guidance for central lung tumours. *Phys. Imaging Radiat. Oncol.* **2022**, *23*, 24–31. [CrossRef] [PubMed]
53. Finazzi, T.; Haasbeek, C.J.A.; Spoelstra, F.O.B.; Palacios, M.A.; Admiraal, M.A.; Bruynzeel, A.M.E.; Slotman, B.J.; Lagerwaard, F.J.; Senan, S. Clinical Outcomes of Stereotactic MR-Guided Adaptive Radiation Therapy for High-Risk Lung Tumors. *Int. J. Radiat. Oncol. Biol. Phys.* **2020**, *107*, 270–278. [CrossRef] [PubMed]
54. Henke, L.E.; Olsen, J.R.; Contreras, J.A.; Curcuru, A.; DeWees, T.A.; Green, O.L.; Michalski, J.; Mutic, S.; Roach, M.C.; Bradley, J.D.; et al. Stereotactic MR-Guided Online Adaptive Radiation Therapy (SMART) for Ultracentral Thorax Malignancies: Results of a Phase 1 Trial. *Adv. Radiat. Oncol.* **2019**, *4*, 201–209. [CrossRef] [PubMed]
55. Bryant, J.M.; Sim, A.J.; Feygelman, V.; Latifi, K.; Rosenberg, S.A. Adaptive hypofractionted and stereotactic body radiotherapy for lung tumors with real-time MRI guidance. *Front. Oncol.* **2023**, *13*, 1061854. [CrossRef]
56. Sandoval, M.L.; Sim, A.J.; Bryant, J.M.; Bhandari, M.; Wuthrick, E.J.; Perez, B.A.; Dilling, T.J.; Redler, G.; Andreozzi, J.; Nardella, L.; et al. MR-Guided SBRT/Hypofractionated RT for Metastatic and Primary Central and Ultracentral Lung Lesions. *JTO Clin. Res. Rep.* **2023**, 100488. [CrossRef]
57. Reardon, M.J.; Walkes, J.C.; Benjamin, R. Therapy insight: Malignant primary cardiac tumors. *Nat. Clin. Pract. Cardiovasc. Med.* **2006**, *3*, 548–553. [CrossRef]
58. Hudzik, B.; Miszalski-Jamka, K.; Glowacki, J.; Lekston, A.; Gierlotka, M.; Zembala, M.; Polonski, L.; Gasior, M. Malignant tumors of the heart. *Cancer Epidemiol.* **2015**, *39*, 665–672. [CrossRef]
59. Goldberg, A.D.; Blankstein, R.; Padera, R.F. Tumors metastatic to the heart. *Circulation* **2013**, *128*, 1790–1794. [CrossRef]
60. Wolchok, J.D.; Chiarion-Sileni, V.; Gonzalez, R.; Rutkowski, P.; Grob, J.J.; Cowey, C.L.; Lao, C.D.; Wagstaff, J.; Schadendorf, D.; Ferrucci, P.F.; et al. Overall Survival with Combined Nivolumab and Ipilimumab in Advanced Melanoma. *N. Engl. J. Med.* **2017**, *377*, 1345–1356. [CrossRef]
61. Murphy, M.C.; Sweeney, M.S.; Putnam, J.B., Jr.; Walker, W.E.; Frazier, O.H.; Ott, D.A.; Cooley, D.A. Surgical treatment of cardiac tumors: A 25-year experience. *Ann. Thorac. Surg.* **1990**, *49*, 612–617; discussion 617–618. [CrossRef]
62. Cham, W.C.; Freiman, A.H.; Carstens, P.H.; Chu, F.C. Radiation therapy of cardiac and pericardial metastases. *Radiology* **1975**, *114*, 701–704. [CrossRef]

63. Bonomo, P.; Livi, L.; Rampini, A.; Meattini, I.; Agresti, B.; Simontacchi, G.; Paiar, F.; Mangoni, M.; Bonucci, I.; Greto, D.; et al. Stereotactic body radiotherapy for cardiac and paracardiac metastases: University of Florence experience. *Radiol. Med.* **2013**, *118*, 1055–1065. [CrossRef] [PubMed]
64. Sim, A.J.; Palm, R.F.; DeLozier, K.B.; Feygelman, V.; Latifi, K.; Redler, G.; Washington, I.R.; Wuthrick, E.J.; Rosenberg, S.A. MR-guided stereotactic body radiation therapy for intracardiac and pericardial metastases. *Clin. Transl. Radiat. Oncol.* **2020**, *25*, 102–106. [CrossRef] [PubMed]
65. Katz, M.H.G.; Shi, Q.; Meyers, J.P.; Herman, J.M.; Choung, M.; Wolpin, B.M.; Ahmad, S.; Marsh, R.d.W.; Schwartz, L.H.; Behr, S.; et al. Alliance A021501: Preoperative mFOLFIRINOX or mFOLFIRINOX plus hypofractionated radiation therapy (RT) for borderline resectable (BR) adenocarcinoma of the pancreas. *J. Clin. Oncol.* **2021**, *39*, 377. [CrossRef]
66. Chang, D.T.; Schellenberg, D.; Shen, J.; Kim, J.; Goodman, K.A.; Fisher, G.A.; Ford, J.M.; Desser, T.; Quon, A.; Koong, A.C. Stereotactic radiotherapy for unresectable adenocarcinoma of the pancreas. *Cancer* **2009**, *115*, 665–672. [CrossRef] [PubMed]
67. Hammel, P.; Huguet, F.; van Laethem, J.L.; Goldstein, D.; Glimelius, B.; Artru, P.; Borbath, I.; Bouche, O.; Shannon, J.; Andre, T.; et al. Effect of Chemoradiotherapy vs Chemotherapy on Survival in Patients with Locally Advanced Pancreatic Cancer Controlled after 4 Months of Gemcitabine with or without Erlotinib: The LAP07 Randomized Clinical Trial. *JAMA* **2016**, *315*, 1844–1853. [CrossRef]
68. Koong, A.C.; Le, Q.T.; Ho, A.; Fong, B.; Fisher, G.; Cho, C.; Ford, J.; Poen, J.; Gibbs, I.C.; Mehta, V.K.; et al. Phase I study of stereotactic radiosurgery in patients with locally advanced pancreatic cancer. *Int. J. Radiat. Oncol. Biol. Phys.* **2004**, *58*, 1017–1021. [CrossRef]
69. Koong, A.C.; Christofferson, E.; Le, Q.T.; Goodman, K.A.; Ho, A.; Kuo, T.; Ford, J.M.; Fisher, G.A.; Greco, R.; Norton, J.; et al. Phase II study to assess the efficacy of conventionally fractionated radiotherapy followed by a stereotactic radiosurgery boost in patients with locally advanced pancreatic cancer. *Int. J. Radiat. Oncol. Biol. Phys.* **2005**, *63*, 320–323. [CrossRef]
70. Hoyer, M.; Roed, H.; Sengelov, L.; Traberg, A.; Ohlhuis, L.; Pedersen, J.; Nellemann, H.; Kiil Berthelsen, A.; Eberholst, F.; Engelholm, S.A.; et al. Phase-II study on stereotactic radiotherapy of locally advanced pancreatic carcinoma. *Radiother. Oncol.* **2005**, *76*, 48–53. [CrossRef]
71. Schellenberg, D.; Goodman, K.A.; Lee, F.; Chang, S.; Kuo, T.; Ford, J.M.; Fisher, G.A.; Quon, A.; Desser, T.S.; Norton, J.; et al. Gemcitabine chemotherapy and single-fraction stereotactic body radiotherapy for locally advanced pancreatic cancer. *Int. J. Radiat. Oncol. Biol. Phys.* **2008**, *72*, 678–686. [CrossRef]
72. Schellenberg, D.; Kim, J.; Christman-Skieller, C.; Chun, C.L.; Columbo, L.A.; Ford, J.M.; Fisher, G.A.; Kunz, P.L.; Van Dam, J.; Quon, A.; et al. Single-fraction stereotactic body radiation therapy and sequential gemcitabine for the treatment of locally advanced pancreatic cancer. *Int. J. Radiat. Oncol. Biol. Phys.* **2011**, *81*, 181–188. [CrossRef]
73. Zhu, X.; Ju, X.; Cao, Y.; Shen, Y.; Cao, F.; Qing, S.; Fang, F.; Jia, Z.; Zhang, H. Patterns of Local Failure after Stereotactic Body Radiation Therapy and Sequential Chemotherapy as Initial Treatment for Pancreatic Cancer: Implications of Target Volume Design. *Int. J. Radiat. Oncol. Biol. Phys.* **2019**, *104*, 101–110. [CrossRef] [PubMed]
74. Bernard, V.; Herman, J.M. Pancreas SBRT: Who, What, When, Where, and How. *Pract. Radiat. Oncol.* **2020**, *10*, 183–185. [CrossRef] [PubMed]
75. Arcelli, A.; Guido, A.; Buwenge, M.; Simoni, N.; Mazzarotto, R.; Macchia, G.; Deodato, F.; Cilla, S.; Bonomo, P.; Scotti, V.; et al. Higher Biologically Effective Dose Predicts Survival in SBRT of Pancreatic Cancer: A Multicentric Analysis (PAULA-1). *Anticancer Res.* **2020**, *40*, 465–472. [CrossRef]
76. Krishnan, S.; Chadha, A.S.; Suh, Y.; Chen, H.C.; Rao, A.; Das, P.; Minsky, B.D.; Mahmood, U.; Delclos, M.E.; Sawakuchi, G.O.; et al. Focal Radiation Therapy Dose Escalation Improves Overall Survival in Locally Advanced Pancreatic Cancer Patients Receiving Induction Chemotherapy and Consolidative Chemoradiation. *Int. J. Radiat. Oncol. Biol. Phys.* **2016**, *94*, 755–765. [CrossRef] [PubMed]
77. Ma, S.J.; Prezzano, K.M.; Hermann, G.M.; Singh, A.K. Dose escalation of radiation therapy with or without induction chemotherapy for unresectable locally advanced pancreatic cancer. *Radiat. Oncol.* **2018**, *13*, 214. [CrossRef]
78. Reyngold, M.; O'Reilly, E.M.; Varghese, A.M.; Fiasconaro, M.; Zinovoy, M.; Romesser, P.B.; Wu, A.; Hajj, C.; Cuaron, J.J.; Tuli, R.; et al. Association of Ablative Radiation Therapy with Survival Among Patients with Inoperable Pancreatic Cancer. *JAMA Oncol.* **2021**, *7*, 735–738. [CrossRef] [PubMed]
79. Tchelebi, L.T.; Zaorsky, N.G.; Rosenberg, J.C.; Sharma, N.K.; Tuanquin, L.C.; Mackley, H.B.; Ellis, R.J. Reducing the Toxicity of Radiotherapy for Pancreatic Cancer With Magnetic Resonance-guided Radiotherapy. *Toxicol. Sci.* **2020**, *175*, 19–23. [CrossRef]
80. Bohoudi, O.; Bruynzeel, A.M.E.; Senan, S.; Cuijpers, J.P.; Slotman, B.J.; Lagerwaard, F.J.; Palacios, M.A. Fast and robust online adaptive planning in stereotactic MR-guided adaptive radiation therapy (SMART) for pancreatic cancer. *Radiother. Oncol.* **2017**, *125*, 439–444. [CrossRef]
81. Rudra, S.; Jiang, N.; Rosenberg, S.A.; Olsen, J.R.; Roach, M.C.; Wan, L.; Portelance, L.; Mellon, E.A.; Bruynzeel, A.; Lagerwaard, F.; et al. Using adaptive magnetic resonance image-guided radiation therapy for treatment of inoperable pancreatic cancer. *Cancer Med.* **2019**, *8*, 2123–2132. [CrossRef]
82. Chuong, M.D.; Bryant, J.; Mittauer, K.E.; Hall, M.; Kotecha, R.; Alvarez, D.; Romaguera, T.; Rubens, M.; Adamson, S.; Godley, A.; et al. Ablative 5-Fraction Stereotactic Magnetic Resonance-Guided Radiation Therapy with On-Table Adaptive Replanning and Elective Nodal Irradiation for Inoperable Pancreas Cancer. *Pract. Radiat. Oncol.* **2021**, *11*, 134–147. [CrossRef]

83. Hassanzadeh, C.; Rudra, S.; Bommireddy, A.; Hawkins, W.G.; Wang-Gillam, A.; Fields, R.C.; Cai, B.; Park, J.; Green, O.; Roach, M.; et al. Ablative Five-Fraction Stereotactic Body Radiation Therapy for Inoperable Pancreatic Cancer Using Online MR-Guided Adaptation. *Adv. Radiat. Oncol.* **2021**, *6*, 100506. [CrossRef] [PubMed]
84. Bryant, J.; Palm, R.F.; Herrera, R.; Rubens, M.; Hoffe, S.E.; Kim, D.W.; Kaiser, A.; Ucar, A.; Fleming, J.; De Zarraga, F.; et al. Multi-Institutional Outcomes of Patients Aged 75 years and Older with Pancreatic Ductal Adenocarcinoma Treated with 5-Fraction Ablative Stereotactic Magnetic Resonance Image-Guided Adaptive Radiation Therapy (A-SMART). *Cancer Control* **2023**, *30*, 10732748221150228. [CrossRef] [PubMed]
85. Heerkens, H.D.; van Vulpen, M.; Erickson, B.; Reerink, O.; Intven, M.P.; van den Berg, C.A.; Molenaar, I.Q.; Vleggaar, F.P.; Meijer, G.J. MRI guided stereotactic radiotherapy for locally advanced pancreatic cancer. *Br. J. Radiol.* **2018**, *91*, 20170563. [CrossRef] [PubMed]
86. Henke, L.; Kashani, R.; Robinson, C.; Curcuru, A.; DeWees, T.; Bradley, J.; Green, O.; Michalski, J.; Mutic, S.; Parikh, P.; et al. Phase I trial of stereotactic MR-guided online adaptive radiation therapy (SMART) for the treatment of oligometastatic or unresectable primary malignancies of the abdomen. *Radiother. Oncol.* **2018**, *126*, 519–526. [CrossRef] [PubMed]
87. Hall, W.A.; Straza, M.W.; Chen, X.; Mickevicius, N.; Erickson, B.; Schultz, C.; Awan, M.; Ahunbay, E.; Li, X.A.; Paulson, E.S. Initial clinical experience of Stereotactic Body Radiation Therapy (SBRT) for liver metastases, primary liver malignancy, and pancreatic cancer with 4D-MRI based online adaptation and real-time MRI monitoring using a 1.5 Tesla MR-Linac. *PLoS ONE* **2020**, *15*, e0236570. [CrossRef]
88. Bryant, J.M.; Palm, R.F.; Liveringhouse, C.; Boyer, E.; Hodul, P.; Malafa, M.; Denbo, J.; Kim, D.; Carballido, E.; Fleming, J.B.; et al. Surgical and Pathologic Outcomes of Pancreatic Adenocarcinoma (PA) After Preoperative Ablative Stereotactic Magnetic Resonance Image Guided Adaptive Radiation Therapy (A-SMART). *Adv. Radiat. Oncol.* **2022**, *7*, 101045. [CrossRef] [PubMed]
89. Parikh, P.J.; Lee, P.; Low, D.; Kim, J.; Mittauer, K.E.; Bassetti, M.F.; Glide-Hurst, C.; Raldow, A.; Yang, Y.; Portelance, L.; et al. Stereotactic MR-Guided On-Table Adaptive Radiation Therapy (SMART) for Patients with Borderline or Locally Advanced Pancreatic Cancer: Primary Endpoint Outcomes of a Prospective Phase II Multi-Center International Trial. *Int. J. Radiat. Oncol.* **2022**, *114*, 1062–1063. [CrossRef]
90. Benson, A.B.; D'Angelica, M.I.; Abbott, D.E.; Anaya, D.A.; Anders, R.; Are, C.; Bachini, M.; Borad, M.; Brown, D.; Burgoyne, A.; et al. Hepatobiliary Cancers, Version 2.2021, NCCN Clinical Practice Guidelines in Oncology. *J. Natl. Compr. Cancer Netw.* **2021**, *19*, 541–565. [CrossRef]
91. Adam, R.; Chiche, L.; Aloia, T.; Elias, D.; Salmon, R.; Rivoire, M.; Jaeck, D.; Saric, J.; Le Treut, Y.P.; Belghiti, J.; et al. Hepatic resection for noncolorectal nonendocrine liver metastases: Analysis of 1452 patients and development of a prognostic model. *Ann. Surg.* **2006**, *244*, 524–535. [CrossRef] [PubMed]
92. Nordlinger, B.; Sorbye, H.; Glimelius, B.; Poston, G.J.; Schlag, P.M.; Rougier, P.; Bechstein, W.O.; Primrose, J.N.; Walpole, E.T.; Finch-Jones, M.; et al. Perioperative FOLFOX4 chemotherapy and surgery versus surgery alone for resectable liver metastases from colorectal cancer (EORTC 40983): Long-term results of a randomised, controlled, phase 3 trial. *Lancet Oncol.* **2013**, *14*, 1208–1215. [CrossRef]
93. Smith, J.J.; D'Angelica, M.I. Surgical management of hepatic metastases of colorectal cancer. *Hematol. Oncol. Clin. N. Am.* **2015**, *29*, 61–84. [CrossRef]
94. Ruers, T.; Van Coevorden, F.; Punt, C.J.; Pierie, J.E.; Borel-Rinkes, I.; Ledermann, J.A.; Poston, G.; Bechstein, W.; Lentz, M.A.; Mauer, M.; et al. Local Treatment of Unresectable Colorectal Liver Metastases: Results of a Randomized Phase II Trial. *JNCI J. Natl. Cancer Inst.* **2017**, *109*, djx015. [CrossRef]
95. Rim, C.H.; Lee, J.S.; Kim, S.Y.; Seong, J. Comparison of radiofrequency ablation and ablative external radiotherapy for the treatment of intrahepatic malignancies: A hybrid meta-analysis. *JHEP Rep.* **2023**, *5*, 100594. [CrossRef] [PubMed]
96. Dawson, L.A.; Winter, K.A.; Knox, J.J.; Zhu, A.X.; Krishnan, S.; Guha, C.; Kachnic, L.A.; Gillin, M.; Hong, T.S.; Craig, T.; et al. NRG/RTOG 1112: Randomized Phase III Study of Sorafenib vs. Stereotactic Body Radiation Therapy (SBRT) Followed by Sorafenib in Hepatocellular Carcinoma (HCC) (NCT01730937). In Proceedings of the ASTRO's 64th Annual Meeting, San Antonio, TX, USA, 23–26 October 2022; p. 1057.
97. Ohri, N.; Tome, W.A.; Mendez Romero, A.; Miften, M.; Ten Haken, R.K.; Dawson, L.A.; Grimm, J.; Yorke, E.; Jackson, A. Local Control After Stereotactic Body Radiation Therapy for Liver Tumors. *Int. J. Radiat. Oncol. Biol. Phys.* **2021**, *110*, 188–195. [CrossRef]
98. Pan, C.C.; Kavanagh, B.D.; Dawson, L.A.; Li, X.A.; Das, S.K.; Miften, M.; Ten Haken, R.K. Radiation-associated liver injury. *Int. J. Radiat. Oncol. Biol. Phys.* **2010**, *76*, S94–S100. [CrossRef] [PubMed]
99. Sterzing, F.; Brunner, T.B.; Ernst, I.; Baus, W.W.; Greve, B.; Herfarth, K.; Guckenberger, M. Stereotactic body radiotherapy for liver tumors: Principles and practical guidelines of the DEGRO Working Group on Stereotactic Radiotherapy. *Strahlenther. Onkol.* **2014**, *190*, 872–881. [CrossRef] [PubMed]
100. Feldman, A.M.; Modh, A.; Glide-Hurst, C.; Chetty, I.J.; Movsas, B. Real-time Magnetic Resonance-guided Liver Stereotactic Body Radiation Therapy: An Institutional Report Using a Magnetic Resonance-Linac System. *Cureus* **2019**, *11*, e5774. [CrossRef] [PubMed]
101. Rosenberg, S.A.; Henke, L.E.; Shaverdian, N.; Mittauer, K.; Wojcieszynski, A.P.; Hullett, C.R.; Kamrava, M.; Lamb, J.; Cao, M.; Green, O.L.; et al. A Multi-Institutional Experience of MR-Guided Liver Stereotactic Body Radiation Therapy. *Adv. Radiat. Oncol.* **2019**, *4*, 142–149. [CrossRef] [PubMed]

102. Boldrini, L.; Cellini, F.; Manfrida, S.; Chiloiro, G.; Teodoli, S.; Cusumano, D.; Fionda, B.; Mattiucci, G.C.; De Gaetano, A.M.; Azario, L.; et al. Use of Indirect Target Gating in Magnetic Resonance-guided Liver Stereotactic Body Radiotherapy: Case Report of an Oligometastatic Patient. *Cureus* **2018**, *10*, e2292. [CrossRef]
103. Moreno, P.; de la Quintana Basarrate, A.; Musholt, T.J.; Paunovic, I.; Puccini, M.; Vidal, O.; Ortega, J.; Kraimps, J.L.; Bollo Arocena, E.; Rodriguez, J.M.; et al. Adrenalectomy for solid tumor metastases: Results of a multicenter European study. *Surgery* **2013**, *154*, 1215–1222; discussion 1222–1223. [CrossRef] [PubMed]
104. Planchard, D.; Popat, S.; Kerr, K.; Novello, S.; Smit, E.F.; Faivre-Finn, C.; Mok, T.S.; Reck, M.; Van Schil, P.E.; Hellmann, M.D.; et al. Metastatic non-small cell lung cancer: ESMO Clinical Practice Guidelines for diagnosis, treatment and follow-up. *Ann. Oncol.* **2018**, *29*, iv192–iv237. [CrossRef] [PubMed]
105. Yaney, A.; Stevens, A.; Monk, P.; Martin, D.; Diaz, D.A.; Wang, S.J. Radiotherapy in Oligometastatic, Oligorecurrent and Oligoprogressive Prostate Cancer: A Mini-Review. *Front. Oncol.* **2022**, *12*, 932637. [CrossRef] [PubMed]
106. Scorsetti, M.; Alongi, F.; Filippi, A.R.; Pentimalli, S.; Navarria, P.; Clerici, E.; Castiglioni, S.; Tozzi, A.; Reggiori, G.; Mancosu, P.; et al. Long-term local control achieved after hypofractionated stereotactic body radiotherapy for adrenal gland metastases: A retrospective analysis of 34 patients. *Acta Oncol.* **2012**, *51*, 618–623. [CrossRef] [PubMed]
107. Alexandrescu, S.T.; Croitoru, A.E.; Grigorie, R.T.; Tomescu, D.R.; Droc, G.; Grasu, M.C.; Popescu, I. Aggressive surgical approach in patients with adrenal-only metastases from hepatocellular carcinoma enables higher survival rates than standard systemic therapy. *Hepatobiliary Pancreat. Dis. Int.* **2021**, *20*, 28–33. [CrossRef]
108. Gunjur, A.; Duong, C.; Ball, D.; Siva, S. Surgical and ablative therapies for the management of adrenal 'oligometastases'—A systematic review. *Cancer Treat. Rev.* **2014**, *40*, 838–846. [CrossRef] [PubMed]
109. Holy, R.; Piroth, M.; Pinkawa, M.; Eble, M.J. Stereotactic body radiation therapy (SBRT) for treatment of adrenal gland metastases from non-small cell lung cancer. *Strahlenther. Onkol.* **2011**, *187*, 245–251. [CrossRef] [PubMed]
110. Rudra, S.; Malik, R.; Ranck, M.C.; Farrey, K.; Golden, D.W.; Hasselle, M.D.; Weichselbaum, R.R.; Salama, J.K. Stereotactic body radiation therapy for curative treatment of adrenal metastases. *Technol. Cancer Res. Treat.* **2013**, *12*, 217–224. [CrossRef]
111. Chance, W.W.; Nguyen, Q.N.; Mehran, R.; Welsh, J.W.; Gomez, D.R.; Balter, P.; Komaki, R.; Liao, Z.; Chang, J.Y. Stereotactic ablative radiotherapy for adrenal gland metastases: Factors influencing outcomes, patterns of failure, and dosimetric thresholds for toxicity. *Pract. Radiat. Oncol.* **2017**, *7*, e195–e203. [CrossRef]
112. Wysocka, B.; Kassam, Z.; Lockwood, G.; Brierley, J.; Dawson, L.A.; Buckley, C.A.; Jaffray, D.; Cummings, B.; Kim, J.; Wong, R.; et al. Interfraction and respiratory organ motion during conformal radiotherapy in gastric cancer. *Int. J. Radiat. Oncol. Biol. Phys.* **2010**, *77*, 53–59. [CrossRef]
113. Knybel, L.; Cvek, J.; Otahal, B.; Jonszta, T.; Molenda, L.; Czerny, D.; Skacelikova, E.; Rybar, M.; Dvorak, P.; Feltl, D. The analysis of respiration-induced pancreatic tumor motion based on reference measurement. *Radiat. Oncol.* **2014**, *9*, 192. [CrossRef] [PubMed]
114. Chen, B.; Hu, Y.; Liu, J.; Cao, A.N.; Ye, L.X.; Zeng, Z.C. Respiratory motion of adrenal gland metastases: Analyses using four-dimensional computed tomography images. *Phys. Med.* **2017**, *38*, 54–58. [CrossRef] [PubMed]
115. Desai, A.; Rai, H.; Haas, J.; Witten, M.; Blacksburg, S.; Schneider, J.G. A Retrospective Review of CyberKnife Stereotactic Body Radiotherapy for Adrenal Tumors (Primary and Metastatic): Winthrop University Hospital Experience. *Front. Oncol.* **2015**, *5*, 185. [CrossRef] [PubMed]
116. Palacios, M.A.; Bohoudi, O.; Bruynzeel, A.M.E.; van Sorsen de Koste, J.R.; Cobussen, P.; Slotman, B.J.; Lagerwaard, F.J.; Senan, S. Role of Daily Plan Adaptation in MR-Guided Stereotactic Ablative Radiation Therapy for Adrenal Metastases. *Int. J. Radiat. Oncol. Biol. Phys.* **2018**, *102*, 426–433. [CrossRef]
117. Michalet, M.; Bettaieb, O.; Khalfi, S.; Ghorbel, A.; Valdenaire, S.; Debuire, P.; Ailleres, N.; Draghici, R.; De Meric De Bellefon, M.; Charissoux, M.; et al. Stereotactic MR-Guided Radiotherapy for Adrenal Gland Metastases: First Clinical Results. *J. Clin. Med.* **2022**, *12*, 291. [CrossRef]
118. Motzer, R.J.; Jonasch, E.; Agarwal, N.; Alva, A.; Baine, M.; Beckermann, K.; Carlo, M.I.; Choueiri, T.K.; Costello, B.A.; Derweesh, I.H.; et al. Kidney Cancer, Version 3.2022, NCCN Clinical Practice Guidelines in Oncology. *J. Natl. Compr. Cancer Netw.* **2022**, *20*, 71–90. [CrossRef]
119. Siva, S.; Correa, R.J.M.; Warner, A.; Staehler, M.; Ellis, R.J.; Ponsky, L.; Kaplan, I.D.; Mahadevan, A.; Chu, W.; Gandhidasan, S.; et al. Stereotactic Ablative Radiotherapy for >/=T1b Primary Renal Cell Carcinoma: A Report from the International Radiosurgery Oncology Consortium for Kidney (IROCK). *Int. J. Radiat. Oncol. Biol. Phys.* **2020**, *108*, 941–949. [CrossRef]
120. Siva, S.; Ali, M.; Correa, R.J.M.; Muacevic, A.; Ponsky, L.; Ellis, R.J.; Lo, S.S.; Onishi, H.; Swaminath, A.; McLaughlin, M.; et al. 5-year outcomes after stereotactic ablative body radiotherapy for primary renal cell carcinoma: An individual patient data meta-analysis from IROCK (the International Radiosurgery Consortium of the Kidney). *Lancet Oncol.* **2022**, *23*, 1508–1516. [CrossRef]
121. Sonier, M.; Chu, W.; Lalani, N.; Erler, D.; Cheung, P.; Korol, R. Implementation of a volumetric modulated arc therapy treatment planning solution for kidney and adrenal stereotactic body radiation therapy. *Med. Dosim.* **2016**, *41*, 323–328. [CrossRef] [PubMed]
122. Prins, F.M.; Stemkens, B.; Kerkmeijer, L.G.W.; Barendrecht, M.M.; de Boer, H.J.; Vonken, E.P.A.; Lagendijk, J.J.W.; Tijssen, R.H.N. Intrafraction Motion Management of Renal Cell Carcinoma With Magnetic Resonance Imaging-Guided Stereotactic Body Radiation Therapy. *Pract. Radiat. Oncol.* **2019**, *9*, e55–e61. [CrossRef] [PubMed]
123. Keller, B.; Bruynzeel, A.M.E.; Tang, C.; Swaminath, A.; Kerkmeijer, L.; Chu, W. Adaptive Magnetic Resonance-Guided Stereotactic Body Radiotherapy: The Next Step in the Treatment of Renal Cell Carcinoma. *Front. Oncol.* **2021**, *11*, 634830. [CrossRef]

124. Rudra, S.; Fischer-Valuck, B.; Pachynski, R.; Daly, M.; Green, O. Magnetic Resonance Image Guided Stereotactic Body Radiation Therapy to the Primary Renal Mass in Metastatic Renal Cell Carcinoma. *Adv. Radiat. Oncol.* **2019**, *4*, 566–570. [CrossRef]
125. Tetar, S.U.; Bohoudi, O.; Senan, S.; Palacios, M.A.; Oei, S.S.; Wel, A.M.V.; Slotman, B.J.; Moorselaar, R.; Lagerwaard, F.J.; Bruynzeel, A.M.E. The Role of Daily Adaptive Stereotactic MR-Guided Radiotherapy for Renal Cell Cancer. *Cancers* **2020**, *12*, 2763. [CrossRef] [PubMed]
126. Lalani, A.-K.A.; Swaminath, A.; Pond, G.R.; Morgan, S.C.; Azad, A.; Chu, W.; Winquist, E.; Kapoor, A.; Bonert, M.; Bramson, J.L.; et al. Phase II trial of cytoreductive stereotactic hypofractionated radiotherapy with combination ipilimumab/nivolumab for metastatic kidney cancer (CYTOSHRINK). *J. Clin. Oncol.* **2022**, *40*, TPS398. [CrossRef]
127. Siva, S.; Chesson, B.; Bressel, M.; Pryor, D.; Higgs, B.; Reynolds, H.M.; Hardcastle, N.; Montgomery, R.; Vanneste, B.; Khoo, V.; et al. TROG 15.03 phase II clinical trial of Focal Ablative STereotactic Radiosurgery for Cancers of the Kidney—FASTRACK II. *BMC Cancer* **2018**, *18*, 1030. [CrossRef]
128. Early Stage Breast Cancer. Consent Statement. 1990. Available online: https://consensus.nih.gov/1990/1990earlystagebreastcancer081html.htm (accessed on 12 March 2023).
129. Acharya, S.; Hsieh, S.; Michalski, J.M.; Shinohara, E.T.; Perkins, S.M. Distance to Radiation Facility and Treatment Choice in Early-Stage Breast Cancer. *Int. J. Radiat. Oncol. Biol. Phys.* **2016**, *94*, 691–699. [CrossRef] [PubMed]
130. Joo, J.H.; Ki, Y.; Jeon, H.; Kim, D.W.; Jung, J.; Kim, S.S. Who are the optimal candidates for partial breast irradiation? *Asia Pac. J. Clin. Oncol.* **2021**, *17*, 305–311. [CrossRef] [PubMed]
131. Meattini, I.; Marrazzo, L.; Saieva, C.; Desideri, I.; Scotti, V.; Simontacchi, G.; Bonomo, P.; Greto, D.; Mangoni, M.; Scoccianti, S.; et al. Accelerated Partial-Breast Irradiation Compared With Whole-Breast Irradiation for Early Breast Cancer: Long-Term Results of the Randomized Phase III APBI-IMRT-Florence Trial. *J. Clin. Oncol.* **2020**, *38*, 4175–4183. [CrossRef] [PubMed]
132. Galalae, R.; Hannoun-Levi, J.M. Accelerated partial breast irradiation by brachytherapy: Present evidence and future developments. *Jpn. J. Clin. Oncol.* **2020**, *50*, 743–752. [CrossRef]
133. Livi, L.; Meattini, I.; Marrazzo, L.; Simontacchi, G.; Pallotta, S.; Saieva, C.; Paiar, F.; Scotti, V.; De Luca Cardillo, C.; Bastiani, P.; et al. Accelerated partial breast irradiation using intensity-modulated radiotherapy versus whole breast irradiation: 5-year survival analysis of a phase 3 randomised controlled trial. *Eur. J. Cancer* **2015**, *51*, 451–463. [CrossRef]
134. Whelan, T.J.; Julian, J.A.; Berrang, T.S.; Kim, D.H.; Germain, I.; Nichol, A.M.; Akra, M.; Lavertu, S.; Germain, F.; Fyles, A.; et al. External beam accelerated partial breast irradiation versus whole breast irradiation after breast conserving surgery in women with ductal carcinoma in situ and node-negative breast cancer (RAPID): A randomised controlled trial. *Lancet* **2019**, *394*, 2165–2172. [CrossRef] [PubMed]
135. Kennedy, W.R.; Roach, M.C.; Thomas, M.A.; Ochoa, L.; Altman, M.B.; Hernandez-Aya, L.F.; Cyr, A.E.; Margenthaler, J.A.; Zoberi, I. Long-Term Outcomes with 3-Dimensional Conformal External Beam Accelerated Partial Breast Irradiation. *Pract. Radiat. Oncol.* **2020**, *10*, e128–e135. [CrossRef] [PubMed]
136. Acharya, S.; Fischer-Valuck, B.W.; Mazur, T.R.; Curcuru, A.; Sona, K.; Kashani, R.; Green, O.; Ochoa, L.; Mutic, S.; Zoberi, I.; et al. Magnetic Resonance Image Guided Radiation Therapy for External Beam Accelerated Partial-Breast Irradiation: Evaluation of Delivered Dose and Intrafractional Cavity Motion. *Int. J. Radiat. Oncol. Biol. Phys.* **2016**, *96*, 785–792. [CrossRef] [PubMed]
137. Price, A.T.; Kennedy, W.R.; Henke, L.E.; Brown, S.R.; Green, O.L.; Thomas, M.A.; Ginn, J.; Zoberi, I. Implementing stereotactic accelerated partial breast irradiation using magnetic resonance guided radiation therapy. *Radiother. Oncol.* **2021**, *164*, 275–281. [CrossRef]
138. Crivellari, D.; Sun, Z.; Coates, A.S.; Price, K.N.; Thurlimann, B.; Mouridsen, H.; Mauriac, L.; Forbes, J.F.; Paridaens, R.J.; Castiglione-Gertsch, M.; et al. Letrozole compared with tamoxifen for elderly patients with endocrine-responsive early breast cancer: The BIG 1-98 trial. *J. Clin. Oncol.* **2008**, *26*, 1972–1979. [CrossRef] [PubMed]
139. Schaeffer, E.; Srinivas, S.; Antonarakis, E.S.; Armstrong, A.J.; Bekelman, J.E.; Cheng, H.; D'Amico, A.V.; Davis, B.J.; Desai, N.; Dorff, T.; et al. NCCN Guidelines Insights: Prostate Cancer, Version 1.2021. *J. Natl. Compr. Cancer Netw.* **2021**, *19*, 134–143. [CrossRef] [PubMed]
140. Baker, B.R.; Basak, R.; Mohiuddin, J.J.; Chen, R.C. Use of stereotactic body radiotherapy for prostate cancer in the United States from 2004 through 2012. *Cancer* **2016**, *122*, 2234–2241. [CrossRef]
141. Widmark, A.; Gunnlaugsson, A.; Beckman, L.; Thellenberg-Karlsson, C.; Hoyer, M.; Lagerlund, M.; Kindblom, J.; Ginman, C.; Johansson, B.; Bjornlinger, K.; et al. Ultra-hypofractionated versus conventionally fractionated radiotherapy for prostate cancer: 5-year outcomes of the HYPO-RT-PC randomised, non-inferiority, phase 3 trial. *Lancet* **2019**, *394*, 385–395. [CrossRef] [PubMed]
142. Katz, A.; Ferrer, M.; Suarez, J.F.; Multicentric Spanish Group of Clinically Localized Prostate Cancer. Comparison of quality of life after stereotactic body radiotherapy and surgery for early-stage prostate cancer. *Radiat. Oncol.* **2012**, *7*, 194. [CrossRef] [PubMed]
143. Brand, D.H.; Tree, A.C.; Ostler, P.; van der Voet, H.; Loblaw, A.; Chu, W.; Ford, D.; Tolan, S.; Jain, S.; Martin, A.; et al. Intensity-modulated fractionated radiotherapy versus stereotactic body radiotherapy for prostate cancer (PACE-B): Acute toxicity findings from an international, randomised, open-label, phase 3, non-inferiority trial. *Lancet Oncol.* **2019**, *20*, 1531–1543. [CrossRef]
144. Nicosia, L.; Mazzola, R.; Rigo, M.; Figlia, V.; Giaj-Levra, N.; Napoli, G.; Ricchetti, F.; Corradini, S.; Ruggieri, R.; Alongi, F. Moderate versus extreme hypofractionated radiotherapy: A toxicity comparative analysis in low- and favorable intermediate-risk prostate cancer patients. *J. Cancer Res. Clin. Oncol.* **2019**, *145*, 2547–2554. [CrossRef]

145. Kasivisvanathan, V.; Rannikko, A.S.; Borghi, M.; Panebianco, V.; Mynderse, L.A.; Vaarala, M.H.; Briganti, A.; Budaus, L.; Hellawell, G.; Hindley, R.G.; et al. MRI-Targeted or Standard Biopsy for Prostate-Cancer Diagnosis. *N. Engl. J. Med.* **2018**, *378*, 1767–1777. [CrossRef]
146. Sidaway, P. MRI improves diagnosis. *Nat. Rev. Clin. Oncol.* **2018**, *15*, 345. [CrossRef] [PubMed]
147. Wibmer, A.G.; Vargas, H.A.; Hricak, H. Role of MRI in the diagnosis and management of prostate cancer. *Future Oncol.* **2015**, *11*, 2757–2766. [CrossRef]
148. Teunissen, F.R.; Wortel, R.C.; Hes, J.; Willigenburg, T.; de Groot-van Breugel, E.N.; de Boer, J.C.; van Melick, H.H.; Verkooijen, H.M. Adaptive magnetic resonance-guided neurovascular-sparing radiotherapy for preservation of erectile function in prostate cancer patients. *Phys. Imaging Radiat. Oncol.* **2021**, *20*, 5–10. [CrossRef] [PubMed]
149. Kerkmeijer, L.G.; Groen, V.H.; Pos, F.J.; Haustermans, K.; Monninkhof, E.M.; Smeenk, R.J.; Kunze-Busch, M.C.; den Boer, J.C.; Zijp, J.V.; Vulpen, M.V.; et al. Focal Boost to the Intraprostatic Tumor in External Beam Radiotherapy for Patients with Localized Prostate Cancer: Results from the FLAME Randomized Phase III Trial. *J. Clin. Oncol.* **2021**, *39*, 787–796. [CrossRef]
150. Tocco, B.R.; Kishan, A.U.; Ma, T.M.; Kerkmeijer, L.G.W.; Tree, A.C. MR-Guided Radiotherapy for Prostate Cancer. *Front. Oncol.* **2020**, *10*, 616291. [CrossRef]
151. Cuccia, F.; Corradini, S.; Mazzola, R.; Spiazzi, L.; Rigo, M.; Bonu, M.L.; Ruggieri, R.; Buglione di Monale, E.B.M.; Magrini, S.M.; Alongi, F. MR-Guided Hypofractionated Radiotherapy: Current Emerging Data and Promising Perspectives for Localized Prostate Cancer. *Cancers* **2021**, *13*, 1791. [CrossRef]
152. Fawaz, Z.S.; Yassa, M.; Nguyen, D.H.; Vavassis, P. Fiducial marker implantation in prostate radiation therapy: Complication rates and technique. *Cancer Radiother.* **2014**, *18*, 736–739. [CrossRef]
153. Gill, S.; Li, J.; Thomas, J.; Bressel, M.; Thursky, K.; Styles, C.; Tai, K.H.; Duchesne, G.M.; Foroudi, F. Patient-reported complications from fiducial marker implantation for prostate image-guided radiotherapy. *Br. J. Radiol.* **2012**, *85*, 1011–1017. [CrossRef] [PubMed]
154. Dunlop, A.; Mitchell, A.; Tree, A.; Barnes, H.; Bower, L.; Chick, J.; Goodwin, E.; Herbert, T.; Lawes, R.; McNair, H.; et al. Daily adaptive radiotherapy for patients with prostate cancer using a high field MR-linac: Initial clinical experiences and assessment of delivered doses compared to a C-arm linac. *Clin. Transl. Radiat. Oncol.* **2020**, *23*, 35–42. [CrossRef]
155. Tetar, S.U.; Bruynzeel, A.M.E.; Oei, S.S.; Senan, S.; Fraikin, T.; Slotman, B.J.; Moorselaar, R.; Lagerwaard, F.J. Magnetic Resonance-guided Stereotactic Radiotherapy for Localized Prostate Cancer: Final Results on Patient-reported Outcomes of a Prospective Phase 2 Study. *Eur. Urol. Oncol.* **2021**, *4*, 628–634. [CrossRef] [PubMed]
156. Alongi, F.; Rigo, M.; Figlia, V.; Cuccia, F.; Giaj-Levra, N.; Nicosia, L.; Ricchetti, F.; Sicignano, G.; De Simone, A.; Naccarato, S.; et al. 1.5 T MR-guided and daily adapted SBRT for prostate cancer: Feasibility, preliminary clinical tolerability, quality of life and patient-reported outcomes during treatment. *Radiat. Oncol.* **2020**, *15*, 69. [CrossRef] [PubMed]
157. Bruynzeel, A.M.E.; Tetar, S.U.; Oei, S.S.; Senan, S.; Haasbeek, C.J.A.; Spoelstra, F.O.B.; Piet, A.H.M.; Meijnen, P.; Bakker van der Jagt, M.A.B.; Fraikin, T.; et al. A Prospective Single-Arm Phase 2 Study of Stereotactic Magnetic Resonance Guided Adaptive Radiation Therapy for Prostate Cancer: Early Toxicity Results. *Int. J. Radiat. Oncol. Biol. Phys.* **2019**, *105*, 1086–1094. [CrossRef] [PubMed]
158. Ma, T.M.; Ballas, L.K.; Wilhalme, H.; Sachdeva, A.; Chong, N.; Sharma, S.; Yang, T.; Basehart, V.; Reiter, R.E.; Saigal, C.; et al. Quality-of-Life Outcomes and Toxicity Profile among Patients with Localized Prostate Cancer after Radical Prostatectomy Treated with Stereotactic Body Radiation: The SCIMITAR Multicenter Phase 2 Trial. *Int. J. Radiat. Oncol. Biol. Phys.* **2023**, *115*, 142–152. [CrossRef]
159. Kishan, A.U.; Ma, T.M.; Lamb, J.M.; Casado, M.; Wilhalme, H.; Low, D.A.; Sheng, K.; Sharma, S.; Nickols, N.G.; Pham, J.; et al. Magnetic Resonance Imaging-Guided vs Computed Tomography-Guided Stereotactic Body Radiotherapy for Prostate Cancer: The MIRAGE Randomized Clinical Trial. *JAMA Oncol.* **2023**. [CrossRef] [PubMed]
160. Redmond, K.J.; Robertson, S.; Lo, S.S.; Soltys, S.G.; Ryu, S.; McNutt, T.; Chao, S.T.; Yamada, Y.; Ghia, A.; Chang, E.L.; et al. Consensus Contouring Guidelines for Postoperative Stereotactic Body Radiation Therapy for Metastatic Solid Tumor Malignancies to the Spine. *Int. J. Radiat. Oncol. Biol. Phys.* **2017**, *97*, 64–74. [CrossRef] [PubMed]
161. Redler, G.; Stevens, T.; Cammin, J.; Malin, M.; Green, O.; Mutic, S.; Pitroda, S.; Aydogan, B. Dosimetric Feasibility of Utilizing the ViewRay Magnetic Resonance Guided Linac System for Image-guided Spine Stereotactic Body Radiation Therapy. *Cureus* **2019**, *11*, e6364. [CrossRef]
162. Stradiotti, P.; Curti, A.; Castellazzi, G.; Zerbi, A. Metal-related artifacts in instrumented spine. Techniques for reducing artifacts in CT and MRI: State of the art. *Eur. Spine J.* **2009**, *18* (Suppl. 1), 102–108. [CrossRef] [PubMed]
163. Paulson, E.S.; Erickson, B.; Schultz, C.; Allen Li, X. Comprehensive MRI simulation methodology using a dedicated MRI scanner in radiation oncology for external beam radiation treatment planning. *Med. Phys.* **2015**, *42*, 28–39. [CrossRef]
164. Spieler, B.; Samuels, S.E.; Llorente, R.; Yechieli, R.; Ford, J.C.; Mellon, E.A. Advantages of Radiation Therapy Simulation with 0.35 Tesla Magnetic Resonance Imaging for Stereotactic Ablation of Spinal Metastases. *Pract. Radiat. Oncol.* **2020**, *10*, 339–344. [CrossRef] [PubMed]
165. Weichselbaum, R.R.; Hellman, S. Oligometastases revisited. *Nat. Rev. Clin. Oncol.* **2011**, *8*, 378–382. [CrossRef] [PubMed]
166. Gomez, D.R.; Tang, C.; Zhang, J.; Blumenschein, G.R., Jr.; Hernandez, M.; Lee, J.J.; Ye, R.; Palma, D.A.; Louie, A.V.; Camidge, D.R.; et al. Local Consolidative Therapy vs. Maintenance Therapy or Observation for Patients with Oligometastatic Non-Small-Cell Lung Cancer: Long-Term Results of a Multi-Institutional, Phase II, Randomized Study. *J. Clin. Oncol.* **2019**, *37*, 1558–1565. [CrossRef] [PubMed]

167. Phillips, R.; Shi, W.Y.; Deek, M.; Radwan, N.; Lim, S.J.; Antonarakis, E.S.; Rowe, S.P.; Ross, A.E.; Gorin, M.A.; Deville, C.; et al. Outcomes of Observation vs Stereotactic Ablative Radiation for Oligometastatic Prostate Cancer: The ORIOLE Phase 2 Randomized Clinical Trial. *JAMA Oncol.* **2020**, *6*, 650–659. [CrossRef] [PubMed]
168. Palma, D.A.; Olson, R.; Harrow, S.; Gaede, S.; Louie, A.V.; Haasbeek, C.; Mulroy, L.; Lock, M.; Rodrigues, G.B.; Yaremko, B.P.; et al. Stereotactic Ablative Radiotherapy for the Comprehensive Treatment of Oligometastatic Cancers: Long-Term Results of the SABR-COMET Phase II Randomized Trial. *J. Clin. Oncol.* **2020**, *38*, 2830–2838. [CrossRef]
169. Chmura, S.; Winter, K.A.; Robinson, C.; Pisansky, T.M.; Borges, V.; Al-Hallaq, H.; Matuszak, M.; Park, S.S.; Yi, S.; Hasan, Y.; et al. Evaluation of Safety of Stereotactic Body Radiotherapy for the Treatment of Patients With Multiple Metastases: Findings from the NRG-BR001 Phase 1 Trial. *JAMA Oncol.* **2021**, *7*, 845–852. [CrossRef]
170. Derynda, B.R.; Liveringhouse, C.L.; Bryant, J.M.; Rosenberg, S.A. MR-Guided Radiation Therapy for Oligometastatic Malignancies. *Appl. Rad. Oncol.* **2021**, *10*, 25–32.
171. Tyran, M.; Cao, M.; Raldow, A.C.; Dang, A.; Lamb, J.; Low, D.A.; Steinberg, M.L.; Lee, P. Stereotactic Magnetic Resonance-guided Online Adaptive Radiotherapy for Oligometastatic Breast Cancer: A Case Report. *Cureus* **2018**, *10*, e2368. [CrossRef]
172. Haque, W.; Crane, C.H.; Krishnan, S.; Delclos, M.E.; Javle, M.; Garrett, C.R.; Wolff, R.A.; Das, P. Reirradiation to the abdomen for gastrointestinal malignancies. *Radiat. Oncol.* **2009**, *4*, 55. [CrossRef]
173. Valentini, V.; Morganti, A.G.; Gambacorta, M.A.; Mohiuddin, M.; Doglietto, G.B.; Coco, C.; De Paoli, A.; Rossi, C.; Di Russo, A.; Valvo, F.; et al. Preoperative hyperfractionated chemoradiation for locally recurrent rectal cancer in patients previously irradiated to the pelvis: A multicentric phase II study. *Int. J. Radiat. Oncol. Biol. Phys.* **2006**, *64*, 1129–1139. [CrossRef]
174. Hunt, A.; Das, P.; Minsky, B.D.; Koay, E.J.; Krishnan, S.; Herman, J.M.; Taniguchi, C.; Koong, A.; Smith, G.L.; Holliday, E.B. Hyperfractionated abdominal reirradiation for gastrointestinal malignancies. *Radiat. Oncol.* **2018**, *13*, 143. [CrossRef] [PubMed]
175. Koom, W.S.; Choi, Y.; Shim, S.J.; Cha, J.; Seong, J.; Kim, N.K.; Nam, K.C.; Keum, K.C. Reirradiation to the pelvis for recurrent rectal cancer. *J. Surg. Oncol.* **2012**, *105*, 637–642. [CrossRef]
176. Tao, R.; Tsai, C.J.; Jensen, G.; Eng, C.; Kopetz, S.; Overman, M.J.; Skibber, J.M.; Rodriguez-Bigas, M.; Chang, G.J.; You, Y.N.; et al. Hyperfractionated accelerated reirradiation for rectal cancer: An analysis of outcomes and toxicity. *Radiother. Oncol.* **2017**, *122*, 146–151. [CrossRef]
177. Chuong, M.D.; Bryant, J.M.; Herrera, R.; McCulloch, J.; Contreras, J.; Kotecha, R.; Romaguera, T.; Alvarez, D.; Hall, M.D.; Rubens, M.; et al. Dose-Escalated Magnetic Resonance Image-Guided Abdominopelvic Reirradiation With Continuous Intrafraction Visualization, Soft Tissue Tracking, and Automatic Beam Gating. *Adv. Radiat. Oncol.* **2022**, *7*, 100840. [CrossRef] [PubMed]
178. Cuccia, F.; Rigo, M.; Figlia, V.; Giaj-Levra, N.; Mazzola, R.; Nicosia, L.; Ricchetti, F.; Trapani, G.; De Simone, A.; Gurrera, D.; et al. 1.5T MR-Guided Daily Adaptive Stereotactic Body Radiotherapy for Prostate Re-Irradiation: A Preliminary Report of Toxicity and Clinical Outcomes. *Front. Oncol.* **2022**, *12*, 858740. [CrossRef] [PubMed]
179. Wang, J.; Weygand, J.; Hwang, K.P.; Mohamed, A.S.; Ding, Y.; Fuller, C.D.; Lai, S.Y.; Frank, S.J.; Zhou, J. Magnetic Resonance Imaging of Glucose Uptake and Metabolism in Patients with Head and Neck Cancer. *Sci. Rep.* **2016**, *6*, 30618. [CrossRef]
180. Salzillo, T.C.; Mawoneke, V.; Weygand, J.; Shetty, A.; Gumin, J.; Zacharias, N.M.; Gammon, S.T.; Piwnica-Worms, D.; Fuller, G.N.; Logothetis, C.J.; et al. Measuring the Metabolic Evolution of Glioblastoma throughout Tumor Development, Regression, and Recurrence with Hyperpolarized Magnetic Resonance. *Cells* **2021**, *10*, 2621. [CrossRef] [PubMed]
181. Dutta, P.; Perez, M.R.; Lee, J.; Kang, Y.; Pratt, M.; Salzillo, T.C.; Weygand, J.; Zacharias, N.M.; Gammon, S.T.; Koay, E.J.; et al. Combining Hyperpolarized Real-Time Metabolic Imaging and NMR Spectroscopy to Identify Metabolic Biomarkers in Pancreatic Cancer. *J. Proteome Res.* **2019**, *18*, 2826–2834. [CrossRef]
182. Maziero, D.; Straza, M.W.; Ford, J.C.; Bovi, J.A.; Diwanji, T.; Stoyanova, R.; Paulson, E.S.; Mellon, E.A. MR-Guided Radiotherapy for Brain and Spine Tumors. *Front. Oncol.* **2021**, *11*, 626100. [CrossRef] [PubMed]
183. Le Bihan, D.; Breton, E.; Lallemand, D.; Grenier, P.; Cabanis, E.; Laval-Jeantet, M. MR imaging of intravoxel incoherent motions: Application to diffusion and perfusion in neurologic disorders. *Radiology* **1986**, *161*, 401–407. [CrossRef] [PubMed]
184. Sugahara, T.; Korogi, Y.; Kochi, M.; Ikushima, I.; Shigematu, Y.; Hirai, T.; Okuda, T.; Liang, L.; Ge, Y.; Komohara, Y.; et al. Usefulness of diffusion-weighted MRI with echo-planar technique in the evaluation of cellularity in gliomas. *J. Magn. Reson. Imaging* **1999**, *9*, 53–60. [CrossRef]
185. Ellingson, B.M.; Malkin, M.G.; Rand, S.D.; Connelly, J.M.; Quinsey, C.; LaViolette, P.S.; Bedekar, D.P.; Schmainda, K.M. Validation of functional diffusion maps (fDMs) as a biomarker for human glioma cellularity. *J. Magn. Reson. Imaging* **2010**, *31*, 538–548. [CrossRef] [PubMed]
186. Hein, P.A.; Eskey, C.J.; Dunn, J.F.; Hug, E.B. Diffusion-weighted imaging in the follow-up of treated high-grade gliomas: Tumor recurrence versus radiation injury. *AJNR Am. J. Neuroradiol.* **2004**, *25*, 201–209.
187. Decker, G.; Murtz, P.; Gieseke, J.; Traber, F.; Block, W.; Sprinkart, A.M.; Leitzen, C.; Buchstab, T.; Lutter, C.; Schuller, H.; et al. Intensity-modulated radiotherapy of the prostate: Dynamic ADC monitoring by DWI at 3.0 T. *Radiother. Oncol.* **2014**, *113*, 115–120. [CrossRef] [PubMed]
188. Bains, L.J.; Zweifel, M.; Thoeny, H.C. Therapy response with diffusion MRI: An update. *Cancer Imaging* **2012**, *12*, 395–402. [CrossRef] [PubMed]
189. McGarry, S.D.; Hurrell, S.L.; Kaczmarowski, A.L.; Cochran, E.J.; Connelly, J.; Rand, S.D.; Schmainda, K.M.; LaViolette, P.S. Magnetic Resonance Imaging-Based Radiomic Profiles Predict Patient Prognosis in Newly Diagnosed Glioblastoma before Therapy. *Tomography* **2016**, *2*, 223–228. [CrossRef] [PubMed]

190. Park, J.E.; Kim, H.S.; Jo, Y.; Yoo, R.E.; Choi, S.H.; Nam, S.J.; Kim, J.H. Radiomics prognostication model in glioblastoma using diffusion- and perfusion-weighted MRI. *Sci. Rep.* **2020**, *10*, 4250. [CrossRef] [PubMed]
191. Kooreman, E.S.; van Houdt, P.J.; Nowee, M.E.; van Pelt, V.W.J.; Tijssen, R.H.N.; Paulson, E.S.; Gurney-Champion, O.J.; Wang, J.; Koetsveld, F.; van Buuren, L.D.; et al. Feasibility and accuracy of quantitative imaging on a 1.5 T MR-linear accelerator. *Radiother. Oncol.* **2019**, *133*, 156–162. [CrossRef]
192. Thorwarth, D.; Ege, M.; Nachbar, M.; Monnich, D.; Gani, C.; Zips, D.; Boeke, S. Quantitative magnetic resonance imaging on hybrid magnetic resonance linear accelerators: Perspective on technical and clinical validation. *Phys. Imaging Radiat. Oncol.* **2020**, *16*, 69–73. [CrossRef] [PubMed]
193. Habrich, J.; Boeke, S.; Nachbar, M.; Nikolaou, K.; Schick, F.; Gani, C.; Zips, D.; Thorwarth, D. Repeatability of diffusion-weighted magnetic resonance imaging in head and neck cancer at a 1.5 T MR-Linac. *Radiother. Oncol.* **2022**, *174*, 141–148. [CrossRef] [PubMed]
194. Kooreman, E.S.; van Houdt, P.J.; Keesman, R.; Pos, F.J.; van Pelt, V.W.J.; Nowee, M.E.; Wetscherek, A.; Tijssen, R.H.N.; Philippens, M.E.P.; Thorwarth, D.; et al. ADC measurements on the Unity MR-linac—A recommendation on behalf of the Elekta Unity MR-linac consortium. *Radiother. Oncol.* **2020**, *153*, 106–113. [CrossRef] [PubMed]
195. Yang, Y.; Cao, M.; Sheng, K.; Gao, Y.; Chen, A.; Kamrava, M.; Lee, P.; Agazaryan, N.; Lamb, J.; Thomas, D.; et al. Longitudinal diffusion MRI for treatment response assessment: Preliminary experience using an MRI-guided tri-cobalt 60 radiotherapy system. *Med. Phys.* **2016**, *43*, 1369–1373. [CrossRef] [PubMed]
196. Shaverdian, N.; Yang, Y.; Hu, P.; Hart, S.; Sheng, K.; Lamb, J.; Cao, M.; Agazaryan, N.; Thomas, D.; Steinberg, M.; et al. Feasibility evaluation of diffusion-weighted imaging using an integrated MRI-radiotherapy system for response assessment to neoadjuvant therapy in rectal cancer. *Br. J. Radiol.* **2017**, *90*, 20160739. [CrossRef]
197. Kalbasi, A.; Kamrava, M.; Chu, F.I.; Telesca, D.; Van Dams, R.; Yang, Y.; Ruan, D.; Nelson, S.D.; Dry, S.M.; Hernandez, J.; et al. A Phase II Trial of 5-Day Neoadjuvant Radiotherapy for Patients with High-Risk Primary Soft Tissue Sarcoma. *Clin. Cancer Res.* **2020**, *26*, 1829–1836. [CrossRef] [PubMed]
198. Gao, Y.; Ghodrati, V.; Kalbasi, A.; Fu, J.; Ruan, D.; Cao, M.; Wang, C.; Eilber, F.C.; Bernthal, N.; Bukata, S.; et al. Prediction of soft tissue sarcoma response to radiotherapy using longitudinal diffusion MRI and a deep neural network with generative adversarial network-based data augmentation. *Med. Phys.* **2021**, *48*, 3262–3372. [CrossRef]
199. Lewis, B.; Guta, A.; Mackey, S.; Gach, H.M.; Mutic, S.; Green, O.; Kim, T. Evaluation of diffusion-weighted MRI and geometric distortion on a 0.35T MR-LINAC at multiple gantry angles. *J. Appl. Clin. Med. Phys.* **2021**, *22*, 118–125. [CrossRef]
200. Weygand, J.; Armstrong, T.; Bryant, J.M.; Andreozzi, J.; Oraiqat, I.M.; Liveringhouse, C.L.; Latifi, K.; Yamoah, K.; Costello, J.R.; Frakes, J.M.; et al. Accurate, repeatable, and geometrically precise diffusion-weighted imaging on a 0.35 T MRI-guided linear accelerator. In Proceedings of the Annual European Society for Radiotherapy and Oncology (ESTRO) Meeting, Vienna, Austria, 24–28 March 2023.
201. Oderinde, O.M.; Shirvani, S.M.; Olcott, P.D.; Kuduvalli, G.; Mazin, S.; Larkin, D. The technical design and concept of a PET/CT linac for biology-guided radiotherapy. *Clin. Transl. Radiat. Oncol.* **2021**, *29*, 106–112. [CrossRef]
202. Warburg, O. The Metabolism of Carcinoma Cells. *J. Cancer Res.* **1925**, *9*, 148–163. [CrossRef]
203. Sullivan, L.B.; Gui, D.Y.; Vander Heiden, M.G. Altered metabolite levels in cancer: Implications for tumour biology and cancer therapy. *Nat. Rev. Cancer* **2016**, *16*, 680–693. [CrossRef]
204. Phelps, M.E.; Hoffman, E.J.; Mullani, N.A.; Ter-Pogossian, M.M. Application of annihilation coincidence detection to transaxial reconstruction tomography. *J. Nucl. Med.* **1975**, *16*, 210–224.
205. Ter-Pogossian, M.M.; Phelps, M.E.; Hoffman, E.J.; Mullani, N.A. A positron-emission transaxial tomograph for nuclear imaging (PETT). *Radiology* **1975**, *114*, 89–98. [CrossRef] [PubMed]
206. Phelps, M.E.; Huang, S.C.; Hoffman, E.J.; Selin, C.; Sokoloff, L.; Kuhl, D.E. Tomographic measurement of local cerebral glucose metabolic rate in humans with (F-18)2-fluoro-2-deoxy-D-glucose: Validation of method. *Ann. Neurol.* **1979**, *6*, 371–388. [CrossRef] [PubMed]
207. Posse, S.; Otazo, R.; Dager, S.R.; Alger, J. MR spectroscopic imaging: Principles and recent advances. *J. Magn. Reson. Imaging* **2013**, *37*, 1301–1325. [CrossRef]
208. Van Zijl, P.C.; Yadav, N.N. Chemical exchange saturation transfer (CEST): What is in a name and what isn't? *Magn. Reson. Med.* **2011**, *65*, 927–948. [CrossRef]
209. Wu, B.; Warnock, G.; Zaiss, M.; Lin, C.; Chen, M.; Zhou, Z.; Mu, L.; Nanz, D.; Tuura, R.; Delso, G. An overview of CEST MRI for non-MR physicists. *EJNMMI Phys.* **2016**, *3*, 19. [CrossRef] [PubMed]
210. Ardenkjaer-Larsen, J.H.; Fridlund, B.; Gram, A.; Hansson, G.; Hansson, L.; Lerche, M.H.; Servin, R.; Thaning, M.; Golman, K. Increase in signal-to-noise ratio of >10,000 times in liquid-state NMR. *Proc. Natl. Acad. Sci. USA* **2003**, *100*, 10158–10163. [CrossRef]
211. Salzillo, T.C.; Hu, J.; Nguyen, L.; Whiting, N.; Lee, J.; Weygand, J.; Dutta, P.; Pudakalakatti, S.; Millward, N.Z.; Gammon, S.T.; et al. Interrogating Metabolism in Brain Cancer. *Magn. Reson. Imaging Clin. N. Am.* **2016**, *24*, 687–703. [CrossRef] [PubMed]
212. Bogner, W.; Gruber, S.; Trattnig, S.; Chmelik, M. High-resolution mapping of human brain metabolites by free induction decay (1)H MRSI at 7 T. *NMR Biomed.* **2012**, *25*, 873–882. [CrossRef] [PubMed]
213. Hangel, G.; Cadrien, C.; Lazen, P.; Furtner, J.; Lipka, A.; Heckova, E.; Hingerl, L.; Motyka, S.; Gruber, S.; Strasser, B.; et al. High-resolution metabolic imaging of high-grade gliomas using 7T-CRT-FID-MRSI. *Neuroimage Clin.* **2020**, *28*, 102433. [CrossRef]

214. De Feyter, H.M.; Behar, K.L.; Corbin, Z.A.; Fulbright, R.K.; Brown, P.B.; McIntyre, S.; Nixon, T.W.; Rothman, D.L.; de Graaf, R.A. Deuterium metabolic imaging (DMI) for MRI-based 3D mapping of metabolism in vivo. *Sci. Adv.* **2018**, *4*, eaat7314. [CrossRef]
215. Korzowski, A.; Weinfurtner, N.; Mueller, S.; Breitling, J.; Goerke, S.; Schlemmer, H.P.; Ladd, M.E.; Paech, D.; Bachert, P. Volumetric mapping of intra- and extracellular pH in the human brain using (31) P MRSI at 7T. *Magn. Reson. Med.* **2020**, *84*, 1707–1723. [CrossRef] [PubMed]
216. Bogner, W.; Otazo, R.; Henning, A. Accelerated MR spectroscopic imaging-a review of current and emerging techniques. *NMR Biomed.* **2021**, *34*, e4314. [CrossRef] [PubMed]
217. Henning, A.; Fuchs, A.; Murdoch, J.B.; Boesiger, P. Slice-selective FID acquisition, localized by outer volume suppression (FIDLOVS) for (1)H-MRSI of the human brain at 7 T with minimal signal loss. *NMR Biomed.* **2009**, *22*, 683–696. [CrossRef] [PubMed]
218. Hovener, J.B.; Schwaderlapp, N.; Lickert, T.; Duckett, S.B.; Mewis, R.E.; Highton, L.A.; Kenny, S.M.; Green, G.G.; Leibfritz, D.; Korvink, J.G.; et al. A hyperpolarized equilibrium for magnetic resonance. *Nat. Commun.* **2013**, *4*, 2946. [CrossRef]
219. Nelson, S.J.; Kurhanewicz, J.; Vigneron, D.B.; Larson, P.E.; Harzstark, A.L.; Ferrone, M.; van Criekinge, M.; Chang, J.W.; Bok, R.; Park, I.; et al. Metabolic imaging of patients with prostate cancer using hyperpolarized[1-(1)(3)C]pyruvate. *Sci. Transl. Med.* **2013**, *5*, 198ra108. [CrossRef] [PubMed]
220. Zhou, J.; van Zijl, P.C. Chemical exchange saturation transfer imaging and spectroscopy. *Prog. Nucl. Magn. Reson. Spectrosc.* **2006**, *48*, 109–136. [CrossRef]
221. Meissner, J.E.; Korzowski, A.; Regnery, S.; Goerke, S.; Breitling, J.; Floca, R.O.; Debus, J.; Schlemmer, H.P.; Ladd, M.E.; Bachert, P.; et al. Early response assessment of glioma patients to definitive chemoradiotherapy using chemical exchange saturation transfer imaging at 7 T. *J. Magn. Reson. Imaging* **2019**, *50*, 1268–1277. [CrossRef] [PubMed]
222. Regnery, S.; Adeberg, S.; Dreher, C.; Oberhollenzer, J.; Meissner, J.E.; Goerke, S.; Windschuh, J.; Deike-Hofmann, K.; Bickelhaupt, S.; Zaiss, M.; et al. Chemical exchange saturation transfer MRI serves as predictor of early progression in glioblastoma patients. *Oncotarget* **2018**, *9*, 28772–28783. [CrossRef]
223. Cusumano, D.; Boldrini, L.; Dhont, J.; Fiorino, C.; Green, O.; Gungor, G.; Jornet, N.; Kluter, S.; Landry, G.; Mattiucci, G.C.; et al. Artificial Intelligence in magnetic Resonance guided Radiotherapy: Medical and physical considerations on state of art and future perspectives. *Phys. Med.* **2021**, *85*, 175–191. [CrossRef]
224. Bryant, J.M.; Saghand, P.G.; Latifi, K.; Frakes, J.; Hoffe, S.A.; Moros, E.; Mittauer, K.E.; Kotecha, R.; El Naqa, I.; Rosenberg, S.A. A novel multi-task hybrid deep neural network (DNN) predicts tumor progression during MRgRT. In Proceedings of the Annual European Society for Radiotherapy and Oncology (ESTRO) Meeting, Vienna, Austria, 24 March–28 March 2023.
225. Botman, R.; Tetar, S.U.; Palacios, M.A.; Slotman, B.J.; Lagerwaard, F.J.; Bruynzeel, A.M.E. The clinical introduction of MR-guided radiation therapy from a RTT perspective. *Clin. Transl. Radiat. Oncol.* **2019**, *18*, 140–145. [CrossRef]
226. Mittauer, K.; Paliwal, B.; Hill, P.; Bayouth, J.E.; Geurts, M.W.; Baschnagel, A.M.; Bradley, K.A.; Harari, P.M.; Rosenberg, S.; Brower, J.V.; et al. A New Era of Image Guidance with Magnetic Resonance-guided Radiation Therapy for Abdominal and Thoracic Malignancies. *Cureus* **2018**, *10*, e2422. [CrossRef] [PubMed]
227. Kueng, R.; Guyer, G.; Volken, W.; Frei, D.; Stabel, F.; Stampanoni, M.F.M.; Manser, P.; Fix, M.K. Development of an extended Macro Monte Carlo method for efficient and accurate dose calculation in magnetic fields. *Med. Phys.* **2020**, *47*, 6519–6530. [CrossRef] [PubMed]

Disclaimer/Publisher's Note: The statements, opinions and data contained in all publications are solely those of the individual author(s) and contributor(s) and not of MDPI and/or the editor(s). MDPI and/or the editor(s) disclaim responsibility for any injury to people or property resulting from any ideas, methods, instructions or products referred to in the content.

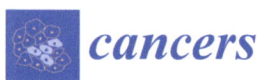 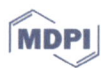

Article

Online Adaptive MRI-Guided Stereotactic Body Radiotherapy for Pancreatic and Other Intra-Abdominal Cancers

Danny Lee [1,2,*], Paul Renz [1], Seungjong Oh [1,2], Min-Sig Hwang [1,2], Daniel Pavord [1,2], Kyung Lim Yun [1], Colleen Collura [1], Mary McCauley [1], Athanasios (Tom) Colonias [1], Mark Trombetta [1,2] and Alexander Kirichenko [1,2]

[1] Radiation Oncology, Allegheny Health Network, Pittsburgh, PA 15212, USA; paul.renz@ahn.org (P.R.); seungjong.oh@ahn.org (S.O.); min-sig.hwang@ahn.org (M.-S.H.); daniel.pavord@ahn.org (D.P.); kyunglim.yun@ahn.org (K.L.Y.); colleen.collura@ahn.org (C.C.); mary.mccauley@ahn.org (M.M.); mark.trombetta@ahn.org (M.T.); alexander.kirichenko@ahn.org (A.K.)

[2] College of Medicine, Radiologic Sciences/Drexel University, Philadelphia, PA 19129, USA

* Correspondence: danny.lee@ahn.org; Tel.: +1-412-359-4589

Simple Summary: MRI can provide better visualization of tumors and nearby organs at risk (OAR) than CT for fast and accurate contouring during online adaptive MRI-guided stereotactic body radiation treatment (MRI-guided SBRT) for pancreatic and other intra-abdominal cancers. Pre-set MRI sequences provided in a 1.5T MRI scanner hybrid with a linear accelerator can be used during MRI-guided SBRT, but they often limit tumor and OAR visualization and require a long image acquisition time. This study retrospectively analyzed 26 patients with pancreatic and intra-abdominal cancers that underwent CT and MR simulations and 3–5 fractionated MRI-guided SBRT. The visualization of tumors and OAR was improved with T1W imaging, which is essential for online adaptive planning and resulted in fast and accurate contouring in a shorter imaging time.

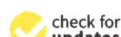

Citation: Lee, D.; Renz, P.; Oh, S.; Hwang, M.-S.; Pavord, D.; Yun, K.L.; Collura, C.; McCauley, M.; Colonias, A.; Trombetta, M.; et al. Online Adaptive MRI-Guided Stereotactic Body Radiotherapy for Pancreatic and Other Intra-Abdominal Cancers. Cancers 2023, 15, 5272. https://doi.org/10.3390/cancers15215272

Academic Editors: Sam Beddar and Michael D. Chuong

Received: 29 September 2023
Revised: 31 October 2023
Accepted: 1 November 2023
Published: 3 November 2023

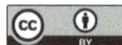

Copyright: © 2023 by the authors. Licensee MDPI, Basel, Switzerland. This article is an open access article distributed under the terms and conditions of the Creative Commons Attribution (CC BY) license (https://creativecommons.org/licenses/by/4.0/).

Abstract: A 1.5T MRI combined with a linear accelerator (Unity®, Elekta; Stockholm, Sweden) is a device that shows promise in MRI-guided stereotactic body radiation treatment (SBRT). Previous studies utilized the manufacturer's pre-set MRI sequences (i.e., T2 Weighted (T2W)), which limited the visualization of pancreatic and intra-abdominal tumors and organs at risk (OAR). Here, a T1 Weighted (T1W) sequence was utilized to improve the visualization of tumors and OAR for online adapted-to-position (ATP) and adapted-to-shape (ATS) during MRI-guided SBRT. Twenty-six patients, 19 with pancreatic and 7 with intra-abdominal cancers, underwent CT and MRI simulations for SBRT planning before being treated with multi-fractionated MRI-guided SBRT. The boundary of tumors and OAR was more clearly seen on T1W image sets, resulting in fast and accurate contouring during online ATP/ATS planning. Plan quality in 26 patients was dependent on OAR proximity to the target tumor and achieved 96 ± 5% and 92 ± 9% in gross tumor volume $D_{90\%}$ and planning target volume $D_{90\%}$. We utilized T1W imaging (about 120 s) to shorten imaging time by 67% compared to T2W imaging (about 360 s) and improve tumor visualization, minimizing target/OAR delineation uncertainty and the treatment margin for sparing OAR. The average time-consumption of MRI-guided SBRT for the first 21 patients was 55 ± 15 min for ATP and 79 ± 20 min for ATS.

Keywords: MRI in RT; MRI-Linac; MRI-guided SBRT; adapt-to-position; adapt-to-shape; pancreatic cancers; abdominal cancers; online adaptive planning; Unity®; stereotactic body radiation treatment

1. Introduction

Magnetic resonance imaging (MRI) combined with a linear accelerator (MRI-Linac) [1–4] yields a technique that shows promise in MRI-guided stereotactic body radiotherapy (SBRT) [5]. MRI-Linac [6] provides superior visualization of target tumors and surrounding organs at risk (OAR) to improve delineation accuracy; MRI-guidance accounts for position, size, and shape changes during online adaptive SBRT planning [7]. Therefore, MRI-guided SBRT [8–10] is increasingly used for pancreatic and other intra-abdominal cancers using currently two clinically available MRI-Linacs [11].

True fast imaging with steady state precession (TrueFISP) combined with breath holding (BH) is possible on the first MRI-Linac, a 0.35T MRI combined with a linear accelerator (MRIdian®, ViewRay Inc., Mountain View, CA, USA) [12–14]. A T2-Weighted with exhalation-navigating (T2W + Nav) MRI scan with the second MRI-Linac is acquired on a 1.5T MRI combined with a linear accelerator (Unity®, Elekta; Stockholm, Sweden) [15]. In each fraction of MRI-guided SBRT on these MRI-Linacs, one (or more) TrueFISP or T2W + Nav image sets are acquired as daily-MRIs to account for inter-fractional changes of targets and OAR. The contours can be adjusted during online adaptive planning, and patient setup can be verified before and after beam delivery while patients are on the treatment couch.

Online adaptive planning heavily relies on the image quality of daily-MRIs, which requires superior soft-tissue contrast for fast and accurate contour adjusting of the target tumor and OAR [8,16–18]. An MRI scan with BH acquires a 3D volume in a short period of time (i.e., 17 s with TrueFISP + BH) [19], but pancreatic tumors can move more than 4 mm during the scan [20]. On the other hand, an MRI scan with exhalation-navigating acquires a 3D volume in a longer period of time but is dependent on the breathing period and regularity in individual patients (i.e., up to 882 s with T2W + Nav) [21]. In terms of the target motion, a gating technique, which measures real-time target motion by deformably registering fast cine images to daily-MRI, is utilized to account for the respiratory-induced target motion during beam delivery [13,19]. As an alternative, T2W with a compression belt in free-breathing significantly reduced the range of target motion [22–24]. However, it could still include respiratory-induced motion blurring artifacts, which leads to some degree of difficulty in adjusting with daily-MRI. Therefore, fast and precise online adaptive planning requires high-quality images from the daily-MRI with minimal or no blurring artifacts. The changing positions of the patient and their internal anatomy must also be accounted for during online adaptive planning for both adapt-to-position (ATP) and adapt-to-shape (ATS) [7,25].

Pancreatic and intra-abdominal malignancies are challenging to treat with SBRT [16,26], and require high-quality imaging with appropriate motion management [27,28]. However, most studies of online adaptive MRI-guided SBRT on clinical MRI-Lianc(s) used the pre-set MRI sequences provided by the manufacturer [11–15], which limited the visualization of the target and OAR on MR image sets. Furthermore, the pre-set daily-MRI required a long imaging time and had poor visualization of the target and OAR, causing difficulties in fusion, contouring [21], and fraction-to-fraction contour propagation using a rigid or deformable algorithm [29,30]. Therefore, our clinic utilized a customized T1W MRI sequence to achieve rapid imaging with superior visualization of the target and OAR and improve contouring accuracy during online adaptive planning. This study retrospectively analyzed and compared visualizing tumors and OAR on T1W image sets and pre-set T2W image sets. We also evaluated the treatment data produced in multi-fractionated MRI-guided SBRT.

2. Materials and Methods

In this institutional review board-approved study, multiple MR image sets were acquired from patients with pancreatic and intra-abdominal tumors before undergoing multi-fractionated online adaptive MRI-guided SBRT. All MR image sets were inspected to determine which set would be used as an MRI sequence to acquire daily-MRI for superior visualization of tumors and OAR.

2.1. The Workflow of CT and MRI Simulations, and MRI-Guided SBRT

Our workflow comprised 4 steps (Figure 1). First, selected patients were asked to complete the first MRI screening sheet (Figure 1a). Then, each patient underwent CT and MRI simulations (Figure 1b), where free-breathing CT (FB-CT) was used to develop a CT reference plan for online adaptive MRI-guided SBRT. Four-dimensional CT (4D-CT) image sets with an abdominal compression belt (ZiFix^{TM}, Qfix, PA, USA) were used to measure tumor motion range [22]. If tumor motion was equal to or less than 0.5 cm, the patient was eligible for MRI-guided SBRT and was asked to complete the second MRI screening sheet for MRI safety before the MRI simulation [31,32]. On the same day as the CT simulation, MR image sets of T2W + Nav, T1-Weighted (T1W), and T1W + Fat Saturated (FS) were acquired using a 1.5T Unity®, and one of them was chosen (typically T1W) to contour the target tumor and use it as a sequence of daily-MRI. The third step was SBRT planning (Figure 1c), during which a FB-CT was rigidly registered to a chosen T1W, and target tumors and OAR were contoured on a chosen T1W and FB-CT image set, respectively. A CT reference plan ($_{CT}$Ref) was then developed on a FB-CT for all patients. Additionally, an MRI reference plan ($_{MR}$Ref) was developed on a T1W for the first few patients.

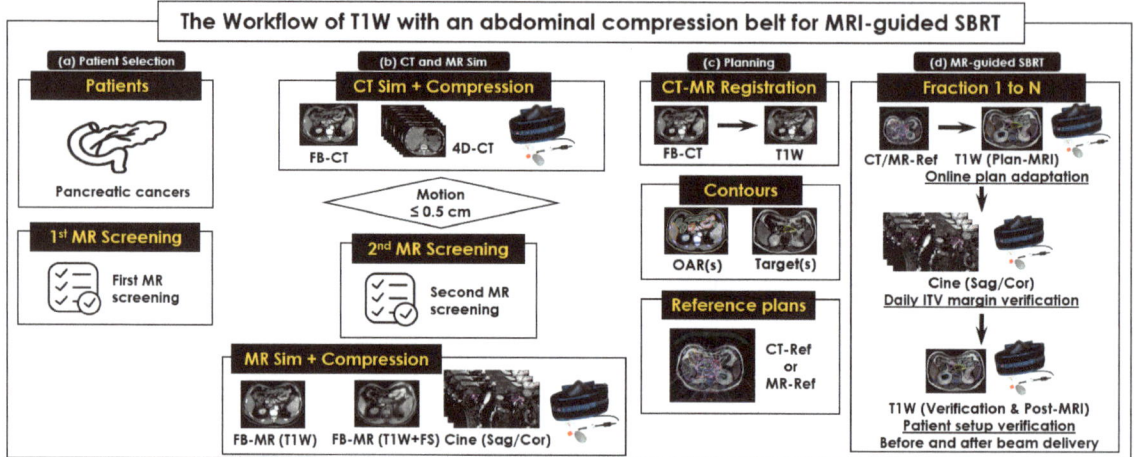

Figure 1. The workflow of simulations and multi-fractionated stereotactic body radiotherapy for pancreatic and intra-abdominal cancers (MRI-guided SBRT) on a 1.5T Unity®. (**a**) Patient selection and 1st MRI screening to check the eligibility of each patient; (**b**) CT and MRI simulations with an abdominal compression belt to acquire CT and MR image sets; (**c**) contouring organs at risk (OAR) on FB-CT images and target tumors on T1W images to develop a CT reference plan ($_{CT}$Ref) and an MRI reference plan ($_{MR}$Ref); and (**d**) MRI-guided SBRT in 3–5 fractions. An identical Unity® couch top and the same abdominal compression belt were used in CT and MRI simulations and across all SBRT fractions. Orthogonal sagittal and coronal 2D cine images were acquired to measure the range of target motion induced by respiration for determining an internal target volume (ITV) margin.

The fourth step was treating the patient with online adaptive MRI-guided SBRT. In each fraction of MRI-guided SBRT (Figure 1d), 3 image sets for daily-MRI were acquired: 1 set for online adaptive planning (plan-MRI) and 2 sets for patient setup verifications before (verification-MRI) and after beam delivery (post-MRI). Orthogonal, sagittal, and coronal cine images were acquired to verify internal target volume (ITV) by measuring target motion range on MiM (v7.0.6, MiM Software Inc, Cleveland, OH, USA). In this study, the patient setup was maintained by using the same Unity® couch top and MRI-safe or conditional immobilization devices during each CT and MRI simulation and multi-fractionated MRI-guided SBRT.

2.2. Patients

Patients were usually treated every other day using a 1.5T Unity®. The imaging, planning, and treatment data of each patient's CT and MRI simulation and consecutive 3–5 fractionated MRI-guided SBRT were retrospectively analyzed.

2.3. CT and MRI Simulations with Immobilization Devices

On the same day, all patients underwent both a CT and an MRI simulation to acquire FB-CT images with and without a gadolinium-based contrast agent for OAR contouring, 4D-CT images for measuring target motion range, and multiple MR image sets of T2W + Nav, T1W, and T1W + FS for target tumor contouring. In addition, a 2D orthogonal coronal and sagittal image set (2D-Cine) was acquired to manually measure the range of target motion for individual patients and determine the margin of ITV. The target motion range was used to verify and adjust the initial target motion range measured in 4D-CT. An abdominal compression belt, which is safe for both CT and MRI scanning, was used for abdominal imaging to manage target and organ motion up to 0.5 cm in all directions induced by respiration [22]. The pressure level of an abdominal compression belt for each patient, measured in a CT simulation, was used to set up that patient in an MRI simulation and throughout the entire MRI-guided SBRT. Two patients were scanned without the abdominal compression belt due to their discomfort.

Imaging parameters of the T1W and T1W + FS sequences were optimized during scans of volunteers and the first few patients in the study. The optimized MRI sequences were then used for all patients. For the MRI simulation, we used a T2W + Nav with a 3D turbo spin echo (TSE) MRI pulse sequence and a T1W and T1W + FS of a 3D turbo field echo (TFE) MRI pulse sequence on a 1.5T Unity®, with 2 MRI receiver coils (a 4-channel anterior coil and a 4-channel posterior coil). Imaging parameters of T2W + Nav were repetition time (TR)/echo time (TE) = 1800/205 ms, field of view (FOV) = 400 × 400 mm^2, pixel size = 1.56 × 1.56 mm^2, image matrix = 480 × 480, thickness = 2.4 mm, flip angle = 90°, bandwidth = 727 Hz, and number of signals (average = 5). Each MR image set took approximately 228 to 410 s; 233 images were acquired in total. A navigating window was set at the liver dome scout (1/3 on the lung side and 2/3 on the liver side).

Imaging parameters of T1W were TR/TE = 4.5/2.2 ms, FOV = 400 × 400 mm^2, pixel size = 1.1 × 1.1 mm^2, image matrix = 280 × 280, thickness = 2 mm, flip angle = 10°, bandwidth = 383, Hz and number of signal average = 5. Each MR image set took approximately 120 s; 161 images were acquired in total. All image sets acquired during the CT and MRI simulations were transferred to MiM in a Digital Imaging and Communications in Medicine format.

2.4. SBRT Planning

CT and MRI simulation image sets were used to develop 1 or more $_{CT}$Ref or $_{MR}$Ref plans for each patient. For the first 5 patients in the study, we developed both a $_{CT}$Ref and a $_{MR}$Ref, but we developed only a $_{CT}$Ref for the rest of the patients. The T1W image sets were used to develop $_{MR}$Ref plans through off-line adaptive ATS planning from the $_{CT}$Ref plans. Average electron densities of the tumor and OAR from the $_{CT}$Ref were assigned to corresponding contours in the $_{MR}$Ref. Both $_{CT}$Ref and $_{MR}$Ref plans were developed to meet the dose constraints listed in Table 1. One of the $_{CT}$Ref and $_{MR}$Ref plans was peer-reviewed in the department chart round at Radiation Oncology, Allegheny Health Network Cancer Center.

On the MiM software, the OAR delineated on a FB-CT image set were heart, kidneys, liver, spinal cord, duodenum, small bowel, stomach, jejunum, colon, bone, body, spleen, and extras (i.e., air, contrast, vein, and celiac). Gross tumor volume (GTV), delineated on a T1W (or T1W + FS) MR image set, was determined for pancreatic tumors, left adrenal tumors, and pancreatic lymph nodes. The GTV contour was transferred from the T1W image set to the FB-CT image set for addition to the OAR contours. A FB-CT image set with all contours was exported to the treatment planning system (TPS, MR-Linac Monaco v5.51.11, CMS; St. Louis, MO, USA), and a patient-specific SBRT plan was developed. Each SBRT plan with 15–45 Gy in 3–5 fractions (Table 1) was calculated using Monte Carlo® and used 7–14 beams delivered in a step-and-shoot intensity-modulated radiation therapy (IMRT) technique with 7FFF (flattening filter-free) photons. A reference plan developed on the FB-CT was exported to the oncology system (Mosaiq v2.8.3, CMS; St. Louis, MO, USA) for a treatment schedule every other day.

Table 1. The dose constraints of planning target volume (PTV) and organs at risk for stereotactic body radiotherapy for pancreatic and other intra-abdominal cancers. This is an example of 40 Gy in 5 fractions, so the dose constraints varied on the prescription dose (15 Gy to 45 Gy).

Organs	Dose Constraints (5 Fractions) of 40 Gy in 8 Gy × 5 Fractions
PTV (or PTV_eval)	>90% coverage
GTV	90–95% Rx to cover 90–95%
Cord	$V_{20Gy} < 0.03$ cc
Liver	$V_{12Gy} < 50\%$
Bilat kidneys	$V_{12Gy} < 50\%$
Stomach PRV (2 mm)	$V_{40Gy} < 0.5$ cc, $V_{35Gy} < 1$ cc, $V_{30Gy} < 2$ cc
Duodenum PRV (2 mm)	$V_{40Gy} < 0.5$ cc, $V_{35Gy} < 1$ cc, $V_{30Gy} < 2$ cc
Small bowel PRV (2 mm)	$V_{40Gy} < 0.5$ cc, $V_{35Gy} < 1$ cc, $V_{30Gy} < 2$ cc
Colon PRV (2 mm)	$V_{40Gy} < 0.5$ cc, $V_{35Gy} < 1$ cc, $V_{30Gy} < 2$ cc
Jejunum PRV (2 mm)	$V_{40Gy} < 0.5$ cc, $V_{35Gy} < 1$ cc, $V_{30Gy} < 2$ cc
Spleen	< 4 Gy
Heart	Dmax ≤ 20 Gy

GTV: Gross tumor volume; PRV: Planning of organ at-risk volume.

A patient-specific quality assurance (QA) was performed for $_{CT}$Ref and $_{MR}$Ref plans and the first adaptive ATS plan ($_{MR}$ATS) to verify the applicability and deliverability of these QA plans on the Unity®. This QA test was performed using an ion chamber (Exradin A1SLMR, Standard Imaging, Inc., Middleton, WI, USA) [33] and using an MRI-conditional cylindrical diode array dosimeter (ArcCHECK-MR, Sun Nuclear Corporation, Melbourne, FL, USA) [34].

2.5. Online Adaptive MRI-Guided SBRT

Patients were treated with 3–5 fractionated MRI-guided SBRT, using our Unity®, between May 2020 and May 2023. For each fraction, 1 $_{CT}$Ref or $_{MR}$Ref plan was chosen for online adaptive ATP or ATS MRI-guided SBRT, and 1 or more $_{MR}$ATS(s) was added to the list of reference plans for the next online adaptive MRI-guided SBRT. Three T1W (or T1W + FS) image sets were acquired during each fraction. The first T1W image set, the plan-MRI, was used to account for inter-fraction changes of targets and OAR shape, position, and size. After image fusion between the $_{CT}$Ref (or $_{MR}$Ref) and plan-MRI by a physicist (or a therapist), an attending physician determined ATP or ATS for further online adaptive planning. Then, GTV and OAR contours, rigidly or deformably transferred from the $_{CT}$Ref (or $_{MR}$Ref), were adjusted to match the plan-MRI. For ATS, GTV and the contours of the stomach, duodenum, small bowel, colon, and jejunum were usually adjusted or re-delineated by an attending physician, and the contours of the air and body were adjusted or removed by an attending physicist.

Next, 2 T1W image sets, the verification-MRI and post-MRI images, were acquired before and after the beam delivery to verify patient setup. Once the patient setup was verified, the target motion, moving within the planning target volume (PTV), was visually evaluated by the attending physician prior to the beam delivery. If there were patient setup differences between the plan-MRI and verification-MRI in GTV and OAR contours, the verification-MRI was used as the new plan-MRI to repeat online adaptive planning. A little over 10% of the fractions in all patients enrolled in this study experienced the changes in anatomical position and size found in the verification-MRI.

2.6. Statistical Analysis of Plan Quality

For each patient, we compared the image quality of T1W, FB-CT, and T2W + Nav image sets by inspecting tumor and OAR visualization on the plan-MRI acquired during 3–5 fractionated MRI-guided SBRT. The changes in tumor and OAR contours adjusted during ATS were quantified as a function of their variability in volume. Next, the quality of online adaptive SBRT plans was evaluated by quantifying the coverage of radiation dose to tumors and OAR. Both image quality and plan quality were evaluated for all patients using MiM. Lastly, the time-consumption of each step in our workflow was analyzed in individual, online adaptive ATP/ATS plans to determine our workflow's efficiency.

3. Results

All patients successfully completed CT and MRI simulations to acquire planning image sets and were treated with 3–5 fractionated online adaptive MRI-guided SBRT.

3.1. Patients

Twenty-six patients with pancreatic (n = 19), left adrenal (n = 3), and lymph node cancer (n = 4), who were treated using Unity® between May 2021 and May 2023, were included in this study. Of the 26 patients, 16 were male and 10 were female, and the cohort had an average age of 71 years [range: 57–95] (Table 2). Average tumor volumes of reference plans ($_{CT}$Ref or $_{MR}$Ref) and adaptive ATP/ATS plans were measured at 37.1 mL [range: 3.4 mL to 105.5 mL] and 35.4 mL [range: 3.4 mL to 106.4 mL], respectively. The same air-pressure of an abdominal compression belt recorded at the CT simulation was reproduced during the MRI simulation and consecutive 3–5 fractionated MRI-guided SBRT.

Table 2. Demographic and disease profiles of 26 patients with pancreatic (n = 19) and intra-abdominal cancers (n = 7). The cohort had an average age of 71 years [range: 57–95]; 16 patients were male and 10 were female. All patients were treated with 126 fractionated MRI-guided SBRT (ATP (n = 49) and ATS (n = 77)) with the SBRT prescription (25 Gy to 45 Gy in 3–5 fractions for 25 patients and 15 Gy in 5 fractions for 1 patient). Patient P09 was treated with the stereotactic boost for the postoperative recurrence of pancreatic cancer after 45 Gy conventional fractionation.

Patient #	Diagnosis	Age	Gender	SBRT Prescription	# of Beams	Type of Adaptive Planning
P01	Pancreatic head	70	M	35 Gy in 5 fractions	13	ATP (n = 0), ATS (n = 5)
P02	Pancreatic head	65	M	40 Gy in 5 fractions	13	ATP (n = 0), ATS (n = 5)
P03	Left adrenal	61	M	30 Gy in 3 fractions	11	ATP (n = 0), ATS (n = 3)
P04	Left pancreatic lymph nodes	72	M	45 Gy in 5 fractions	13	ATP (n = 0), ATS (n = 5)
P05	Left pancreatic lymph nodes	60	F	40 Gy in 5 fractions	8	ATP (n = 0), ATS (n = 5)
P06	Left adrenal gland	63	M	30 Gy in 3 fractions	9	ATP (n = 0), ATS (n = 3)
P07	Pancreatic head	95	M	35 Gy in 5 fractions	12	ATP (n = 0), ATS (n = 5)
P08	Pancreatic head	65	F	45 Gy in 5 fractions	12	ATP (n = 4), ATS (n = 1)
P09	Pancreas Boost	64	F	15 Gy in 5 fractions	12	ATP (n = 0), ATS (n = 5)
P10	Pancreatic tail	67	M	40 Gy in 5 fractions	12	ATP (n = 3), ATS (n = 2)
P11	Pancreas	79	M	35 Gy in 5 fractions	8	ATP (n = 0), ATS (n = 5)
P12	Pancreas head/body	83	M	35 Gy in 5 fractions	11	ATP (n = 0), ATS (n = 5)
P13	Aortocaval lymph nodes	64	M	25 Gy in 5 fractions	11	ATP (n = 4), ATS (n = 1)
P14	Pancreatic body	77	F	45 Gy in 5 fractions	12	ATP (n = 1), ATS (n = 4)
P15	Pancreatic head	57	F	37.5 Gy in 5 fractions	12	ATP (n = 3), ATS (n = 2)
P16	Pancreatic head	67	F	37.5 Gy in 5 fractions	14	ATP (n = 3), ATS (n = 2)
P17	Pancreatic head	74	M	40 Gy in 5 fractions	11	ATP (n = 3), ATS (n = 2)
P18	Pancreatic head	73	F	45 Gy in 5 fractions	7	ATP (n = 4), ATS (n = 1)
P19	Portocaval node	62	M	40 Gy in 5 fractions	10	ATP (n = 5), ATS (n = 0)

Table 2. Cont.

Patient #	Diagnosis	Age	Gender	SBRT Prescription	# of Beams	Type of Adaptive Planning
P20	Pancreas	83	M	40 Gy in 5 fractions	13	ATP (n = 2), ATS (n = 3)
P21	Pancreas	71	M	45 Gy in 5 fractions	10	ATP (n = 3), ATS (n = 2)
P22	Pancreatic tail	72	F	40 Gy in 5 fractions	12	ATP (n = 2), ATS (n = 3)
P23	Pancreatic body mass	79	F	40 Gy in 5 fractions	12	ATP (n = 1), ATS (n = 4)
P24	Pancreatic head	61	F	40 Gy in 5 fractions	8	ATP (n = 4), ATS (n = 1)
P25	Pancreatic head	72	M	45 Gy in 5 fractions	8	ATP (n = 4), ATS (n = 1)
P26	Left adrenal	81	M	32 Gy in 4 fractions	7	ATP (n = 3), ATS (n = 2)
Mean ± STD or Total number		71 ± 9	M (n = 16), F (n = 10)	15 Gy to 45 Gy in 3–5 fractions	7–14	ATP (n = 49), ATS (n = 77)

P = Patient; M = Male; F = Female; ATP = Adapt-to-position; ATS = Adapt-to-shape; STD = Standard deviation.

3.2. CT and MR Image Sets and Target Contouring

Figure 2 shows an example of pancreatic tumor and OAR visualization on FB-CT, T2W + Nav, and T1W image sets. Like FB-CT, the boundaries of a pancreatic tumor and OAR were well visualized on T1W, but not on T2W + Nav. Regarding tumor and OAR contouring, T1W images more clearly showed the boundaries of tumors in all 26 patients than the T2W + Nav images (Figure 3). The clear interface of organs required for higher accuracy and precision of SBRT planning was shown in T1W images, but it was unclear in T2W + Nav images.

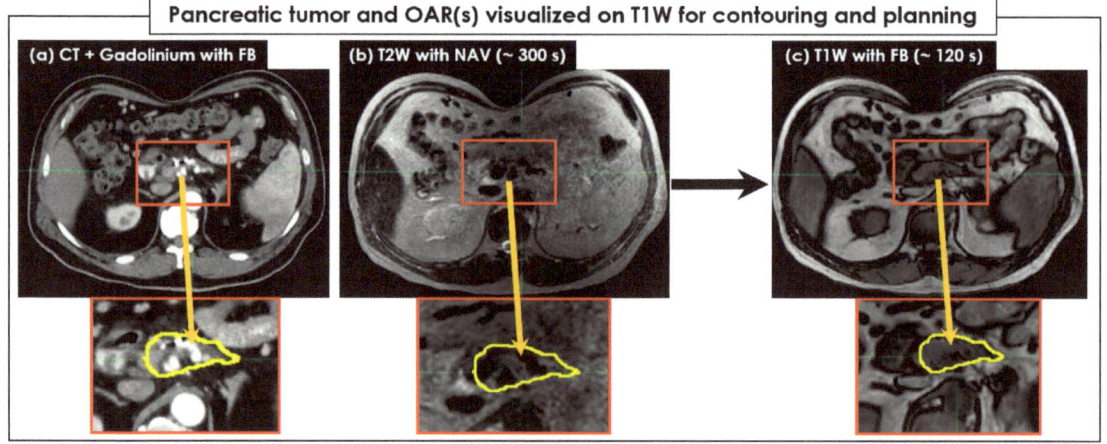

Figure 2. The pancreatic tumor and organs at risk (OAR) visualized on T1W for contouring and further SBRT planning. A CT image set (**a**) acquired in free-breathing (FB) with Gadolinium was compared to a T2W with exhalation-navigating (+Nav) image set (**b**) and a T1W image set (**c**). The target tumor areas were magnified, and the target tumors were contoured on a CT image set with the yellow color and copied to MR image sets. The boundary of the target tumor was clearly visible on the T1W image set acquired in a short period of time, but it was unclear on the T2W + Nav image set. The body shape due to the use of an abdominal compression belt was identical across all FB-CT, T2W + Nav, and T1W image sets.

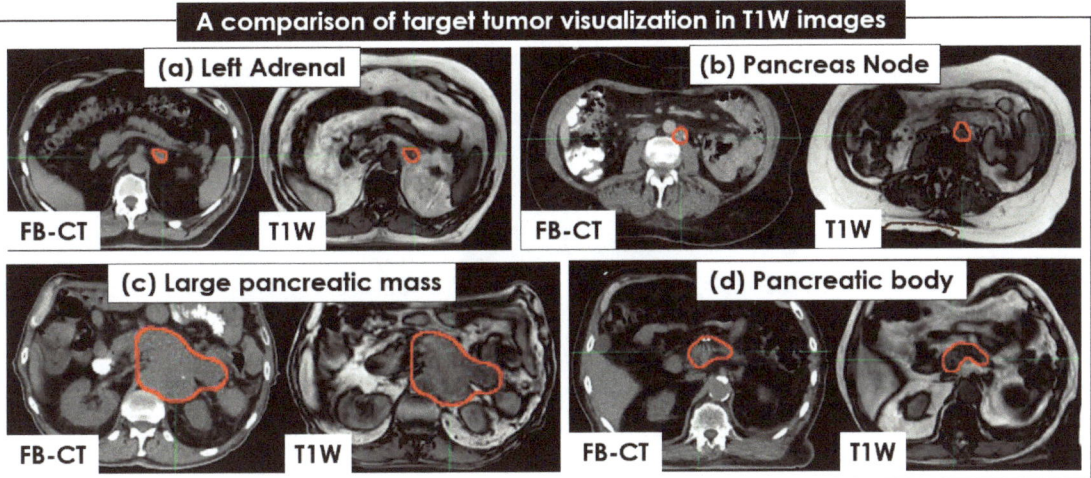

Figure 3. Comparison of tumor visualization between CT and 4 T1W image sets. The same target tumors of 4 patients, colored in red, are shown in free-breathing (FB)-CT and T1W: (**a**) left adrenal, (**b**) pancreatic node, (**c**) large pancreatic mass, and (**d**) pancreatic body. The target tumors are clearly seen in both the FB-CT and T1W image sets.

The average GTV and PTV, measured in the $_{CT}$Ref or $_{MR}$Ref across all 26 patients, were 36.6 mL (range: 3.4 mL to 106.4 mL) and 74.9 mL (range: 7.1 mL to 181.4 mL), respectively. A target motion of 0.2–0.4 cm was measured with 4D-CT or 2D-Cine and added to the GTV as a margin along all directions for ITV, accounting for respiratory-induced target motion when using the abdominal compression belt.

3.3. Plan Quality of Reference SBRT Plans

Figure 4 shows 2 examples of patient $_{CT}$Ref and $_{MR}$Ref plans. All QA testing $_{CT}$Ref, $_{MR}$Ref, and $_{MR}$ATS plans showed a >95% passing rate for the 3%-3mm gamma analysis and a <2% point dose difference between data measured by an ion chamber and data calculated by TPS.

3.4. Online Adaptive MRI-Guided SBRT

Superior visualization of tumors and OAR on T1W image sets contributed to minimizing contouring uncertainty and improving the efficiency of image fusion between a chosen reference plan and plan-MRI. Furthermore, the total acquisition time of plan-MRI, verification-MRI, and post-MRI was reduced three times from 360 s for T2W + Nav to 120 s for T1W (a 67% reduction of the total acquisition time). Figure 5 shows the visualization of tumors and OAR on 5 $_{MR}$ATS plans created with 5 fractioned online adaptive plans.

The difference in GTV and PTV contours in all $_{MR}$ATS(s), compared to $_{CT}$Ref (or $_{MR}$Ref), was minimal. The average GTV was 37.1 mL in all $_{CT}$Ref(s) and $_{MR}$Ref and 35.4 mL in all $_{MR}$ATS(s). Similarly, the average PTV was 74.1 mL in all $_{CT}$Ref(s) and $_{MR}$Ref and 72.1 mL in all $_{MR}$ATS(s). In addition, the dose coverages of GTV $D_{95\%}$ and $D_{90\%}$ for all $_{CT}$Ref(s) were 94.2% [range: 78.8% to 100.0%] and 96.9% [range: 86.1% to 100.0%], respectively. The dose coverages of PTV $D_{95\%}$ and $D_{90\%}$ were slightly lower at 89.7% [range: 69.3% to 99.7%] and 94% [range: 78.8% to 100%], respectively. For all $_{MR}$ATS(s), GTV/PTV $D_{95\%}$ and $D_{90\%}$ were approximately at 83.7% [range: 16.8% to 100.0%]/91.6% [range: 52.8% to 100.0%], respectively. The dose coverages of GTV and PTV were mainly dependent on the locations of OAR, such as duodenum or jejunum (n = 10), stomach (n = 7), small bowel or colon (n = 9), and spleen (n = 11). Other OAR, such as the liver, kidneys, and spinal cords, had a negligible effect on GTV and PTV dose coverages since the beams' gantry angles avoided these OAR.

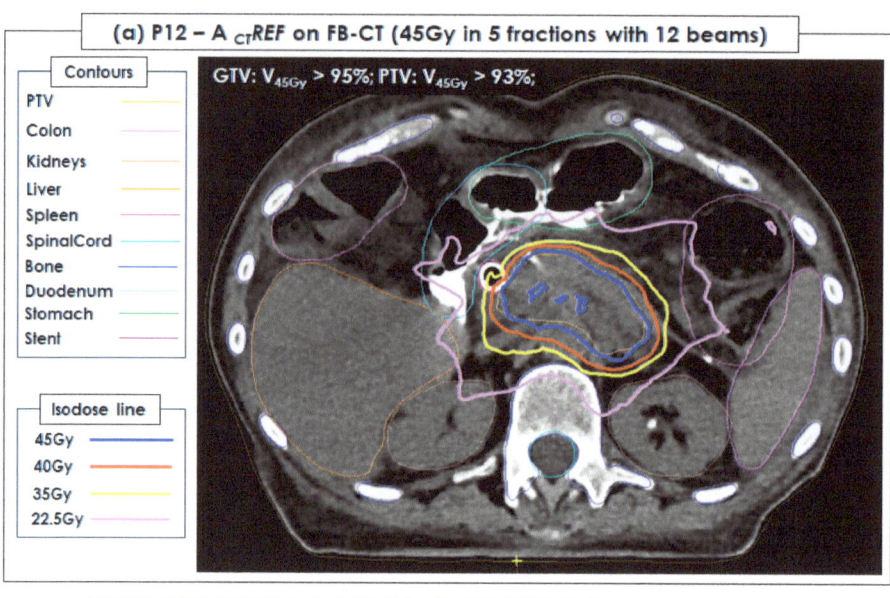
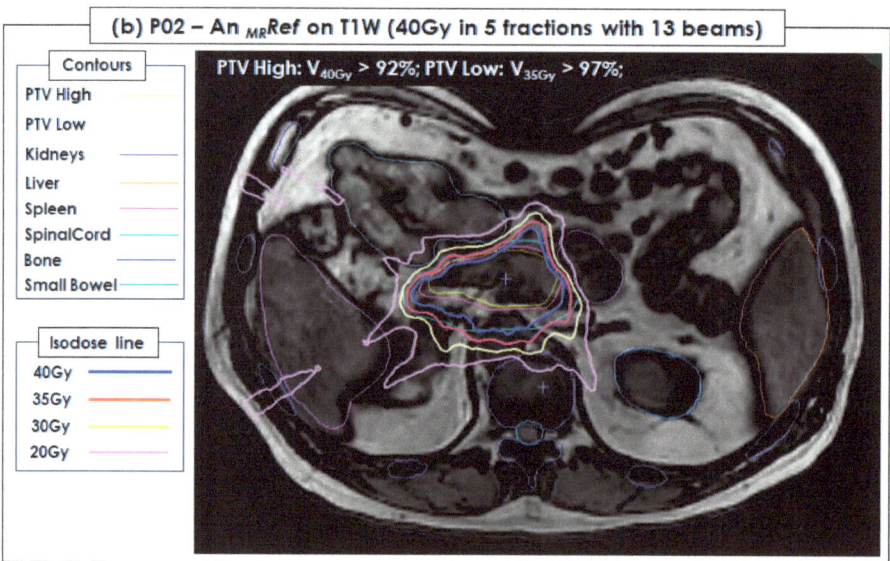

Figure 4. A CT reference plan ($_{CT}$Ref) of P12 and an MRI reference plan ($_{MR}$Ref) of P02 developed in a free-breathing (FB) CT image set (45 Gy = 9 Gy × 5 fractions with 12 beams) and a T1W image set (40 Gy = 8 Gy × 5 fractions with 13 beams), respectively. PTV and OAR (kidneys, liver, spleen, spinal cord, duodenum, bone, body (external), and small bowel) were contoured and shown in the FB-CT and T1W image sets. Both were successfully used for pancreatic and intra-abdominal cancers during 5 fractionated MRI-guided stereotactic body radiotherapy (SBRT). (**a**) The dose coverage of gross tumor volume (GTV) and planning target volume (PTV) in $_{CT}$Ref achieved $V_{45Gy} > 95\%$ and $V_{45Gy} > 93\%$, respectively. (**b**) The dose coverage of PTV High and PTV Low in $_{MR}$Ref achieved $V_{40Gy} > 92\%$ and $V_{35Gy} > 97\%$, respectively.

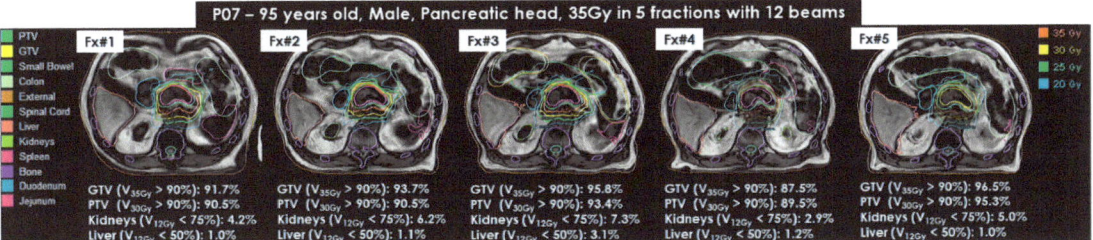

Figure 5. Online adaptive MRI-guided stereotactic body radiotherapy for pancreatic and intra-abdominal cancers of (MRI-guided SBRT) for P07 using 35Gy in 5 fractions with 12 beams (95 years old, male, pancreas head). All MRI adapt-to-shape ($_{MR}$ATS) plans were created on T1W image sets. The target coverages of gross tumor volume (GTV) and planning target volume (PTV) were greater than 90% in 4 fractions (Fx#1, Fx#2, Fx#3, and Fx#5), except for Fx#4. Organs at risk (OAR), the duodenum and jejunum, were very close to the target tumor and resulted in less than 90% in Fx#4. All OAR coverages were achieved in all $_{MR}$ATS(s).

3.5. Overall Time-Consumption of Online MRI-Guided SBRT in 10 Steps

The average time-consumption of online MRI-guided SBRT for the first 21 patients was 55 min for ATP and 79 min for ATS (Table 3). The most time-consuming steps were fusion/contouring and beam delivery (5 Gy to 9 Gy in each fraction with 7–13 beams), followed by patient setup, plan optimization, and plan QA/approval.

Table 3. Time-consumption of online adaptive MRI-guided stereotactic body radiotherapy for pancreatic and intra-abdominal cancers (SBRT) in 10 steps. The step of fusion and contouring included some waiting time of attending physicians. The step of plan QA and approval included an independent dose verification and a visual inspection of the target tumor moving within the PTV contour.

Adaptive	MRI Screening	Patient Setup	Imaging Plan-MRI	Fusion/ Contouring	Plan Optimization	Plan Review	Plan QA/Approval	Therapist Check	BEAM Delivery	Imaging Post-MRI	Seconds	Minutes
					Imaging Verification-MRI							
ATP	81 ± 35	493 ± 144	276 ± 99	763 ± 546	330 ± 180	264 ± 328	248 ± 113	17 ± 17	725 ± 238	97 ± 14	3296 ± 925	54.9 ± 15.4
ATS	77 ± 39	622 ± 254	238 ± 90	1629 ± 739	545 ± 545	337 ± 271	337 ± 396	26 ± 45	850 ± 261	98 ± 17	4759 ± 1243	79.3 ± 20.7

4. Discussion

SBRT planning requires that the tumor be superiorly visualized in CT or MR image sets to determine the radiation dose limit for OAR in patients with pancreatic and intra-abdominal caners [5,9,12–14]. In this study, we utilized T1W imaging (about 120 s) to reduce the imaging time of plan-MRI, verification-MRI, and post-MRI by approximately 67%, compared to T2W + Nav imaging (about 360 s). T1W imaging also improved tumor visualization to (1) minimize delineation uncertainty, (2) reduce GTV, and (3) spare OAR during MRI-guided SBRT. We demonstrated the efficiency of T1W imaging by inspecting all images within the clear boundaries of contoured tumors and OAR.

Intra- and inter-fractional changes in a tumor's anatomical position and shape and a patient's setup are often found in image-guided radiotherapy, required re-planning, or online adaptive planning [35–37]. To account for an inter-fractional change between a reference plan ($_{CT}$Ref, $_{MR}$Ref, or $_{MR}$ATS) and the plan-MRI, we performed online adaptive ATP or ATS planning, and we repeated adaptive planning within a fraction if we found an intra-fractional change between the plan-MRI and verification-MRI. To repeat adaptive planning, the latest verification-MRI was used as the plan-MRI and fused to a reference plan or the latest $_{MR}$ATS, followed by contouring and/or plan optimization. More than one adaptive planning was required in 10% of all fractions, which could be improved by increasing patient comfort [38]. For example, we minimized the time patients stayed on the treatment couch during online adaptive planning. T1W imaging can achieve fast imaging and efficient contouring of tumors and OAR, but it still requires patient setup for those with pre-existing health conditions, causing discomfort and pain (i.e., surgery, injury, and claustrophobia), eliminating (or minimizing) the idle waiting time for the attending physician, and reducing the delivery time of uncomplicated SBRT plans [39–41].

The tumor contours delineated on T1W image sets matched the contours in FB-CT image sets because they account for the respiratory-induced motion during image acquisition. However, T2W + Nav image sets were acquired at exhalation in Unity®, so the contour size of tumors was slightly smaller than it was in T1W image sets [42]. Our ITV was determined at every fraction by encompassing GTV delineated on a T1W image set and motion range measured on orthogonal, sagittal, and coronal cine images in between inhalation and exhalation over the multiple breathing cycles (i.e., about 5–7 breathing cycles). This helps to clarify fractional breathing patterns for increasing the reliability of ITV margins in the presence of inter-fractional breathing variability [43].

Patient immobilization is critical for maintaining patient setup and preventing changes in target/OAR position and shape [32,44]. A thin or medium-sized vac-bag was tested with the first 5 patients during patient setup, but this required a long setup time. The vac-bag also required the patient to rotate so that the ATS could be achieved during the long treatment time. Instead of a vac-bag, we used an abdominal compression belt to control the target motion moving within 5 mm [22]. The setup consistency of an abdominal compression belt was dependent on the level of experience of individual therapists, and it was more consistent when the same therapist set it up every time across all simulations and multi-fractionated MRI-guided SBRT.

Our study has limitations. Limitations of this study include the basic analysis of image and plan quality using T1W imaging. However, our clinical protocol is continuously being improved to increase workflow efficiency using immobilization devices, MRI sequences, and auto-contouring and planning. Compared to our T1W sequence, the newly released MRI sequence (b3DVaneXD) and research sequences (compressed sensing and mDIXON) were not tested to compare tumor and OAR visualization. The present manual measurement of ITV margin may not be required when using a respiratory gating technique in the near future.

This is an ongoing project at our institution and will include more quantitative analysis when compared with other MRI sequences, such as b3DVaneXD, compressed sensing, and mDIXON, to provide alternative imaging for less motion-dependent imaging, faster imaging, and fat/water suppression imaging, respectively. In addition, we will assess the complexity and dose coverage of our SBRT plans by comparing them with other plans using other imaging techniques for cross-validation.

5. Conclusions

This was the first study that utilized a customized and optimized T1W sequence to improve the visualization of tumors and OAR for reference planning and online adaptive planning on a 1.5T Unity®. The tumor and OAR boundaries were clearly visible for delineation. Our results can facilitate consistent visualization of pancreatic and other intra-abdominal tumors to achieve fast and accurate MRI-guided SBRT.

Author Contributions: D.L. wrote the manuscript and acquired the T1W and T2W + Nav image sets. P.R. recruited the patients with pancreatic and intra-abdominal cancers. P.R., A.K., M.T. and A.C. worked as attending physicians. S.O., M.-S.H., K.L.Y., D.P. and D.L. worked as attending physicists. C.C. and M.M. worked as the attending therapist and dosimetrist. D.L. oversaw statistical analyses. The authors reviewed the final manuscript. All authors have read and agreed to the published version of the manuscript.

Funding: This research received no external funding.

Institutional Review Board Statement: The study was approved by the Institutional Review Board of Allegheny Health Network Cancer Institute (Pittsburgh, PA, USA).

Informed Consent Statement: Patient consent was waived since this was a retrospective study that analyzed imaging and treatment data.

Data Availability Statement: The data can be shared upon request.

Acknowledgments: We thank the physicians, therapists, nurses, dosimetrists, and staff at Allegheny Health Network and the Department of Radiation Oncology for their continuous support. The authors thank Sarah Carey, Jade Chang, and Jacalyn Newman of Allegheny Health Network's Health System Publication Support Office (HSPSO) for their assistance in editing and formatting the manuscript. The HSPSO is funded by Highmark Health (Pittsburgh, PA, United States of America), and all work was performed in accordance with Good Publication Practice (GPP3) guidelines (http://www.ismpp.org/gpp3, accessed on 12 September 2023).

Conflicts of Interest: The authors declare no conflict of interest.

References

1. Mutic, S.; Dempsey, J.F. The ViewRay System: Magnetic Resonance–Guided and Controlled Radiotherapy. *Semin. Radiat. Oncol.* **2014**, *24*, 196–199. [CrossRef]
2. Lagendijk, J.J.W.; Raaymakers, B.W.; van Vulpen, M. The Magnetic Resonance Imaging–Linac System. *Semin. Radiat. Oncol.* **2014**, *24*, 207–209. [CrossRef]
3. Fallone, B.G. The Rotating Biplanar Linac–Magnetic Resonance Imaging System. *Semin. Radiat. Oncol.* **2014**, *24*, 200–202. [CrossRef]
4. Keall, P.J.; Barton, M.; Crozier, S. The Australian Magnetic Resonance Imaging–Linac Program. *Semin. Radiat. Oncol.* **2014**, *24*, 203–206. [CrossRef]
5. Heerkens, H.D.; van Vulpen, M.; Erickson, B.; Reerink, O.; Intven, M.P.; van den Berg, C.A.; Meijer, G.J. MRI guided stereotactic radiotherapy for locally advanced pancreatic cancer. *Br. J. Radiol.* **2018**, *91*, 20170563. [CrossRef]
6. Klüter, S. Technical design and concept of a 0.35 T MR-Linac. *Clin. Transl. Radiat. Oncol.* **2019**, *18*, 98–101. [CrossRef]
7. Winkel, D.; Bol, G.H.; Kroon, P.S.; van Asselen, B.; Hackett, S.S.; Werensteijn-Honingh, A.M.; Intven, M.P.; Eppinga, W.S.; Tijssen, R.H.; Kerkmeijer, L.G.; et al. Adaptive radiotherapy: The Elekta Unity MR-linac concept. *Clin. Transl. Radiat. Oncol.* **2019**, *18*, 54–59. [CrossRef]
8. Hall, W.A.; Small, C.; Paulson, E.; Koay, E.J.; Crane, C.; Intven, M.; Daamen, L.A.; Meijer, G.J.; Heerkens, H.D.; Bassetti, M.; et al. Magnetic Resonance Guided Radiation Therapy for Pancreatic Adenocarcinoma, Advantages, Challenges, Current Approaches, and Future Directions. *Front. Oncol.* **2021**, *11*, 628155. [CrossRef]
9. Rodriguez, L.L.; Kotecha, R.; Tom, M.C.; Chuong, M.D.; Contreras, J.A.; Romaguera, T.; Alvarez, D.; McCulloch, J.; Herrera, R.; Hernandez, R.J.; et al. CT-guided versus MR-guided radiotherapy: Impact on gastrointestinal sparing in adrenal stereotactic body radiotherapy. *Radiother. Oncol.* **2022**, *166*, 101–109. [CrossRef]
10. Hoegen, P.; Katsigiannopulos, E.; Buchele, C.; Regnery, S.; Weykamp, F.; Sandrini, E.; Ristau, J.; Liermann, J.; Meixner, E.; Forster, T.; et al. Stereotactic magnetic resonance-guided online adaptive radiotherapy of adrenal metastases combines high ablative doses with optimized sparing of organs at risk. *Clin. Transl. Radiat. Oncol.* **2023**, *39*, 100567. [CrossRef]
11. Rammohan, N.; Randall, J.W.; Yadav, P. History of Technological Advancements towards MR-Linac: The Future of Image-Guided Radiotherapy. *JCM* **2022**, *11*, 4730. [CrossRef] [PubMed]
12. Luterstein, E.; Cao, M.; Lamb, J.; Raldow, A.C.; Low, D.A.; Steinberg, M.L.; Lee, P. Stereotactic MRI-Guided Adaptive Radiation Therapy (SMART) for Locally Advanced Pancreatic Cancer: A Promising Approach. 2018. Available online: https://www.cureus.com/articles/10922-stereotactic-mri-guided-adaptive-radiation-therapy-smart-for-locally-advanced-pancreatic-cancer-a-promising-approach (accessed on 4 April 2023).
13. Hassanzadeh, C.; Rudra, S.; Bommireddy, A.; Hawkins, W.G.; Wang-Gillam, A.; Fields, R.C.; Cai, B.; Park, J.; Green, O.; Roach, M.; et al. Ablative Five-Fraction Stereotactic Body Radiation Therapy for Inoperable Pancreatic Cancer Using Online MR-Guided Adaptation. *Adv. Radiat. Oncol.* **2021**, *6*, 100506. [CrossRef] [PubMed]
14. Michalet, M.; Bordeau, K.; Cantaloube, M.; Valdenaire, S.; Debuire, P.; Simeon, S.; Portales, F.; Draghici, R.; Ychou, M.; Assenat, E.; et al. Stereotactic MR-Guided Radiotherapy for Pancreatic Tumors: Dosimetric Benefit of Adaptation and First Clinical Results in a Prospective Registry Study. *Front. Oncol.* **2022**, *12*, 842402. [CrossRef] [PubMed]
15. Bordeau, K.; Michalet, M.; Keskes, A.; Valdenaire, S.; Debuire, P.; Cantaloube, M.; Caballé, M.; Portales, F.; Draghici, R.; Ychou, M.; et al. Stereotactic MR-Guided Adaptive Radiotherapy for Pancreatic Tumors: Updated Results of the Montpellier Prospective Registry Study. *Cancers* **2022**, *15*, 7. [CrossRef]
16. Heerkens, H.; Hall, W.; Li, X.; Knechtges, P.; Dalah, E.; Paulson, E.; Berg, C.v.D.; Meijer, G.; Koay, E.; Crane, C.; et al. Recommendations for MRI-based contouring of gross tumor volume and organs at risk for radiation therapy of pancreatic cancer. *Pract. Radiat. Oncol.* **2017**, *7*, 126–136. [CrossRef]
17. Hall, W.A.; Heerkens, H.D.; Paulson, E.S.; Meijer, G.J.; Kotte, A.N.; Knechtges, P.; Parikh, P.J.; Bassetti, M.F.; Lee, P.; Aitken, K.L.; et al. Pancreatic gross tumor volume contouring on computed tomography (CT) compared with magnetic resonance imaging (MRI): Results of an international contouring conference. *Pract. Radiat. Oncol.* **2018**, *8*, 107–115. [CrossRef]

18. Rhee, H.; Park, M.S. The Role of Imaging in Current Treatment Strategies for Pancreatic Adenocarcinoma. *Korean J. Radiol.* **2021**, *22*, 23. [CrossRef]
19. Chuong, M.D.; Bryant, J.; Mittauer, K.E.; Hall, M.; Kotecha, R.; Alvarez, D.; Romaguera, T.; Rubens, M.; Adamson, S.; Godley, A.; et al. Ablative 5-Fraction Stereotactic Magnetic Resonance–Guided Radiation Therapy With On-Table Adaptive Replanning and Elective Nodal Irradiation for Inoperable Pancreas Cancer. *Pract. Radiat. Oncol.* **2021**, *11*, 134–147. [CrossRef]
20. Lens, E.; van der Horst, A.; Versteijne, E.; Bel, A.; van Tienhoven, G. Considerable pancreatic tumor motion during breath-holding. *Acta Oncol.* **2016**, *55*, 1360–1368. [CrossRef]
21. Lee, D.; Greer, P.B.; Arm, J.; Keall, P.; Kim, T. Audiovisual biofeedback improves image quality and reduces scan time for respiratory-gated 3D MRI. *J. Phys. Conf. Ser.* **2014**, *489*, 012033. [CrossRef]
22. Tyagi, N.; Liang, J.; Burleson, S.; Subashi, E.; Scripes, P.G.; Tringale, K.R.; Romesser, P.B.; Reyngold, M.; Crane, C.H. Feasibility of ablative stereotactic body radiation therapy of pancreas cancer patients on a 1.5 Tesla magnetic resonance-linac system using abdominal compression. *Phys. Imaging Radiat Oncol.* **2021**, *19*, 53–59. [CrossRef] [PubMed]
23. Lee, M.; Simeonov, A.; Stanescu, T.; Dawson, L.A.; Brock, K.K.; Velec, M. MRI evaluation of normal tissue deformation and breathing motion under an abdominal compression device. *J. Appl. Clin. Med. Phys.* **2021**, *22*, 90–97. [CrossRef] [PubMed]
24. Alam, S.; Veeraraghavan, H.; Tringale, K.; Amoateng, E.; Subashi, E.; Wu, A.J.; Crane, C.H.; Tyagi, N. Inter-and intrafraction motion assessment and accumulated dose quantification of upper gastrointestinal organs during magnetic resonance-guided ablative radiation therapy of pancreas patients. *Phys. Imaging Radiat Oncol.* **2022**, *21*, 54–61. [CrossRef] [PubMed]
25. Axford, A.; Dikaios, N.; Roberts, D.A.; Clark, C.H.; Evans, P.M. An end-to-end assessment on the accuracy of adaptive radiotherapy in an MR-linac. *Phys. Med. Biol.* **2021**, *66*, 055021. [CrossRef]
26. Tirkes, T.; Menias, C.O.; Sandrasegaran, K. MR Imaging Techniques for Pancreas. *Radiol. Clin. North Am.* **2012**, *50*, 379–393. [CrossRef]
27. Keall, P.J.; Mageras, G.S.; Balter, J.M.; Emery, R.S.; Forster, K.M.; Jiang, S.B.; Kapatoes, J.M.; Low, M.J.; Murphy, S.B.; Murray, B.R.; et al. The management of respiratory motion in radiation oncology report of AAPM Task Group 76a): Respiratory motion in radiation oncology. *Med. Phys.* **2006**, *33*, 3874–3900. [CrossRef]
28. Grimbergen, G.; Eijkelenkamp, H.; Heerkens, H.D.; Raaymakers, B.W.; Intven, M.P.W.; Meijer, G.J. Intrafraction pancreatic tumor motion patterns during ungated magnetic resonance guided radiotherapy with an abdominal corset. *Phys. Imaging Radiat. Oncol.* **2022**, *21*, 1–5. [CrossRef]
29. Oh, S.; Kim, S. Deformable image registration in radiation therapy. *Radiat Oncol. J.* **2017**, *35*, 101–111. [CrossRef]
30. Rong, Y.; Rosu-Bubulac, M.; Benedict, S.H.; Cui, Y.; Ruo, R.; Connell, T.; Kashani, R.; Latifi, K.; Chen, Q.; Geng, H.; et al. Rigid and Deformable Image Registration for Radiation Therapy: A Self-Study Evaluation Guide for NRG Oncology Clinical Trial Participation. *Pr. Radiat. Oncol.* **2021**, *11*, 282–298. [CrossRef]
31. Expert Panel on MR Safety: Kanal, E.; Barkovich, A.J.; Bell, C.; Borgstede, J.P.; Bradley, W.G., Jr.; Froelich, J.W.; Gimbel, J.R.; Gosbee, J.W.; Kuhni-Kaminski, E.; et al. ACR guidance document on MR safe practices. *J. Magn. Reson. Imaging* **2013**, *37*, 501–530.
32. Glide-Hurst, C.K.; Paulson, E.S.; McGee, K.; Tyagi, N.; Hu, Y.; Balter, J.; Bayouth, J. Task group 284 report: Magnetic resonance imaging simulation in radiotherapy: Considerations for clinical implementation, optimization, and quality assurance. *Med. Phys.* **2021**, *48*, E636–E670. Available online: https://aapm.onlinelibrary.wiley.com/doi/10.1002/mp.14695 (accessed on 7 September 2023). [CrossRef] [PubMed]
33. Malkov, V.N.; Rogers, D.W.O. Sensitive volume effects on Monte Carlo calculated ion chamber response in magnetic fields. *Med. Phys.* **2017**, *44*, 4854–4858. [CrossRef]
34. Strand, S.; Boczkowski, A.; Smith, B.; E Snyder, J.; Hyer, D.E.; Yaddanapudi, S.; Dunkerley, D.A.P.; St-Aubin, J. Analysis of patient-specific quality assurance for Elekta Unity adaptive plans using statistical process control methodology. *J. Appl. Clin. Med. Phys.* **2021**, *22*, 99–107. [CrossRef] [PubMed]
35. Sonke, J.J.; Aznar, M.; Rasch, C. Adaptive Radiotherapy for Anatomical Changes. *Semin. Radiat. Oncol.* **2019**, *29*, 245–257. [CrossRef] [PubMed]
36. Ashida, R.; Nakamura, M.; Yoshimura, M.; Mizowaki, T. Impact of interfractional anatomical variation and setup correction methods on interfractional dose variation in IMPT and VMAT plans for pancreatic cancer patients: A planning study. *J. Appl. Clin. Med. Phys.* **2020**, *21*, 49–59. [CrossRef]
37. Qiu, Z.; Olberg, S.; Den Hertog, D.; Ajdari, A.; Bortfeld, T.; Pursley, J. Online adaptive planning methods for intensity-modulated radiotherapy. *Phys. Med. Biol.* **2023**, *68*, 10TR01. [CrossRef]
38. Goldsworthy, S.; Latour, J.M.; Palmer, S.; McNair, H.A.; Cramp, M. Patient and therapeutic radiographer experiences of comfort during the radiotherapy pathway: A qualitative study. *Radiography* **2023**, *29*, S24–S31. [CrossRef]
39. Matuszak, M.M.; Larsen, E.W.; Fraass, B.A. Reduction of IMRT beam complexity through the use of beam modulation penalties in the objective function: IMRT beam complexity reduction using modulation penalties. *Med. Phys.* **2007**, *34*, 507–520. [CrossRef]
40. Kamperis, E.; Kodona, C.; Hatziioannou, K.; Giannouzakos, V. Complexity in Radiation Therapy: It's Complicated. *Int. J. Radiat. Oncol. Biol. Phys.* **2020**, *106*, 182–184. [CrossRef]
41. Saroj, D.; Yadav, S.; Paliwal, N. Does fluence smoothing reduce the complexity of the intensity-modulated radiation therapy treatment plan? A dosimetric analysis. *J. Med. Phys.* **2022**, *47*, 336.

42. Prunaretty, J.; Boisselier, P.; Aillères, N.; Riou, O.; Simeon, S.; Bedos, L.; Azria, D.; Fenoglietto, P. Tracking, gating, free-breathing, which technique to use for lung stereotactic treatments? A dosimetric comparison. *Rep. Pract. Oncol. Radiother.* **2019**, *24*, 97–104. [CrossRef] [PubMed]
43. Cusumano, D.; Dhont, J.; Boldrini, L.; Chiloiro, G.; Romano, A.; Votta, C.; Longo, S.; Placidi, L.; Azario, L.; De Spirito, M.; et al. Reliability of ITV approach to varying treatment fraction time: A retrospective analysis based on 2D cine MR images. *Radiat Oncol.* **2020**, *15*, 152. [CrossRef] [PubMed]
44. Dolde, K.; Dávid, C.; Echner, G.; Floca, R.; Hentschke, C.; Maier, F.; Niebuhr, N.I.; Ohmstedt, K.; Saito, N.; Alimusaj, M.; et al. 4DMRI-based analysis of inter—And intrafractional pancreas motion and deformation with different immobilization devices. *Biomed Phys. Eng. Express* **2019**, *5*, 025012. [CrossRef]

Disclaimer/Publisher's Note: The statements, opinions and data contained in all publications are solely those of the individual author(s) and contributor(s) and not of MDPI and/or the editor(s). MDPI and/or the editor(s) disclaim responsibility for any injury to people or property resulting from any ideas, methods, instructions or products referred to in the content.

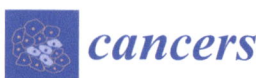 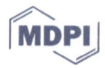

Article

Robotic Stereotactic Radiotherapy for Intracranial Meningiomas—An Opportunity for Radiation Dose De-Escalation

Hanna Grzbiela [1,*], Elzbieta Nowicka [1], Marzena Gawkowska [1], Dorota Tarnawska [2] and Rafal Tarnawski [1]

[1] III Radiotherapy and Chemotherapy Clinic, Maria Sklodowska-Curie National Research Institute of Oncology, Gliwice Branch, Wybrzeze Armii Krajowej 15, 44-100 Gliwice, Poland
[2] Institute of Biomedical Engineering, Faculty of Science and Technology, University of Silesia in Katowice, 75 Pulku Piechoty 1A, 41-500 Chorzow, Poland
* Correspondence: hanna.grzbiela@gliwice.nio.gov.pl

Simple Summary: Meningiomas are among the most common tumors that develop inside the skull. They are often treated with radiotherapy, but there is still no agreement on optimal radiation dose. The aim of our study was to assess the effects of CyberKnife radiotherapy with the total dose of 18 Gy delivered in three fractions. We achieved local control in 91.7% of patients and the results were similar to radiotherapy schemes with greater biologically effective dose, which supports the idea of dose de-escalation in the treatment of meningiomas.

Abstract: Objective: To evaluate the possibility of dose de-escalation, with consideration of the efficacy and safety of robotic stereotactic CyberKnife radiotherapy in patients diagnosed with intracranial meningiomas. Methods: The study group consisted of 172 patients (42 men and 130 women) treated in III Radiotherapy and Chemotherapy Clinic of Maria Sklodowska-Curie National Research Institute of Oncology in Gliwice between January 2011 and July 2018. The qualification for dose de-escalation was based on MRI (magnetic resonance imaging) features: largest tumor diameter less than 5 cm, well-defined tumor margins, no edema, and no brain infiltration. The age of patients was 21–79 years (median 59 years) at diagnosis and 24–80 years (median 62 years) at radiotherapy. Sixty-seven patients (Group A) were irradiated after initial surgery. Histopathological findings were meningioma grade WHO 1 in 51 and WHO 2 in 16 cases. Group B (105 patients) had no prior surgery and the diagnosis was based on the typical features of meningioma on MRI. All patients qualified for the robotic stereotactic CyberKnife radiotherapy, and the total dose received was 18 Gy in three fractions to reference isodose 78–92%. Results: Follow-up period was 18 to 124 months (median 67.5 months). Five- and eight-year progression free survival was 90.3% and 89.4%, respectively. Two patients died during the follow-up period. Progression of tumor after radiotherapy was registered in 16 cases. Four patients required surgery due to progressive disease, and three of them were progression free during further follow-up. Twelve patients received a second course of robotic radiotherapy, 11 of them had stable disease, and one patient showed further tumor growth but died of heart failure. Crude progression free survival after both primary and secondary treatment was 98.8%. Radiotherapy was well-tolerated: acute toxicity grade 1/2 (EORTC-RTOG scale) was seen in 10.5% of patients. We did not observe any late effects of radiotherapy. Conclusion: Stereotactic CyberKnife radiotherapy with total dose of 18 Gy delivered in three fractions showed comparable efficacy to treatment schedules with higher doses. This could support the idea of dose de-escalation in the treatment of intracranial meningiomas.

Keywords: meningiomas; robotic stereotactic radiotherapy; CyberKnife; dose de-escalation

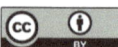

Citation: Grzbiela, H.; Nowicka, E.; Gawkowska, M.; Tarnawska, D.; Tarnawski, R. Robotic Stereotactic Radiotherapy for Intracranial Meningiomas—An Opportunity for Radiation Dose De-Escalation. *Cancers* 2023, *15*, 5436. https://doi.org/10.3390/cancers15225436

Academic Editors: Sam Beddar and Michael D. Chuong

Received: 26 September 2023
Revised: 27 October 2023
Accepted: 14 November 2023
Published: 16 November 2023

Copyright: © 2023 by the authors. Licensee MDPI, Basel, Switzerland. This article is an open access article distributed under the terms and conditions of the Creative Commons Attribution (CC BY) license (https://creativecommons.org/licenses/by/4.0/).

1. Introduction

Up to 30% of all primary intracranial tumors are meningiomas, which makes them the most common non-glial tumors in this location [1–3]. It is difficult to estimate the real prevalence of meningiomas, as many of them are asymptomatic and are found accidentally or during an autopsy, so the incidence is probably much higher than shown in most registries. Meningiomas are mostly benign tumors. They progress very slowly, and only some of them can affect the patient's quality of life. As stated in National Comprehensive Cancer Network (NCCN) Guidelines version 2.2022, small and asymptomatic tumors may be observed using serial imaging [4]. Standard therapy in other cases is usually surgical excision, but not all tumors can be completely removed. Some will recur even after GTR (gross total resection), and for some patients, neurosurgery is impossible (due to tumor location or the patient's poor performance status) [5,6]. For these patients, radiation therapy is a valuable treatment alternative.

Decisions regarding whether the patient requires treatment or can be observed should be made during multidisciplinary board meetings. Factors influencing these decisions are patient-related (age, performance score, comorbidities, personal treatment preferences) or tumor-related (diameter, WHO grade, growth rate, location, proximity to critical structures, presence and severity of symptoms and potential for causing neurological deficits if untreated). Other factors which should be considered are possible neurological complications following surgery or radiotherapy, likelihood of complete resection and/or complete irradiation with stereotactic radiosurgery, further treatment options if progression occurs, and available surgical or radiation oncology expertise and resources.

Radiation therapy is a useful treatment option for benign meningiomas. It should be stressed, however, that in the case of these benign tumors we do not expect a complete response. The main objective of radiation therapy is to stop tumor progression; in some cases, partial response can be achieved. According to NCCN Guidelines, optimal dosing has not been determined [4]. The idea of the current study was thus to set up an observational study using the lowest commonly accepted radiation dose—18 Gy—in three fractions to reference isodose 78–92%.

2. Materials and Methods

2.1. Patient Characteristics

The study group consisted of 172 patients (42 men and 130 women) diagnosed with intracranial meningiomas, treated in the III Radiotherapy and Chemotherapy Clinic of Maria Sklodowska-Curie National Research Institute of Oncology in Gliwice. Between January 2011 and July 2018 all patients received 18 Gy in three fractions (to isodose line 78–92%) using CyberKnife robotic stereotactic radiotherapy. The median age of patients was 59 years (range 21–79 years) at diagnosis and 62 years (range 24–80 years) at radiotherapy. Most patients (57%) belonged to the age group between 51 and 69 years. Baseline ECOG grade was 0 or 1 in 160 patients and 2 in 12 patients. Seventy-two patients suffered from various neurological deficits, such as hemiparesis (18 patients) and visual impairment (36 patients). The most common location (55.2%) was the skull base, including cavernous sinus involvement (Table 1).

Table 1. Topography of meningiomas.

Topography	Number of Patients	%
Skull base	95	55.2
(incl. cavernous sinus)	(42)	(24.4)
Falx or parasagittal	30	17.4
Convexity	28	16.3
Cerebellopontine angle	8	4.7
Optic nerve sheath	6	3.5
Lateral fissure	5	2.9

All cases were discussed during a multidisciplinary board meeting. Patients with lesions less than 5 cm in largest diameter, with a well-defined border, no edema, and no signs of brain infiltration, qualified for radiotherapy with dose de-escalation.

In order to provide more transparency in statistical analysis, two groups were created: 67 patients (20 men and 47 women) in Group A had already undergone surgery as initial treatment before they were qualified for radiotherapy, whereas 105 patients (22 men and 83 women) in Group B were treated by robotic radiotherapy alone.

In Group A, gross total resection (Simpson I–III) was performed in 32 patients. The most common histological subtype was meningothelial meningioma WHO 1, especially in the cavernous sinus region (66%). Most atypical meningiomas were located on cerebral convexity. Table 2 shows the distribution of histological subtypes of tumors. Radiotherapy was implemented at the time of tumor recurrence. Thirty-five patients were irradiated due to subtotal tumor resection or biopsy (Simpson IV–V). The median time from surgery to the start of radiotherapy was 11 months (range 5–56 months) after STR (subtotal resection) and 59.5 months (range 14–211 months) after GTR, and the difference was statistically significant ($p = 0.00000$).

Table 2. Distribution of histological subtypes in Group A.

	Subtype	Number of Patients	%
WHO 1	Meningothelial	32	47.8
	Fibrous	9	13.4
	Angiomatous	2	3
	Psammomatous	2	3
	Transitional	6	8.9
WHO 2	Atypical	15	22.4
	Clear Cell	1	1.5

Group B consisted of 105 patients treated by robotic hfSRT (hypofractionated stereotactic radiation therapy) without initial surgery. The diagnosis of meningioma and the qualification for radiotherapy is based on the tumor's MRI features. The reason for radiotherapy in 41 patients was tumor progression on MRI scans (median time to progression 32 months, range 4–148 months). Sixty-four patients were qualified for radiotherapy shortly after the initial diagnosis because of tumor location (e.g., proximity of eloquent brain structures).

2.2. Radiotherapy Treatment Planning and Delivery

For all patients, a thermoplastic mask dedicated to stereotactic skull radiotherapy was prepared. Following that, thin-slice CT (computed tomography) and MRI with contrast enhancement were performed. Thirty-nine patients with skull base involvement had 68Ga-DOTATATE PET-CT (positron emission tomography-computed tomography) for better tumor visualization. All treatment series were registered using rigid algorithms. Radiotherapy plans were created using CyberKnife treatment planning software for both image registration and treatment planning (Multiplan 4.6 Accuray, Sunnyvale, CA, USA).

Gross Tumor Volume (GTV) was identical with tumor visible on MRI scans. Patients with brain infiltration did not qualify for the current study, so Clinical Target Volume (CTV) was identical with GTV. Due to the high precision of robotic radiotherapy no additional margin was added, and thus Planning Target Volume (PTV) was identical with GTV and CTV. PTV ranged between 0.8 and 29.3 cm^3 (median 6.85 cm^3).

Organs at risk (OAR) were contoured using usually T1 MRI sequence with contrast enhancement, which optimally defines the extension of meningioma (Figure 1). In some cases, other sequences were used for specific tumor location (e.g., T2 with fat saturation images for tumors with orbital involvement). OAR dose constraints were determined according to Timmerman et al.'s criteria as follows (point defined as a volume smaller than 0.035 cm^3): Optic pathway (optic nerves, chiasm, and tracts): maximal point dose 17.4 Gy; 15.3 Gy to volume less than 0.2 cm^3. Cochlea: maximal point dose 14.4 Gy. Brain stem: maximal point dose 23.1 Gy; 15.9 Gy to volume less than 0.35 cm^3. Spinal cord: maximal point dose 22.5 Gy; 15.9 Gy to volume less than 0.35 cm^3 [7].

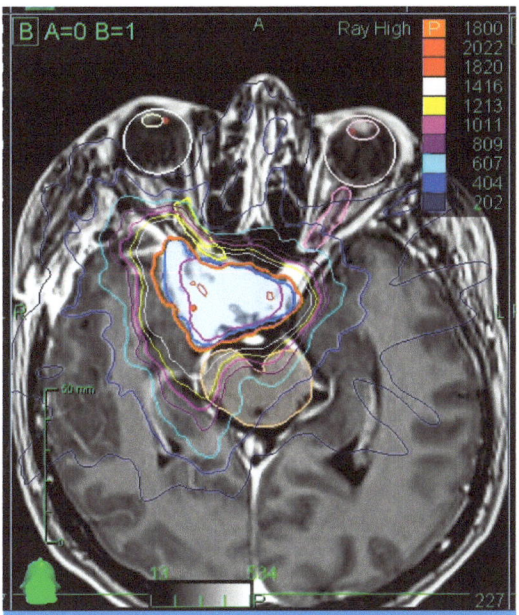

Figure 1. Illustration of GTV and OAR contours and isodoses. Axial view.

As mentioned before, the total dose was 18 Gy delivered in three fractions. The dose was prescribed to the 78–92% isodose line. The minimal PTV dose was 11.8–17.8 Gy (median 17.2 Gy), the maximal PTV dose was 18.82–23.08 (median 20.69 Gy), and the mean dose was 17.05–20.71 Gy. The beam number ranged from 68 to 327 (median 168 beams). Patient positioning and treatment delivery was performed using CyberKnife System (Accuray, Sunnyvale, CA, USA). All patients completed radiotherapy in accordance with the treatment plan.

2.3. Follow-Up

MRI scans and clinical evaluations were obtained at 3, 6, and 12 months after radiotherapy, then yearly and after reaching five years follow-up period every other year. If any new neurological symptoms had appeared, or in the case of any diagnostic uncertainties, additional scans were performed. Twenty-two of the patients with meningiomas located in close proximity to visual pathways had additional detailed ophthalmological examination and follow-up.

2.4. Statistical Analysis

Overall survival (OS) and progression-free survival (PFS) were measured from the time of radiotherapy completion and the analysis was performed using the Kaplan–Meier method. The possible effect of several variables on PFS was determined using Cox regression (p values < 0.05 were considered significant). All statistical analysis was performed using Statistica 13.3 software.

3. Results

3.1. Local Control

Follow-up ranged from 18 to 124 months (median 67.5 months). Local control was achieved in 90.7% of patients—the tumor remained stable in 151 patients (87.8%), whereas five had partial regression (2.9%). Overall survival was 99.3% at 5 years and 98.5% at 8 years

(Figure 2A). Five- and eight-year local control rates were 90.3% and 89.4%, respectively (Figure 2B).

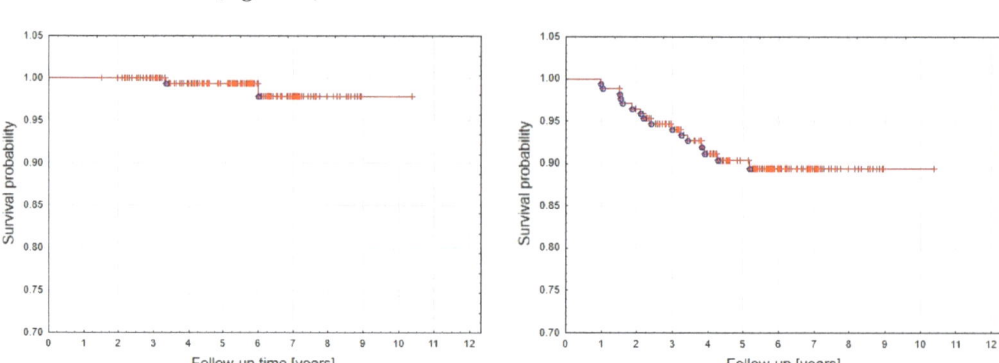

Figure 2. Overall survival (**A**) and local control (**B**) curve.

We analyzed several factors that could potentially influence the outcomes. Five-year PFS was almost equal in all age groups: 24–50 years—91.2%, 51–69 years—90.2%, and 70–80 years—89.2%. Five-year local control rates were higher in women (91.5%) than in men (86.8%), but the difference was not statistically significant.

The worst outcome was observed for cerebral convexity meningiomas—5-year PFS at 75.5%—though it is worth noticing that 25% of tumors in this location were histopathologically confirmed atypical meningiomas. Five-year local control rates for other locations were as follows: 80% for optic nerve sheath meningiomas, 91.2% for skull base meningiomas, 92.8% for cavernous sinus meningiomas, 96.2% for falx meningiomas, and 100% for other locations. Tumor volume had no significant influence on PFS.

Five-year PFS was significantly ($p = 0.01$) higher in Group B (radiotherapy alone) than in Group A (radiotherapy after initial surgery) and the rates were 95.9% and 81.8%, respectively (Figure 3).

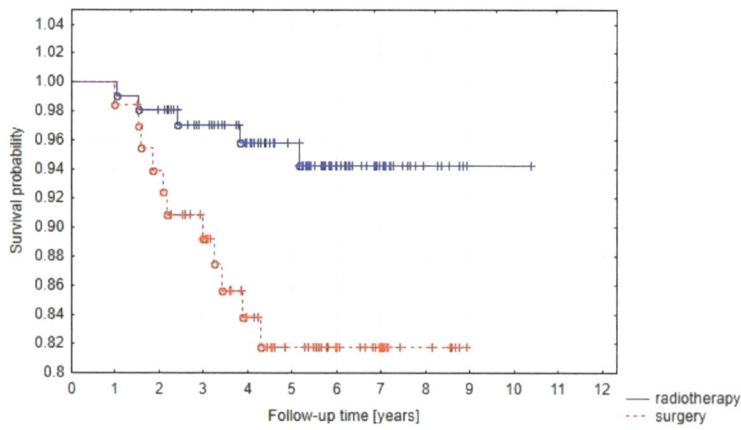

Figure 3. Progression-free survival curve in Group A (prior surgery) and Group B (radiotherapy alone).

In Group A we observed that local control rates at 5 years were higher for benign meningiomas (86.8%) than for atypical meningiomas (66.3%) ($p = 0.03$) (Figure 4). There was no significant difference in PFS between the histological subtypes. Five-year progression-free survival was 100% for angiomatous, transitional, psammomatous, and clear cell meningioma, 82.9% for meningothelial meningioma, 80% for fibrous meningioma, and 63.8% for atypical meningioma ($p = 0.2$). It must be stressed, however, that one of the less common subtypes was found in 11 patients from group A (angiomatous, transitional, psammomatous, or clear cell meningioma). When we only analyzed the three dominant subtypes (meningothelial, fibrous, and atypical), p was 0.07.

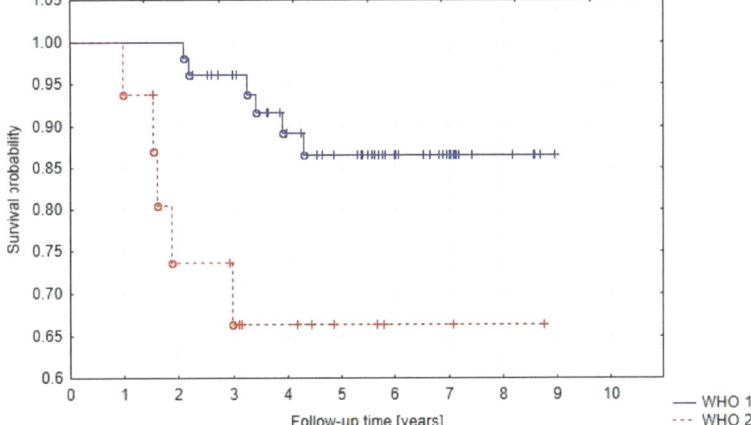

Figure 4. Progression-free survival in Group A related to WHO grade.

3.2. Patients with Tumor Progression

Local failure occurred in 16 patients (9.3%)—10 women and 6 men. The median time to progression was 27.5 months (range 12–62 months). Eleven patients underwent prior surgery (Group A)—four had GTR (and two of them had atypical meningioma) and seven had STR (in three of them meningioma was atypical). Five patients had no prior surgery (Group B) and the tumor progressed before radiotherapy.

After meningioma progression had been diagnosed, four patients were qualified for surgery. Three have stable disease (follow-up range 31–58 months), one patient showed further progression and eventually died 18 months after surgery.

Twelve patients underwent a second course of radiotherapy and were again given 18 Gy in three fractions. Median follow-up in this cohort was 29 months (range 6–54 months). Eleven patients had no progression, and one showed slow progression but died of heart failure 47 months after radiotherapy.

3.3. Tolerance of Treatment

Radiotherapy was very well-tolerated. Eighteen patients (10.5%) reported transient headaches, out of which 10 did not require any treatment (EORTC/RTOG scale grade 1). Only eight patients (4.7%) required small doses of glicocorticosteroids for a short period of time (EORTC/RTOG grade 2); in all those patients tumor volume was greater than 5 cm^3 and the meningioma was localized on the cerebral convexity.

During the treatment planning process special attention was given to the dose to optic apparatus, as many tumors were localized either in the cavernous sinus or the optic nerve sheath. The median dose to the ipsilateral optic nerve was 15.62 Gy (range 3.10–17.33 Gy). In this group, an ophthalmological examination was performed on a regular basis, and 22 patients had extended evaluation, including the assessment of anatomical features (condition of eye surface, central corneal thickness, endothelial cell density, lens densitometry, central macular thickness, and retinal nerve fiber layer) and functional tests (visual acuity, intraocular pressure, visual field, and visual-evoked potentials) [8].

3.4. Clinical Effects of Radiotherapy

As shown in Table 3, 72 patients presented with neurological deficits before radiotherapy. During the follow-up, clinical symptoms were reassessed. After radiotherapy, a substantial improvement was observed in 27 patients (37.5% of those with previous neurological deficits), of which 23 patients reported complete regression of symptoms. Visual impairment had the biggest rate of symptomatic improvement (9 out of 36 patients reported complete regression of symptoms). Forty-three patients (59.7%) reported no change in pre-existing symptoms. Tumor progression only led to the deterioration of their neurological status for two patients (2.8%).

Table 3. Neurological symptoms before radiotherapy and during follow-up.

Symptom	Number of Patients	Complete Regression	Improvement	Worsening
Hemiparesis	18	6	1	2
Visual impairment	36	9	-	-
Hearing impairment	3	-	-	-
Facial nerve palsy	12	7	1	-
Epilepsy	2	-	2	-
Severe headaches	1	1	-	-

We also evaluated the influence of neurological status on treatment outcome and the results were statistically significant—5-year PFS for EORTC/MRC grade 1 (no symptoms), 2 and 3 were 96.8%, 81.9%, and 75.1%, respectively (p = 0.00153) (Figure 5).

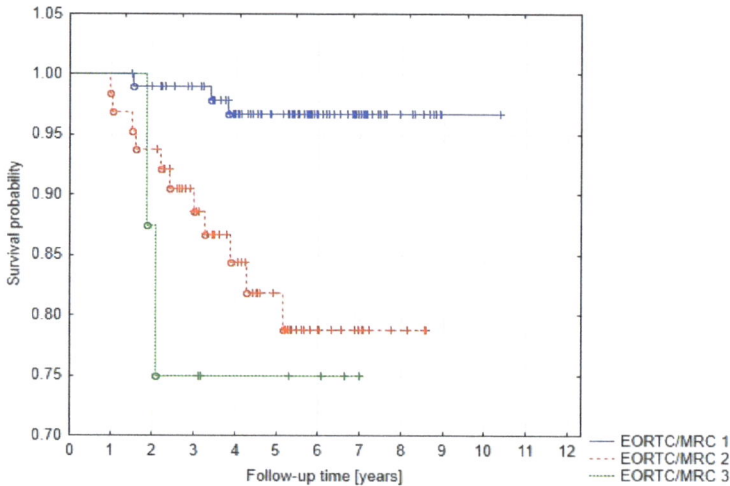

Figure 5. Progression-free survival related to neurological status.

3.5. Other Neoplasms Diagnosed during Follow-Up Period

During the follow-up period, 13 patients were diagnosed with other neoplasms: nine with breast cancer, two with lung cancer, one with colorectal cancer, and one with urinary bladder cancer. All cases of breast cancer were diagnosed as luminal A, with a strong expression of estrogen and progesterone receptors; they all received hormonal therapy, and no meningioma progression was observed in this group.

3.6. Univariate and Multivariate Analysis

We analyzed the influence of demographic, clinical, and histopathological factors on PFS: primary treatment (surgery vs. radiotherapy), age at diagnosis (<50 vs. >50 years), sex (female vs. male), gross tumor volume (<5 cm³ vs. >5 cm³), presence of neurological symptoms (no vs. yes), as well as extent of resection (Simpson I–III vs. IV–V) and histopathological grading (WHO 1 vs. WHO 2) in Group A, and tumor progression before radiotherapy in Group B (yes vs. no).

The univariate Cox regression identified that prior surgery, the presence of neurological deficits and (only in Group A) histopathological grading were associated with poorer outcome. The influence of age, sex, tumor volume, Simpson grade, and progression before radiotherapy was not statistically significant (Table 4). The multivariate Cox regression confirmed that the presence of neurological symptoms was an independent predictive factor of increased recurrence risk (HR 5.54) (Table 5).

Table 4. Univariate Cox regression (PFS).

Prognostic Factor	5-Year PFS	p	HR	CI (95%)
Prior surgery:				
-yes	82%	0.016	3.67	1.27–10.55
-no	96%			
Age at diagnosis:				
<50 years	86%	0.335	0.61	0.22–1.67
>50 years	91%			
Sex:				
-female	92%	0.19	0.51	0.18–1.4
-male	87%			
GTV:				
<5 cm³	92%	0.298	1.82	0.59–5.66
>5 cm³	89%			
Presence of neurological symptoms:				
-no	96%	0.00226	7.09	2.02–24.95
-yes	81%			
Group A				
Simpson Grade:				
I-III	86%	0.34	1.82	0.53–6.22
IV-V	77%			
Histology:				
WHO 1	87%	0.027	3.86	1.17–12.72
WHO 2	66%			
Group B				
Progression prior to radiotherapy:				
-yes	89%	0.089	6.66	0.74–59.63
-no	100%			

Table 5. Multivariate Cox regression (PFS).

Prognostic Factor	p	HR	CI (95%)
Surgery and radiotherapy vs. radiotherapy alone	0.13	2.32	0.78–6.88
No symptoms vs. neurological deficits	0.0095	5.54	1.52–20.23

4. Discussion

Meningiomas are the most common non-glial primary intracranial tumors. Most of them (80–90%) are benign, so the key is to choose a treatment which would lead to the achievement of the best local control rate and keep the morbidity at a low level. There is no general consensus for the total dose and fractionation in radiotherapy of meningiomas. We decided to evaluate the effects of hypofractionated stereotactic radiation therapy with the lowest commonly acceptable dose of 18 Gy in three fractions.

4.1. Study Population

In our study, the majority of patients were women (75.6%), and the female to male ratio was 3.1:1. The same proportion was reported in most studies [2,9–12]. Similar to other analyzed populations, most meningiomas were diagnosed in the sixth or seventh decade of life [2,9–11]. In the literature, atypical meningiomas are reported to be more common in the male population [13]. We also found in Group A that meningiomas WHO 2 accounted for 30% cases in men, but only for 21.3% cases in women.

Park et al. observed the meningothelial subtype to be most common, followed by transitional and fibrous [14]. Almost half of the tumors in our study, after prior surgery (Group A), were meningothelial, followed by fibrous and transitional. When analyzing the relationship between location and histopathological grading, most atypical tumors were located on cerebral convexity and skull base, just as Bhat et al. reported [15].

One patient had the diagnosis of neurofibromatosis 2, and was the youngest of all the patients in our group (21 years at diagnosis); she underwent prior surgery and had a fibrous subtype of the tumor. Meningioma in patients with neurofibromatosis 2 is known to usually be diagnosed at a younger age than in the general population and the histopathological subtype is mostly fibrous or transitional [2,16]. Although some researchers [17] report a more aggressive nature of meningioma in patients with NF2 mutation, in this case we did not observe tumor progression.

In some studies, the coincidence of meningiomas and other neoplasms is described: foremost breast cancer, but also lung and urinary bladder cancer. It has to be stressed, however, that there is no cause-and-effect relationship, but rather those tumors share some risk factors [1,18–21]. Nine of our female patients developed breast cancer and, due to type luminal A, all of them were given hormonal therapy. No meningioma progression was seen in this group; this could support the results of some studies describing the effects of antiestrogenic therapy of meningiomas [22–26].

4.2. Treatment Results

Meningiomas, especially those with the largest diameter smaller than 3 cm which were inoperable due to their location or the patient's performance status, are the ideal target for radiosurgery, whose results, according to some studies, are comparable with radical surgery (Simpson I) [27,28]. Larger tumors or those in proximity to organs at risk (e.g., optic nerves and chiasm) can be treated with hypofractionated stereotactic radiotherapy, which combines the advantages of other treatment modalities: steep dose falloff and short treatment time such as in radiosurgery, and the possibility of repair between fractions and decreased risk of complications, as is typical for conventional radiotherapy [3,29–31].

In our study, all patients underwent hfSRT with CyberKnife and received 18 Gy in three fractions. The location of most meningiomas was the skull base (55.2%). Tumor volume ranged from 0.8 cm^3 to 29.3 cm^3 (median 6.85 cm^3). During the follow-up, local control was achieved in 90.7% of patients. Oh et al. presented the results of large meningiomas treatment in 31 patients. All were greater than 10 cm^3 (range 11.6–58.2 cm^3) and were treated with a dose of 22.6–27.8 Gy in 3–5 fractions. Partial regression was seen in 54.8% [32]. Tuniz et al. treated a variety of tumors (meningiomas, glomerulomas, neuromas) with a volume greater than 15 cm^3. After receiving 18–25 Gy in 2–5 fractions, no patient showed tumor progression during the median follow-up of 31 months (range 12–77 months) [33]. Similarly, local control in 100% of patients was achieved during the median follow-up of 60 months by Conti et al. by using a similar fractionation schedule (18–25 Gy in 2–5 fractions), although the tumors were significantly smaller (median volume 4.95 cm^3) [34]. In 96 patients, Meniai-Merzouki et al. also used various fractionationschemese. The median dose was 25 Gy in five fractions (range 16–40 Gy in 3–10 fractions). Five-year local control was 74%, and in patients who received doses higher than the median dose, 5-year PFS was 88% (median follow-up time was 20.3 months) [35]. Table 6 shows the comparison of treatment outcome achieved in our material and the studies mentioned above, taking into account the biological effective dose

(BED). For the analysis we used the alpha/beta ratio 3.28 and 3.76, calculated by Shrieve and Vernimmen, respectively [36,37].

Table 6. Comparison of different schedules of hypofractionated robotic stereotactic radiotherapy, with regard to BED.

Study	Median Total Dose [Gy]	Number of Fractions	Median Follow-Up [Months]	Local Control [%]	BED Alpha/Beta = 3.28	BED Alpha-Beta = 3.76
Grzbiela et al.	18	3	67.5	90.7	50.9	46.7
Oh et al. [32]	27.8	5	57	90.3	74.9	68.9
Tuniz et al. [33]	24	3	31	100	82.5	75.1
Conti et al. [34]	23	5	60	100	55.3	51.1
Meniai-Merzouki et al. [35]	25	5	20.3	74	63.1	58.2

Seventy-two of our patients presented with neurological deficits and after radiotherapy completion 37.5% experienced symptomatic improvement or complete resolution of symptoms. The results were similar to those reported by Meniai-Merzouki et al. [35], yet our patients reported more positive effects than in the study by Conti et al. [34], despite a similar BED. Oh et al. observed improvement in 95.2% of patients [32], however BED was 47% higher than in our study. Table 7 shows the comparison of clinical effects in our study and in other abovementioned studies.

Table 7. Clinical effect of hypofractionated robotic stereotactic radiotherapy.

Study	Complete Regression [%]	Symptomatic Improvement [%]	Worsening [%]
Grzbiela et al.	31.9	5.6	2.8
Oh et al. [32]		95.2	Not available
Tuniz et al. [33]		21	0
Conti et al. [34]	0	18	0
Meniai-Merzouki et al. [35]	37	14	5

4.3. Treatment Tolerance

Only 10.5% of our patients reported headaches and less than half of them (4.7%) required small doses of corticosteroids for a short period of time (EORTC/RTOG grade 2). We did not observe any late complications. Santacroce et al., analyzing a group of more than four thousand patients treated with GammaKnife radiotherapy (median dose 14 Gy), described early effects in 12.8% of patients and late effects in 4.8% [38]. Similar observations were made by Przybylowski et al.—early effects occurred in 8.3% of patients after a median radiation dose of 15 Gy [39]. Harat et al. treated meningiomas, arteriovenous malformations, and cerebral metastases with a median dose of 16 Gy and described cerebral edema, which lasted up to 6 months, in 17% of patients [40]. It is worth noting that the edema occurred mostly around tumors located above the Frankfurt line; this matches our experience, as patients who required corticosteroids had tumors located on brain convexity. Using a slightly higher radiation dose (21–23 Gy) compared to our study, Meniai-Merzouki et al. observed early effects in 34% and late effects in 2% of patients [35].

4.4. Prognostic Factors

Simpson et al., Narayan et al., Champeaux et al., and other authors view radical neurosurgery as the most important prognostic factor [5,41–44]. In Group A of our study, before the onset of radiotherapy, the difference in progression-free survival between the subgroup after GTR and the subgroup after STR was 48.5 months and was statistically significant ($p = 0.00000$).

Prior to surgery, according to many authors, worse treatment outcomes were forecast [40,44–46]. We observed a significant difference in five-year PFS ($p = 0.016$) between Group A—81.8% and Group B—95.9%.

Age at diagnosis below 50 years seems to be a significant prognostic factor, according to Champeaux et al., Fokas et al., and Zaher et al. [45,47,48], but the differences mainly apply to overall survival. In our study, the differences of PFS rates between particular age groups were smaller than 2%, but due to low mortality (1.2%) we did not compare overall survival in those groups.

In our study, we observed slightly lower PFS rates in the male population. Although the difference was not significant, Solda et al., Santacroce et al., dos Santos et al., and Zhang et al. described male sex as negative prognostic factor [38,44,49,50].

Santacroce et al. and Wang et al. indicated histopathological WHO grade as a prognostic factor in the treatment of meningiomas. We also stated a statistically significant difference in PFS for WHO 1 and WHO 2 meningiomas—86.8% and 66.3%, respectively [38,51].

Five-year PFS for meningiomas greater and smaller than 5 cm^3 was assessed and the difference was 3% and not significant. Kondziolka et al. described a worse outcome for tumor volume greater than 7.5 cm^3, and a similar outcome was observed by Pollock et al. and Zhang et al. [44,52,53].

The presence of neurological symptoms turned out to be an independent prognostic factor, increasing the risk of progression by more than fivefold ($p = 0.0095$). A similar relation was observed by Kondziolka et al. and Kepka et al. [53,54]. Zhang et al. and Soyuera et al. indicated that the performance status of a patient is an important prognostic factor [44,55].

5. Conclusions

Based on the results of our study, robotic stereotactic radiotherapy with a total dose of 18 Gy delivered in three fractions has a similar efficacy to radiotherapy schedules with higher BED, which can support the application of dose de-escalation in the treatment of intracranial meningiomas. By giving a lower radiation dose, it is also possible to administer a second course of radiotherapy in the case of progression. Crude progression free survival after both primary and secondary treatment was 98.8%. The treatment is well-tolerated, with a low risk of early and late effects. The presence of neurological symptoms before the onset of treatment is an independent prognostic factor, increasing the risk of progression.

Author Contributions: Conceptualization, H.G., E.N., M.G., D.T. and R.T.; methodology, H.G., E.N., D.T. and R.T.; validation, H.G., E.N. and R.T.; formal analysis, H.G., E.N. and R.T.; investigation, H.G., E.N., D.T. and R.T; resources, H.G., E.N., M.G. and R.T.; data curation, H.G. and E.N.; writing—original draft preparation, H.G., E.N. and R.T.; writing—review and editing, E.N. and R.T.; supervision, R.T. All authors have read and agreed to the published version of the manuscript.

Funding: This research received no external funding.

Institutional Review Board Statement: The study was conducted in accordance with the Declaration of Helsinki and approved by the Ethics Committee of the Maria Sklodowska-Curie National Research Institute of Oncology (decision code KB/430-03/13 and KB/430-22/23).

Informed Consent Statement: Informed consent was obtained from all subjects involved in the study.

Data Availability Statement: The data are not publicly available due to confidentiality and ethical considerations.

Conflicts of Interest: The authors declare no conflict of interest.

References

1. Marosi, C.; Hassler, M.; Roessler, K.; Reni, M.; Sant, M.; Mazza, E.; Vecht, C. Meningioma. *Crit. Rev. Oncol./Hematol.* **2008**, *67*, 153–171. [PubMed]
2. Riemenschneider, M.; Perry, A.; Reifenberger, G. Histological classification and molecular genetics of meningiomas. *Lancet Neurol.* **2006**, *5*, 1045–1054. [PubMed]

3. Buerki, R.A.; Horbinski, C.M.; Kruser, T.; Horowitz, P.M.; James, C.D.; Lukas, R.V. An overview of meningiomas. *Future Oncol.* **2018**, *14*, 2161–2177.
4. Horbinski, C.; Nabors, L.B.; Portnow, J.; Baehring, J.; Bhatia, A.; Bloch, O.; Brem, S.; Butowski, N.; Cannon, D.M.; Chao, S. NCCN Guidelines Insights: Central Nervous System Cancers; Version 2.2022. *J. Natl. Compr. Canc. Netw.* **2023**, *21*, 12–20. [PubMed]
5. Simpson, D. The recurrence of intracranial meningiomas after surgical treatment. *J. Neurol. Neurosurg. Psychiatry* **1957**, *20*, 22. [CrossRef]
6. Naumann, M.; Meixensberger, J. Factors influencing meningioma recurrence rate. *Acta Neurochir.* **1990**, *107*, 108–111.
7. Timmerman, R.D. An overview of hypofractionation and introduction to this issue of seminars in radiation oncology. *Semin. Radiat. Oncol.* **2008**, *18*, 215–222.
8. Orski, M.; Tarnawski, R.; Wylegala, E.; Tarnawska, D. The Impact of Robotic Fractionated Radiotherapy for Benign Tumors of Parasellar Region on the Eye Structure and Function. *J. Clin. Med.* **2023**, *12*, 404. [CrossRef]
9. Nakasu, S.; Hirano, A.; Shimura, T.; Llena, J.F. Incidental meningiomas in autopsy study. *Surg. Neurol.* **1987**, *27*, 319–322.
10. Klaeboe, L.; Lonn, S.; Scheie, D.; Auvinen, A.; Christensen, H.C.; Feychting, M.; Johansen, C.; Salminen, T.; Tynes, T. Incidence of intracranial meningiomas in Denmark, Finland, Norway, and Sweden, 1968–1997. *Int. J. Cancer* **2005**, *117*, 996–1001. [CrossRef]
11. Radhakrishnan, K.; Mokri, B.; Parisi, J.E.; O'Fallon, W.M.; Sunku, J.; Kurland, L.T. The trends in incidence of primary brain tumors in the population of Rochester, Minnesota. *Ann. Neurol.* **1995**, *37*, 67–73. [CrossRef] [PubMed]
12. Chakravarthy, V.; Kaplan, B.; Gospodarev, V.; Myers, H.; De Los Reyes, K.; Achiriloaie, A. Houdini Tumor: Case Report and Literature Review of Pregnancy-Associated Meningioma. *World Neurosurg.* **2018**, *114*, 1261–1265. [CrossRef] [PubMed]
13. Central Brain Tumor Registry of the United States. *CBTRUS (2009–2010) CDTRUS Statistical Report: Primary Brain and Central nervous System Tumors Diagnosed in Eighteeen States in 2002–2006*; Central Brain Tumor Registry of the United States: Hisdale, IL, USA, 2010.
14. Park, B.J.; Kim, H.K.; Sade, B.; Lee, J.H. *Meningiomas: Diagnosis, Treatment, and Outcome*; Springer: Berlin/Heidelberg, Germany, 2009.
15. Bhat, A.R.; Wani, M.A.; Kirmani, A.R.; Ramzan, A.U. Histological subtypes and anatomical location correlated in meningeal brain tumors (meningiomas). *J. Neurosci. Rural. Pract.* **2014**, *5*, 244–249. [CrossRef] [PubMed]
16. Wellenreuther, R.; Kraus, J.A.; Lenartz, D.; Menon, A.G.; Schramm, J.; Louis, D.N.; Ramesh, V.; Gusella, J.F.; Wiestler, O.D.; von Deimling, A. Analysis of the neurofibromatosis 2 gene reveals molecular variants of meningioma. *Am. J. Pathol.* **1995**, *146*, 827–832. [PubMed]
17. Sahm, F.; Schrimpf, D.; Stichel, D. DNA methylation-based classification and grading system for meningioma: A multi-centre, retrospective analysis. *Lancet Oncol.* **2017**, *17*, 155–159. [CrossRef]
18. Claus, E.B.; Calvocoressi, L.; Bondy, M.L.; Schildkraut, J.M.; Wiemels, J.L.; Wrensch, M. Family and personal medical history and risk of meningioma. *J. Neurosurg.* **2011**, *115*, 1072–1077. [CrossRef]
19. Hill, D.A.; Linet, M.S.; Black, P.M.; Fine, H.A.; Selker, R.G.; Shapiro, W.R.; Inskip, P.D. Meningioma and schwannoma risk in adults in relation to family history of cancer. *Neuro-Oncology* **2004**, *6*, 274–280. [CrossRef]
20. Kirsch, M.; Zhu, J.J.; Black, P.M. Analysis of the BRCA1 and BRCA2 genes in sporadic meningioma. *Genes Chromosomes Cancer* **1997**, *20*, 53–59. [CrossRef]
21. Custer, B.S.; Koepsell, T.D.; Mueller, B.A. The association between breast carcinoma and meningioma in women. *Cancer* **2002**, *94*, 1626–1635. [CrossRef]
22. Markwalder, T.M.; Seiler, R.W.; Zava, D.T. Antiestrogenic therapy of meningiomas—A pilot study. *Surg. Neurol.* **1985**, *24*, 245–249. [CrossRef]
23. Goodwin, J.W.; Crowley, J.; Eyre, H.J.; Stafford, B.; Jaeckle, K.A.; Townsend, J.J. A phase II evaluation of tamoxifen in unresectable or refractory meningiomas: A Southwest Oncology Group study. *J. Neurooncol.* **1993**, *15*, 75–77. [CrossRef] [PubMed]
24. Ji, J.; Sundquist, J.; Sundquist, K. Association of tamoxifen with meningioma: A population-based study in Sweden. *Eur. J. Cancer Prev.* **2016**, *25*, 29–33. [CrossRef] [PubMed]
25. Sun, L.M.; Lin, C.L.; Sun, S.; Hsu, C.Y.; Shae, Z.; Kao, C.H. Long-term use of tamoxifen is associated with a decreased subsequent meningioma risk in patients with breast cancer: A nationwide population-based cohort study. *Front. Pharmacol.* **2019**, *10*, 674. [CrossRef] [PubMed]
26. Champeaux-Depond, C.; Weller, J. Tamoxifen. A treatment for meningioma? *Cancer Treat. Res. Commun.* **2021**, *27*, 100343. [CrossRef]
27. Rogers, L.; Barani, I.; Chamberlain, M.; Kaley, T.; McDermott, M.; Raizer, J.; Schiff, D.; Weber, D.C.; Wen, P.Y.; Vogelbaum, M.A. Meningiomas: Knowledge base, treatment outcomes, and uncertainties: A RANO review. *J. Neurosurg.* **2015**, *122*, 4–23. [CrossRef]
28. Pollock, B.E.; Stafford, S.L.; Utter, A.; Giannini, C.; Schreiner, S.A. Stereotactic radiosurgery provides equivalent tumor control to Simpson Grade 1 resection for patients with small- to medium-size meningiomas. *Int. J. Radiat. Oncol. Biol. Phys.* **2003**, *55*, 1000–1005. [CrossRef]
29. Cohen-Inbar, O.; Lee, C.; Sheehan, J.P. The Contemporary Role of Stereotactic Radiosurgery in the Treatment of Meningiomas. *Neurosurg. Clin. N. Am.* **2016**, *27*, 215–228. [CrossRef]
30. Unger, K.R.; Lominska, C.E.; Chanyasulkit, J.; Randolf-Jackson, P.; White, R.L.; Aulisi, E.; Jacobson, J.; Jean, W.; Gagnon, G.J. Risk factors for posttreatment edema in patients treated with stereotactic radiosurgery for meningiomas. *Neurosurgery* **2012**, *70*, 639–645. [CrossRef]

31. Biswas, T.; Sandhu, A.P.; Singh, D.P.; Schell, M.C.; Maciunas, R.J.; Bakos, R.S.; Muhs, A.G.; Okunieff, P. Low-Dose Radiosurgery for Benign Intracranial Lesions. *Am. J. Clin. Oncol.* **2003**, *26*, 325–331. [CrossRef]
32. Oh, H.J.; Cho, Y.H.; Kim, J.H.; Kim, C.J.; Kwon, D.H.; Lee, D.; Yoon, K.J. Hypofractionated stereotactic radiosurgery for large-sized skull base meningiomas. *J. Neurooncol.* **2020**, *149*, 87–93. [CrossRef]
33. Tuniz, F.; Soltys, S.G.; Choi, C.Y.; Chang, S.D.; Gibbs, I.C.; Fischbein, N.J.; Adler, J.R., Jr. Multisession cyberknife stereotactic radiosurgery of large, benign cranial base tumors: Preliminary study. *Neurosurgery* **2009**, *65*, 898–907. [CrossRef] [PubMed]
34. Conti, A.; Pontoriero, A.; Midili, F.; Iati, G.; Siragusa, C.; Tomasello, C.; La Torre, D.; Cardalli, S.M.; Pergolizzi, S.; De Renzis, C. CyberKnife multisession stereotactic radiosurgery and hypofractionated stereotactic radiotherapy for perioptic meningiomas: Intermediate-term results and radiobiological considerations. *Springerplus* **2015**, *4*, 37. [CrossRef] [PubMed]
35. Meniai-Merzouki, F.; Bernier-Chastagner, V.; Geffrelot, J.; Tresch, E.; Lacornerie, T.; Coche-Dequeant, B.; Lartigau, E.; Pasquier, D. Hypofractionated Stereotactic Radiotherapy for Patients with Intracranial Meningiomas: Impact of radiotherapy regimen on local control. *Sci. Rep.* **2018**, *8*, 13666. [CrossRef] [PubMed]
36. Shrieve, D.C.; Hazard, L.; Boucher, K.; Jensen, R.L. Dose fractionation in stereotactic radiotherapy for parasellar meningiomas: Radiobiological considerations of efficacy and optic nerve tolerance. *J. Neurosurg.* **2004**, *101*, 390–395. [CrossRef]
37. Vernimmen, F.J.; Slabbert, J.P. Assessment of the alpha/beta ratios for arteriovenous malformations, meningiomas, acoustic neuromas, and the optic chiasma. *Int. J. Radiat. Biol.* **2010**, *86*, 486–498. [CrossRef]
38. Santacroce, A.; Walier, M.; Régis, J.; Liščak, R.; Motti, E.; Lindquist, C.; Kemeny, A.; Kitz, K.; Lippitz, B.; Álvarez, R.M.; et al. Long-term tumor control of benign intracranial meningiomas after radiosurgery in a series of 4565 patients. *Neurosurgery* **2012**, *70*, 32–39. [CrossRef]
39. Przybylowski, C.J.; Raper, D.M.; Starke, R.M.; Xu, Z.; Liu, K.C.; Sheehan, J.P. Stereotactic radiosurgery of meningiomas following resection: Predictors of progression. *J. Clin. Neurosci.* **2015**, *22*, 161–165. [CrossRef]
40. Harat, M.; Lebioda, A.; Lasota, J.; Makarewicz, R. Evaluation of brain edema formation defined by MRI after LINAC-based stereotactic radiosurgery. *Radiol. Oncol.* **2017**, *51*, 137–141. [CrossRef]
41. Gallagher, M.J.; Jenkinson, M.D.; Brodbelt, A.R.; Mills, S.J.; Chavredakis, E. WHO grade I meningioma recurrence: Are location and Simpson grade still relevant? *Clin. Neurol. Neurosurg.* **2016**, *141*, 117–121. [CrossRef]
42. Narayan, V.; Bir, S.C.; Mohammed, N.; Savardekar, A.R.; Patra, D.P.; Nanda, A. Surgical Management of Giant Intracranial Meningioma: Operative Nuances, Challenges and Outcome. *World Neurosurg.* **2018**, *110*, 32–41. [CrossRef]
43. Champeaux, C.; Dunn, L. World Health Organization Grade II Meningioma: A 10-Year Retrospective Study for Recurrence and Prognostic Factor Assessment. *World Neurosurg.* **2016**, *89*, 180–186. [CrossRef] [PubMed]
44. Zhang, G.; Zhang, Y.; Zhang, G.; Yan, X.; Li, C.; Zhang, L.; Li, D.; Wu, Z.; Zhang, J. Prognostic Factors, Survival, and Treatment for Intracranial World Health Organization Grade II Chordoid Meningiomas and Clear-Cell Meningiomas. *World Neurosurg.* **2018**, *117*, 57–66. [CrossRef] [PubMed]
45. Fokas, E.; Henzel, M.; Surber, G.; Hamm, K.; Engenhart-Cabillic, R. Stereotactic Radiation Therapy for Benign Meningioma: Long-Term Outcome in 318 Patients. *Int. J. Radiat. Oncol. Biol. Phys.* **2014**, *89*, 569–575. [CrossRef] [PubMed]
46. Kołodziej, I.; Ślosarek, Z.; Blamek, S. Radiochirurgia stereotaktyczna jako leczenie pierwotne lub pooperacyjne u chorych na oponiaki. *Onkol. W Prakt. Klin.* **2017**, *3* (Suppl. C), 23.
47. Champeaux, C.; Houston, D.; Dunn, L. Atypical meningioma. A study on recurrence and disease-specific survival. *Neurochirurgie* **2017**, *63*, 273–281. [CrossRef]
48. Zaher, A.; Mattar, M.A.; Zayed, D.H.; Ellatif, R.A.; Ashamallah, S.A. Atypical meningioma: A Study of Prognostic Factors. *World Neurosurg.* **2013**, *80*, 549–553. [CrossRef]
49. Solda, F.; Wharram, B.; DeIeso, P.B.; Bonner, J.; Ashley, S.; Brada, M. Long-term efficacy of fractionated radiotherapy for benign meningiomas. *Radiother. Oncol.* **2013**, *109*, 330–334. [CrossRef]
50. Dos Santos, M.A.; De Salcedo, J.B.; Gutierrez Diaz, J.A.; Calvo, F.A.; Samblas, J.; Marsiglia, H.; Sallabanda, K. Long-term outcomes of stereotactic radiosurgery for treatment of cavernous sinus meningiomas. *Int. J. Radiat. Oncol. Biol. Phys.* **2011**, *81*, 1436–1441. [CrossRef]
51. Wang, W.H.; Lee, C.C.; Yang, H.C.; Liu, K.D.; Wu, H.M.; Shiau, C.Y.; Guo, W.Y.; Pan, D.H.C.; Chung, W.Y.; Chen, M.T. GammaKnife radiosurgery for atypical and anaplastic meningiomas. *World Neurosurg.* **2016**, *87*, 557–564. [CrossRef]
52. Pollock, B.E.; Stafford, S.L.; Link, M.J.; Garces, Y.I.; Foote, R.L. Single-fraction Radiosurgery for Presumed Intracranial Meningiomas: Efficacy and Complications From a 22-Year Experience. *Int. J. Radiat. Oncol. Biol. Phys.* **2012**, *83*, 1414–1418. [CrossRef]
53. Kondziolka, D.; Flickinger, J.C.; Perez, B. Judicious resection and/or radiosurgery for parasagittal meningioma: Outcomes from a multicenter review. GammaKnife Meningioma Study Group. *Neurosurgery* **1998**, *43*, 405–414. [CrossRef] [PubMed]
54. Kępka, L.; Żółciak, A.; Leszczyk, C.; Fijuth, J. Rola radioterapii w leczeniu chorych na oponiaka mózgu. *Nowotwory* **2000**, *50*, 134–140.
55. Soyuera, S.; Changa, E.L.; Seleka, U.; Shib, W.; Maora, M.H.; DeMonteb, F. Radiotherapy after surgery for benign cerebral meningioma. *Radiother. Oncol.* **2004**, *71*, 85–90. [CrossRef] [PubMed]

Disclaimer/Publisher's Note: The statements, opinions and data contained in all publications are solely those of the individual author(s) and contributor(s) and not of MDPI and/or the editor(s). MDPI and/or the editor(s) disclaim responsibility for any injury to people or property resulting from any ideas, methods, instructions or products referred to in the content.

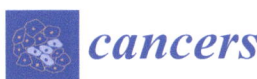

Article

And Yet It Moves: Clinical Outcomes and Motion Management in Stereotactic Body Radiation Therapy (SBRT) of Centrally Located Non-Small Cell Lung Cancer (NSCLC): Shedding Light on the Internal Organ at Risk Volume (IRV) Concept

Felix-Nikolai Oschinka Jegor Habermann [1,2], Daniela Schmitt [1,2], Thomas Failing [1,2,3], David Alexander Ziegler [1,2], Jann Fischer [1,2], Laura Anna Fischer [1,2], Manuel Guhlich [1,2], Stephanie Bendrich [1,2], Olga Knaus [1,2], Tobias Raphael Overbeck [2,4], Hannes Treiber [2,4], Alexander von Hammerstein-Equord [2,5], Raphael Koch [2,4], Rami El Shafie [1,2], Stefan Rieken [1,2], Martin Leu [1,2] and Leif Hendrik Dröge [1,2,*]

1 Department of Radiotherapy and Radiation Oncology, University Medical Center Göttingen, Robert-Koch-Str. 40, 37075 Göttingen, Germany; felix.habermann@med.uni-goettingen.de (F.-N.O.J.H.); daniela.schmitt@med.uni-goettingen.de (D.S.); alexander.ziegler@med.uni-goettingen.de (D.A.Z.); jann.fischer@med.uni-goettingen.de (J.F.); laura-anna.fischer@med.uni-goettingen.de (L.A.F.); manuel.guhlich@med.uni-goettingen.de (M.G.); stephanie.bendrich@med.uni-goettingen.de (S.B.); olga.knaus@med.uni-goettingen.de (O.K.); rami.elshafie@med.uni-goettingen.de (R.E.S.); stefan.rieken@med.uni-goettingen.de (S.R.); martin.leu@med.uni-goettingen.de (M.L.)
2 Göttingen Comprehensive Cancer Center (G-CCC), University Medical Center Göttingen, Von-Bar-Str. 2/4, 37075 Göttingen, Germany; tobias.overbeck@med.uni-goettingen.de (T.R.O.); hannes.treiber@med.uni-goettingen.de (H.T.); alexander.hammerstein@med.uni-goettingen.de (A.v.H.-E.); raphael.koch@med.uni-goettingen.de (R.K.)
3 Institute of Medical Physics and Radiation Protection (IMPS), University of Applied Sciences, Wiesenstr. 14, 35390 Gießen, Germany
4 Department of Hematology and Medical Oncology, University Medical Center Göttingen, Robert-Koch-Str. 40, 37075 Göttingen, Germany
5 Department of Cardio-Thoracic and Vascular Surgery, University Medical Center Göttingen, Robert-Koch-Str. 40, 37075 Göttingen, Germany
* Correspondence: hendrik.droege@med.uni-goettingen.de; Tel.: +49-5513964505

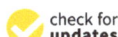

Citation: Habermann, F.-N.O.J.; Schmitt, D.; Failing, T.; Ziegler, D.A.; Fischer, J.; Fischer, L.A.; Guhlich, M.; Bendrich, S.; Knaus, O.; Overbeck, T.R.; et al. And Yet It Moves: Clinical Outcomes and Motion Management in Stereotactic Body Radiation Therapy (SBRT) of Centrally Located Non-Small Cell Lung Cancer (NSCLC): Shedding Light on the Internal Organ at Risk Volume (IRV) Concept. *Cancers* 2024, 16, 231. https://doi.org/10.3390/cancers16010231

Academic Editors: Sam Beddar and Michael D. Chuong

Received: 4 December 2023
Revised: 27 December 2023
Accepted: 28 December 2023
Published: 4 January 2024

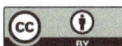

Copyright: © 2024 by the authors. Licensee MDPI, Basel, Switzerland. This article is an open access article distributed under the terms and conditions of the Creative Commons Attribution (CC BY) license (https://creativecommons.org/licenses/by/4.0/).

Simple Summary: We studied clinical aspects in central vs. peripheral tumors (*n* = 78 patients) and applied the internal organ at risk volume (IRV) concept (*n* = 35 patients) in stereotactic body radiation therapy (SBRT) for centrally located non-small cell lung cancer (NSCLC). We found lower biologically effective doses, larger planning target volume sizes, higher lung doses, and worse locoregional control for central tumors when compared with peripheral tumors. We here provide evidence that organ motion/volume changes could be more pronounced in males and tall patients, and less pronounced in cases of higher body mass index. Applying the IRV concept (retrospectively, without new optimization), the normal tissue complication probabilities increased >10% for the bronchial tree in three patients. This study emphasizes the need to optimize methods to balance dose escalation with toxicities in central tumors. Since recent studies have made efforts to further subclassify central tumors to refine treatment, the IRV concept should be considered for optimal risk assessment.

Abstract: The internal organ at risk volume (IRV) concept might improve toxicity profiles in stereotactic body radiation therapy (SBRT) for non-small cell lung cancer (NSCLC). We studied (1) clinical aspects in central vs. peripheral tumors, (2) the IRV concept in central tumors, (3) organ motion, and (4) associated normal tissue complication probabilities (NTCPs). We analyzed patients who received SBRT for NSCLC (clinical aspects, *n* = 78; motion management, *n* = 35). We found lower biologically effective doses, larger planning target volume sizes, higher lung doses, and worse locoregional control for central vs. peripheral tumors. Organ motion was greater in males and tall patients (bronchial tree), whereas volume changes were lower in patients with a high body mass index (BMI) (esophagus). Applying the IRV concept (retrospectively, without new optimization), we found an absolute increase of >10% in NTCPs for the bronchial tree in three patients. This study emphasizes the need to optimize methods to balance dose escalation with toxicities in central tumors. There is evidence that organ motion/volume changes could be more pronounced in males and tall patients, and less pronounced in patients with higher BMI. Since recent studies have made efforts to further subclassify central tumors to refine treatment, the IRV concept should be considered for optimal risk assessment.

Keywords: NSCLC; SBRT; central tumors; clinical outcomes; clinical characteristics; motion management; planning organ at risk volume; PRV; internal organ at risk volume; IRV

1. Introduction

In patients with early-stage non-small cell lung cancer (NSCLC) who are not suitable for surgery or refuse surgery, stereotactic body radiation therapy (SBRT) is an effective treatment option [1]. In stage I patients, SBRT achieves 2-year local control rates of >90% [2].

For SBRT, it has been demonstrated that higher biologically effective doses ($\geq$100–125 Gy, alpha/beta ratio of 10 [BED10]) are crucial to achieve these excellent control rates [3,4]. At the same time, the tumors are located centrally in about 44% [5] of cases. Patients with tumors in central or ultra-central locations are at an increased risk of complications, e.g., bronchial stenosis or esophageal perforation [6–9]. Timmermann et al. reported that 46% of patients with central tumors experienced severe toxicities [10].

Thus, the maintenance of high-quality standards and continuous development of SBRT planning and delivery are required for safe and effective treatment [4,11]. Here, the management of structure motion within the breathing cycle plays a crucial role [11]. A four-dimensional CT scan (4D-CT) with the internal target volume (ITV) concept is widely applied to account for tumor motion [11,12]. The planning organ at risk volume concept (PRV) might help to reduce the probability of organs at risk (OARs) overdosage [13,14]. The concept is less well-studied and rarely used in clinical practice [14,15]. Additionally, intrafractional structure movement is not taken into account [15]. Here, the internal organ at risk volume (IRV) concept might be advantageous [15,16]. Nardone et al. found unacceptable treatment plans in 42% of the cases with central tumors when applying the IRV concept in SBRT for NSCLC [15].

In summary, SBRT in patients with centrally located NSCLC is a substantial challenge for the treatment team [17]. In this study, we compared clinical characteristics and outcomes in peripherally located vs. centrally located tumors in patients who received SBRT in the local radiotherapy department. Additionally, we analyzed the deviation of the geometric centers (OAR vs. IRV) and the volume differences (OAR vs. IRV) in serial OARs (bronchial tree, trachea, esophagus, and spinal canal) throughout the breathing cycle. We tested for an influence of patient-related characteristics on organ motion. Additionally, we evaluated whether the application of the IRV concept (retrospectively, without new optimization) leads to a relevant increase in normal tissue complication probabilities (NTCPs).

2. Patients and Methods

2.1. Study Design

We first identified all the patients in the medical records who were referred to the radiation oncology department for SBRT to the lungs or the mediastinal structures. A total of 151 patients were documented. We previously performed a study as part of the underlying project on patterns of pretreatment diagnostic assessment with a special focus on the COVID-19 pandemic [18]. Here, we present a study that differed in patient selection (Figure 1), methods, and outcome parameters. For the comparison of clinical characteristics and outcomes in centrally vs. peripherally located tumors, only patients with localized NSCLC (n = 78 patients) were included. For the analysis of motion management for OARs, we included all the patients with SBRT for NSCLC in a central tumor position (n = 35). Chang et al. recommended choosing a distance of 2 cm from any critical mediastinal structure as the cut-off for a central position [19]. In this study, we focused on tumors with a distance of ≤2 cm to the serial organs, bronchial tree and trachea (together, central airway), esophagus, and spinal canal. Please see Figure 1 for further details on patient selection. The study was approved by the local ethics committee of the University Medical Center Göttingen (application no. 3/10/20).

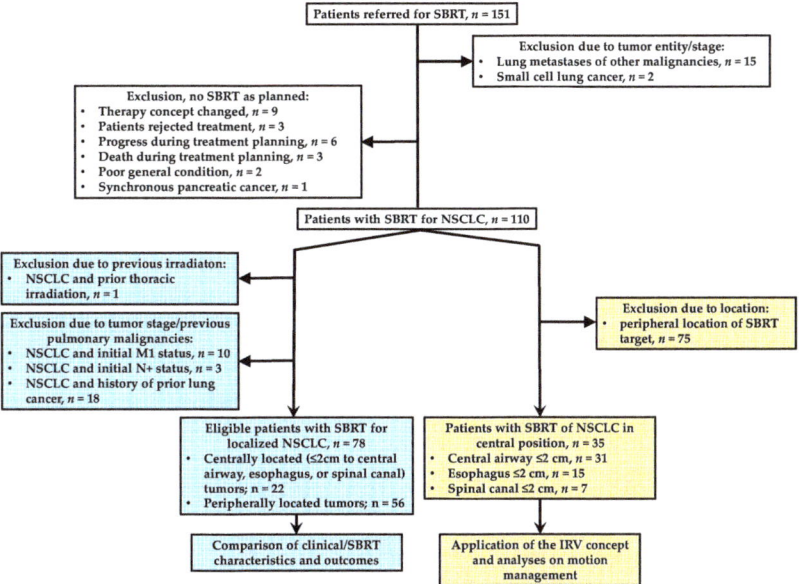

Figure 1. The flow chart illustrates the patient selection for the comparison of clinical characteristics in centrally vs. peripherally located tumors (left side, blue background) and the studies on motion management for OARs (right side, orange background). SBRT: stereotactic body radiation therapy. OARs: organs at risk. IRV: internal organ at risk volume.

2.2. Radiotherapy, Planning and Delivery

Please see Habermann et al. in 2022 for a previous description of SBRT [18]. A 4D-CT with a respiration belt and the patient in a supine position was acquired for treatment planning. For patient positioning, customized devices were used. The ITV concept was used for target volume delineation [11,12]. The gross tumor volume (GTV) was delineated in all of the 10 breathing phases. The ITV was generated by including the GTVs in all the phases. The planning target volume (PTV) was created with individual margins, which were left at the discretion of the treating radiation oncologist (between 3 mm and 10 mm). For treatment planning, the software, Eclipse (Varian Medical Systems, Palo Alto, CA, USA), was used. We applied the Eclipse versions 10.0 (12/2012–09/2013), 11.1 (10/2013–09/2014), 13.5 (10/2014–05/2020), and 15.6 (from 06/2020). Radiotherapy was applied with Varian Clinac 2300 CD linear accelerators (Varian Medical Systems, Palo Alto, CA, USA). Daily cone beam CT was used for image guidance. Please see Sections 2.2.1 and 2.2.2 for further details on the patient cohorts.

2.2.1. Patient Cohort with Analysis of Clinical/SBRT Characteristics and Outcomes

We used the Philips Gemini TF TOF 16 (n = 22 patients), Philips Ingenuity Flex (n = 3 patients), and Philips Brilliance Big Bore (n = 53 patients) for the acquisition of the CT scans (each, Philips Medical Systems, Fitchburg, WI, USA). The slice thicknesses were 2 mm (n = 4 patients) and 3 mm (n = 72 patients). In 2 patients, a larger slice thickness of 5 mm was chosen on an individual basis in the clinical routine. We decided to include these 2 patients in the analysis of clinical outcomes since technical aspects were not the main endpoints in this part of the project. We used the algorithms Acuros ($n = 70$ patients) and AAA ($n = 18$ patients). In 61 patients, the prescription isodose was 80%. In 17 patients, radiotherapy was prescribed homogeneously.

2.2.2. Patient Cohort with Analyses on Motion Management

The CT scanners were the Philips Gemini TF TOF 16 ($n = 11$ patients), Philips Ingenuity Flex ($n = 2$ patients), and Philips Brilliance Big Bore ($n = 22$ patients) (each, Philips Medical Systems, Fitchburg, WI, USA). The slice thickness was 3 mm in all the patients ($n = 35$). We used the algorithm Acuros in all the patients ($n = 35$). The prescription isodose was 80% in 26 patients. In 9 patients, radiotherapy was prescribed homogeneously.

2.3. Endpoints and Statistical Methods

2.3.1. Patient Cohort with Analysis of Clinical/SBRT Characteristics and Outcomes

Please see Habermann et al. in 2022 for a previous description of statistical approaches in the underlying project [18]. We compared characteristics and outcomes between patients with centrally located and peripherally located tumors. When comparing baseline and SBRT characteristics, we used Pearson's Chi-squared test and the Mann–Whitney U test (SPSS v. 27, IBM, Armonk, NY, USA). In survival analyses, the endpoints were overall survival (OS, event: patient death due to any cause), progression-free survival (PFS, event: locoregional or distant progression and patient death), local progression-free survival (LPFS, events: local progression and patient death due to any cause), and locoregional control (LRC, events: local or regional relapse). The survival times were calculated from the first day of SBRT. We used Cox regression analysis (SPSS v. 27, IBM, Armonk, NY, USA). Additionally, the Kaplan–Meier curves with log-rank statistics were generated using the plugin, KMWin v 1.53 [20]. p-values < 0.05 were considered statistically significant.

2.3.2. Patient Cohort with Analyses on Motion Management

In the subset of 35 patients with SBRT of NSCLC in a central position, the IRV concept was applied (retrospectively, without new optimization). The 4D-CTs were used and the OARs (bronchial tree, trachea, esophagus, and spinal canal) were contoured on each of the 10 respiratory phases and the average intensity projection (AIP) CT scan. The OARs were delineated in accordance with the Radiation Therapy Oncology Group guidelines [21]. The bronchial tree was defined as including the distal 2 cm of the trachea, the carina, the main bronchi, the right and left upper lobe bronchi, the bronchus intermedius, the right middle lobe bronchus, the lingular bronchus, and the right and left lower lobe bronchi [21]. The trachea was delineated from the lower edge of the larynx to the bronchial tree. The esophagus was contoured from just below the cricoid to the gastroesophageal junction [21]. The spinal canal was defined based on the surrounding bones [21]. We used the thoracic vertebrae 1–12 as upper and lower limits for the spinal canal. For each of the OARs, we propagated the contours from each of the respiratory phases to the AIP CT scan. Here, an IRV structure was generated.

We aimed to characterize patients with a clinically relevant increase in NTCPs when applying the IRV concept (retrospectively, without new optimization). First, we identified patients with a relevant increase in D1%, D2%, or maximum dose (Dmax) when comparing the dose for the OARs and the corresponding IRVs on the AIP CT scan (an increase of >5 Gy (bronchial tree, esophagus, trachea) or 0.5 Gy (spinal canal)). Please see Supplementary Figure S1 for a graphical presentation of the dose differences between the OARs and IRVs. In the patients with a relevant increase in these dose parameters, we calculated the NTCPs for the OARs and corresponding IRVs. For the spinal canal and the esophagus, we used the software, 'RADBIOMOD' (v.0.3b), with the Lyman–Kutcher–Burman model [22]. Since there is only limited data on NTCP calculations in the trachea and bronchial tree, we estimated the complication risks based on the models by Dujim et al. [23]. For these OARs, we calculated the maximum equivalent dose of 2 Gy per fraction (EQD_2, α/β ratio = 3) and estimated the risks based on the NTCP models for any grade of radiographic toxicity in the lobar bronchi ([23], page 128). In previous studies, the risks (here, for proximal bronchial tree toxicity) were estimated in a similar way [24].

In the analyses on motion management, we compared volumes between the OARs on the AIP CT scan and the IRVs on the AIP CT scans. Additionally, we analyzed the deviation of the geometric centers of the OAR and the IRV structures. Therefore, the coordinates of the centers (x, y, z) were registered for the structures in each of the respiratory phases and the OARs in the AIP CT scan. We calculated the difference between the centers in each of the phases and the center of the IRV structure in the AIP CT scan. For further analysis, we considered the maximum difference for each structure. We tested for an influence of patient-related parameters (e.g., body height) on the volume differences and the distances between the geometric centers. Here, we used the Mann–Whitney U test and Spearman's rank correlation (SPSS v. 27, IBM, Armonk, NY, USA). p-values < 0.05 were considered statistically significant.

3. Results

3.1. Clinical/SBRT Characteristics and Outcomes in Centrally vs. Peripherally Located Tumors

We compared characteristics and outcomes in patients with central and peripheral tumors (cut-off, distance ≤2 cm vs. >2 cm from central OAR (central airways, spinal canal, esophagus)). We found that the applied biologically effective dose (BED, alpha/beta ratio of 10 Gy) was significantly higher in patients with peripheral vs. central tumors (median 115.5 vs. 105 Gy, $p = 0.001$). In patients with central vs. peripheral tumors, a BED < 100 Gy was applied more frequently (27.3% vs. 5.4% of the patients, $p = 0.006$). The PTV volume was significantly higher in patients with central tumors ($p = 0.046$). The doses to lungs–GTV (i.e., the volume created by subtraction of the GTV from both lungs, differences in mean dose, V5Gy, and V20Gy) were higher in patients with central tumors (each, $p < 0.05$). SBRT application was incomplete in two patients (one patient with a central tumor, 7.5/60 Gy; one patient with a peripheral tumor, 52.5/60 Gy). Please see Table 1.

In the whole patient cohort ($n = 78$ patients), the 2-year overall survival rate was 56.8%. There were four patients with local progression, five patients with regional progression, and ten patients with distant progression. The median follow-up was 18.5 months (range, 0.6–65.5 months). At the end of follow-up, 36/78 patients (46.2%) were alive. Death was documented in 42/78 patients (53.8%). The causes of death were unknown in most of the patients (35/42 patients (83.3%)). In 7/42 patients (16.7%), the causes of death were tumor progression ($n = 2$), pneumonitis ($n = 1$), lung infection ($n = 1$), exacerbation of COPD ($n = 1$), cerebral mass with bleeding (potentially metastasis or vascular/ischemic cause, $n = 1$), and pancreatitis ($n = 1$).

When comparing patients with central vs. peripheral tumors, we found worse LRC (2-year LRC: 64.8% vs. 94.4%, log-rank, $p = 0.0051$, Figure 2). When analyzing the differences in outcomes separately for the OARs, we found worse outcomes for central airways (PFS, LPFS (Figure 3), and LRC) and for the esophagus (OS, PFS; LPFS, and LRC), but not for the spinal canal (Please see Supplementary Table S1 for the results of the respective survival analyses).

Table 1. Comparison of clinical/stereotactic body radiation therapy (SBRT) characteristics in patients with centrally vs. peripherally located tumors (distance to OARs (organs at risk): central airways, spinal canal, esophagus, ≤2 cm vs. >2 cm). ECOG: Eastern Cooperative Oncology Group status. UICC: Union Internationale Contre le Cancer, 8th edition. VMAT: volumetric modulated arc therapy. IMRT: intensity-modulated radiotherapy. 3DCRT: 3D conformal radiotherapy. GTV: gross tumor volume. The numbers (% of the patients) are given if not otherwise specified. [1] In one patient, SBRT was applied simultaneously to a central tumor (44 Gy in 8 fractions) and a peripheral tumor (55 Gy in 5 fractions), as described in our previous study [18]. Here, we decided to include this patient in the group with central tumors. The stages were cT1a and cT1b (counted as UICC stage I in the table). The radiotherapy doses (planned/applied/fractions) and GTV/PTV volumes of the central tumor are included in the table and were used for analysis. The technique was VMAT for both tumors. The dose summation for radiotherapy of both tumors was used for lungs–GTV. [2] Since this part of the study mainly focused on clinical outcomes, not on technical analysis of SBRT, we decided to include 3 patients with radiotherapy in 18 fractions [18]. As mentioned in our previous study, formally, the recent literature defines SBRT as radiotherapy in a maximum of 12 fractions [11,18]. [3] Pneumonitis: 9 patients with grade 1, 6 patients with grade 2, and 2 patients with grade 3. [4] Pearson's Chi-squared test. [5] Mann–Whitney U test.

Parameter	Central Tumors (n = 22 Patients)	Peripheral Tumors (n = 56 Patients)	p-Value
Gender			0.32 [4]
Male	16 (72.7)	34 (60.7)	
Female	6 (27.3)	22 (39.3)	
ECOG (median, min, max)	1 (0–2)	1 (0–4)	0.3 [5]
UICC stages [1]			0.96 [4]
I	17 (77.3)	43 (76.8)	
II–III	5 (22.7)	13 (23.2)	
Planned dose [1] [Gy, median, min–max)]	60 (44–60)	55 (54–60)	0.28 [5]
Planned fractions [1,2] (median, min–max)	8 (3–18)	5 (3–18)	0.002 [5]
Planned dose [1] [biologically effective dose, α/β = 10 Gy, Gy, median, min–max]	105 (68.2–151.2)	115.5 (70.2–151.2)	0.001 [5]
Applied dose [1] [biologically effective dose, α/β = 10 Gy, Gy, median, min–max]	105 (13.13–151.2)	115.5 (70.2–151.2)	0.001 [5]
Applied dose < 100 Gy [1] [biologically effective dose, α/β = 10 Gy]	6 (27.3)	3 (5.4)	0.006 [4]
Radiotherapy technique [1]			0.83 [4]
VMAT/IMRT	20 (90.9)	50 (89.3)	
3DCRT	2 (9.1)	6 (10.7)	
GTV volume [1] [cm³, median, min–max]	32.55 (2.7–141.9)	14.8 (1.4–119.4)	0.17 [5]
PTV volume [1] [cm³, median, min–max]	90.26 (11.9–244.9)	45.0 (12.8–329.8)	0.046 [5]
Lungs–GTV [1], Dmean [Gy]	5.8 (1.24–11.3)	3.7 (1.7–10.5)	0.009 [5]
Lungs–GTV [1], V5Gy [%]	26.9 (4.9–56.2)	17.3 (5.9–49.9)	0.003 [5]
Lungs–GTV [1], V20Gy [%]	8.0 (0–15.6)	5.5 (2.0–18.7)	0.02 [5]
Pneumonitis [3]	5 (22.7)	12 (21.4)	0.90 [4]

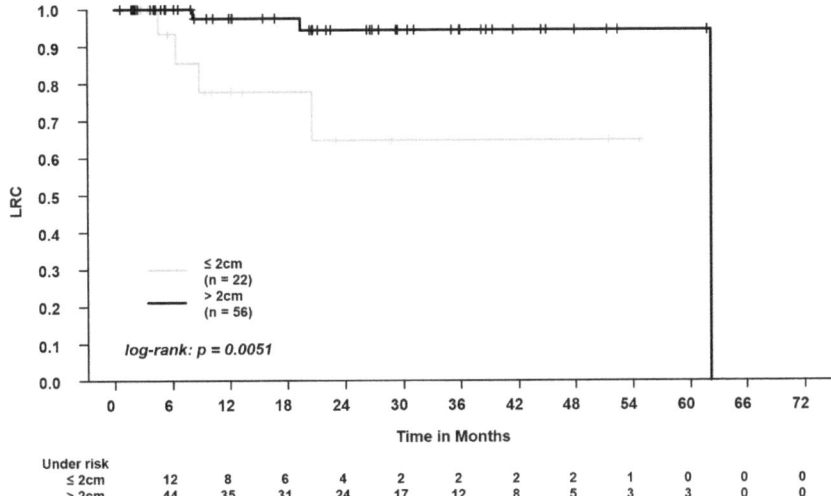

Figure 2. Comparison of locoregional control (LRC) in patients with centrally vs. peripherally located tumors (distance to organs at risk: central airways, spinal canal, esophagus, ≤2 cm vs. >2 cm). The 2-year LRC was 94.4% vs. 64.8%.

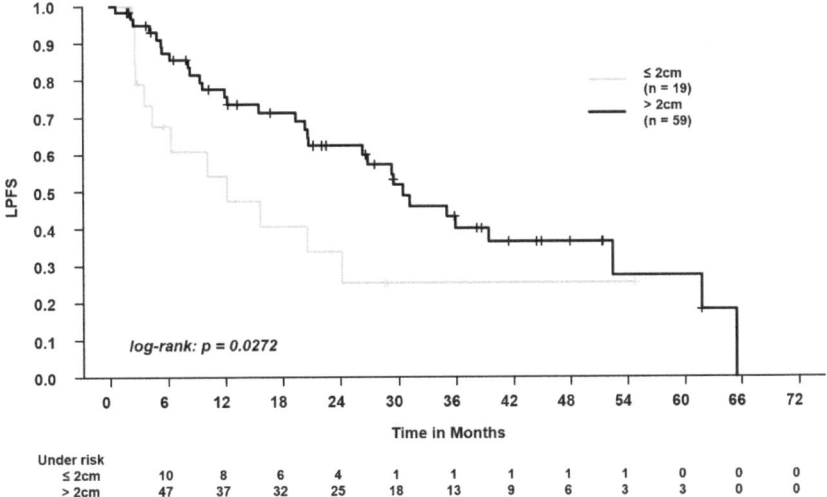

Figure 3. Comparison of locoregional progression-free survival (LPFS) in patients with tumors at a distance ≤2 cm vs. >2 cm from the central airways. The 2-year LPFS was 62.4% vs. 33.8%.

3.2. Structure Movement Amplitudes and Volumes

For analyses on motion management, 35 patients with central tumors were studied. Herein, we present the mean values for the patient cohort. The maximum differences in geometric centers between the OARs in each respiratory phase and the IRVs on the AIP CT scan were 5.2 mm (bronchial tree), 4.2 mm (trachea), 5.5 mm (esophagus), and 4.3 mm (spinal canal). The absolute volume differences between OARs and IRVs were 22.0 cm^3 (bronchial tree), 7.8 cm^3 (trachea), 19.6 cm^3 (esophagus), and 8.2 cm^3 (spinal canal). Please see Table 2 for further details.

Table 2. Structure movement amplitudes and volume differences. Comparison of organs at risk (OARs) volumes in each respiratory phase scan and internal organs at risk volumes (IRVs) on average intensity projection (AIP) CT scan. The mean (min–max) values are presented.

Parameter	Bronchial Tree	Trachea	Esophagus	Spinal Canal
Maximum difference in geometric centers, OAR (each respiratory phase), and IRV on AIP CT scan [mm]	5.2 (2.2–11.1)	4.2 (1.4–14.6)	5.5 (2.0–13.2)	4.3 (1.5–9.7)
OAR volumes on AIP CT scan [cm^3]	54.4 (34.7–85.4)	40.5 (22.3–57.2)	42.0 (25.7–74.2)	57.2 (33.5–90.0)
IRV volumes on AIP CT scan [cm^3]	76.4 (46.8–116.1)	48.3 (27.2–75.7)	61.5 (37.4–103.9)	65.4 (48.9–88.7)
Absolute difference, IRV–OAR volume [cm^3]	22.0 (10.5–35.5)	7.8 (2.7–18.8)	19.6 (11.4–33.7)	8.2 (−1.3–20.2)
Relative difference, IRV–OAR volume [%]	40.9 (26.9–60.4)	19.4 (6.6–53.5)	47.5 (25.4–91.4)	16.1 (−1.4–57.4)

3.3. Influence of Clinical Characteristics on Structure Movement and Volume Changes

Furthermore, we tested for an influence of clinical characteristics on structure movement and volume changes in the 35 patients with central tumors. Here, we considered the patient's age, gender, body height, weight, and body mass index (BMI). In Figure 4a–c, we present the parameters with a significant influence on movement or volume changes. We found a greater maximum vector of movement for the bronchial tree in males (Figure 4a) and in tall patients (Figure 4b, cut-off, median of 1.68 m). Additionally, we found fewer volume changes for the esophagus in patients with high body mass index (BMI, >25 kg/m^2, Figure 4c). Please see Supplementary Table S2 for a detailed analysis of the influence of all the clinical characteristics.

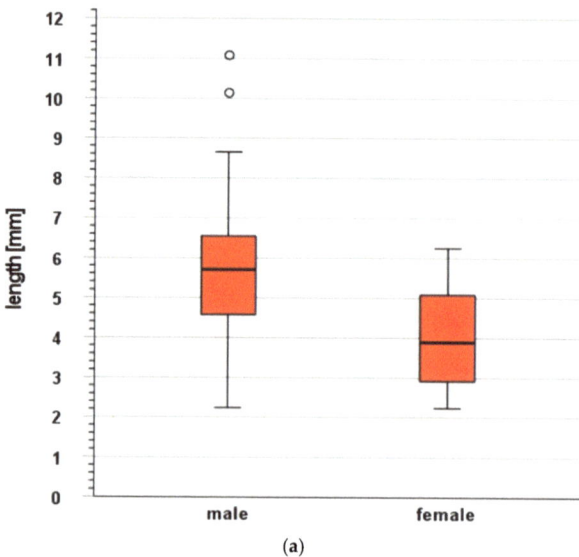

Figure 4. Cont.

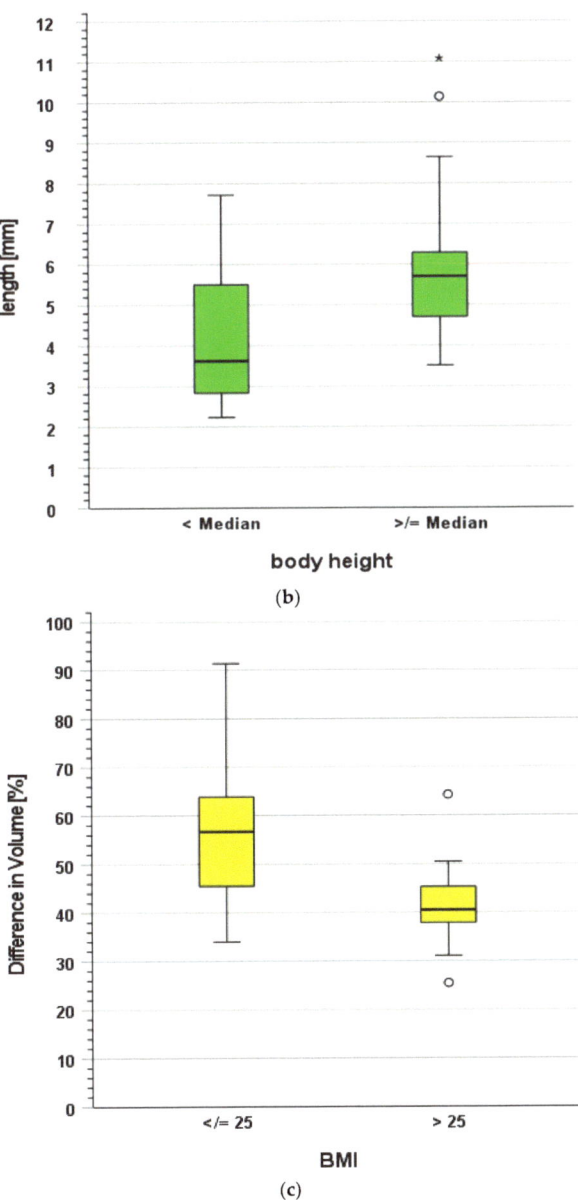

Figure 4. (**a**) Influence of gender on the maximum vector of movement for the bronchial tree (length, mm). Male patients had greater movement (median 5.7 mm vs. 3.9 mm, $p < 0.05$, 21 male patients vs. 14 female patients). (**b**) Influence of body height on the maximum vector of movement for the bronchial tree (length, mm). Tall patients had greater movement (median 5.7 mm vs. 3.6 mm, $p < 0.05$; cut-off median of body height [1.68 m], 16 patients with smaller height vs. 19 patients with height $\geq$ median). * Values that are more than 3x interquartile range below first quartile or above third quartile. (**c**) Influence of the body mass index (BMI) on the volume changes of the esophagus. Here, we compared organs at risk and corresponding internal organs at risk volumes. Patients with high BMI had lower volume changes (median 56.7% vs. 40.5%, $p < 0.05$, cut-off 25 kg/m^2, 13 patients with BMI $\leq$ 25 kg/m^2 vs. 22 patients with higher BMI).

3.4. Influence of the Internal Organ at Risk Volume (IRV) Concept on Normal Tissue Complication Probabilities (NTCPs)

Here, we aimed to characterize patients with a clinically relevant increase in NTCPs among the 35 patients with central tumors when applying the IRV concept (retrospectively, without new optimization). First, we identified 12 patients with a relevant increase in dosimetric parameters when comparing OARs and IRVs (please see Section 2.3.2 and Supplementary Figure S1). In these patients, the NTCPs for OARs and corresponding IRVs were calculated (Supplementary Table S3, differences in maximum doses and NTCPs for these patients). The mean absolute increase in NTCPs was 5.5% (0–22.5%), and the mean relative increase was 54.78% (0–181%). Please see Table 3 and Supplementary Table S3. Please see Figure 5 for an illustration of the respiration-dependent movement of the bronchial tree and its influence on NTCPs.

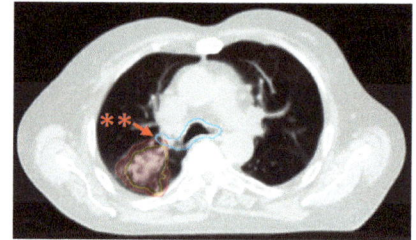

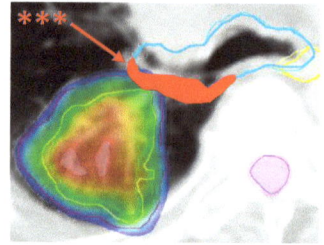

Figure 5. Illustration of the respiration-dependent movement of the bronchial tree. Patient with a stage IIA adenocarcinoma of the right upper lobe. SBRT was applied up to 60 Gy in 8 fractions prescribed on the 80% isodose using VMAT. The images depict the corresponding slices of the 4D-CT scan with maximum inhalation (**A**) and maximum exhalation (**B**). In (**C**) (average intensity projection CT scan), the dose is shown from 60 Gy (blue) to 75 Gy (red) with the contours of the bronchial tree in turquoise (* maximum inhalation, ** maximum exhalation). In the image (**D**) and magnification of image (**C**), the gain in volume between internal organ at risk volume (IRV) and organ at risk (OAR) is marked (***). The distance between the GTV and the bronchial tree was 3 mm. Please note the relevant volume difference between OAR and IRV in proximity to the target volume. The absolute difference in volume between the bronchial tree (59.0 cm^3) and its corresponding IRV (94.4 cm^3) was 35.5 cm^3 (relative increase in volume, 60%). The maximum difference in geometric centers between OAR and IRV was 10.1 mm. The absolute difference in maximum dose was 8.4 Gy (OAR, 62.9 Gy vs. IRV, 71.2 Gy). The absolute increase in normal tissue complication probability, when comparing OAR vs. IRV, was 11.5% (relative increase, 44.2%).

Table 3. Differences in normal tissue complication probabilities (NTCPs) when comparing organs at risk (OARs) and internal organs at risk volumes (IRVs). Please see Section 2.3.2, Supplementary Figure S1 and Supplementary Table S3 for further details. The NTCPs for the bronchial tree and the trachea were estimated using the graphs for the maximum dose (in EQD2) for the bronchial tree by Dujim et al. [23]. The NTCPs for the esophagus and the spinal canal were calculated using the software, 'RADBIOMOD', with the Lyman–Kutcher–Burman model ([22]; please see Section 2.3.2 for further details).

Structure	Patient No.	Distance between Tumor and Structure [cm]	NTCP of OAR [%]	NTCP of IRV [%]	NTCP, Absolute Increase [%]	NTCP, Relative Increase [%]
Bronchial Tree	1	1.4	17.0	34.0	17.0	100.0
	2	0.0	63.0	66.0	3.0	4.8
	3	0.3	26.0	37.5	11.5	44.2
	4	0.0	23.0	32.0	9.0	39.1
	5	0.0	45.0	48.0	3.0	6.7
	6	1.1	35.5	58.0	22.5	63.4
Esophagus	3	2.4	2.1	5.9	3.8	181.0
	7	0.3	1.5	4.0	2.5	166.7
Spinal Canal	1	2.2	0.0	0.0	0.0	0.0
	8	1.8	<0.01	<0.01	0.0	0.0
	9	4.1	<0.01	<0.01	0.0	0.0
Trachea	6	4.1	4.0	5.0	1.0	25.0
	10	1.2	4.0	10.5	6.5	162.5
	11	3.5	4.5	5.5	1.0	22.2
	12	1.0	24.5	26.0	1.5	6.1

4. Discussion

SBRT yields excellent local tumor control in patients with early-stage NSCLC when indicated, e.g., in elderly patients or in patients who refuse surgery [2]. At the same time, treatment can be associated with relevant complications, especially in patients with a central tumor location [10,25]. Previous authors hypothesized that the PRV/IRV concept might improve toxicity profiles [13–15]. Nardone et al. applied the IRV concept in patients with SBRT for NSCLC. When taking the organ motion into account, 42% of the radiotherapy plans were unacceptable [15]. This work aims at (1) comparing clinical aspects in central vs. peripheral tumors, (2) applying the IRV concept in central tumors (retrospectively, without new optimization), (3) analyzing organ motion, and (4) studying associated NTCPs.

We found that, in patients with central tumors, the median BED was significantly lower (central, median 105 Gy vs. peripheral, median 115.5 Gy). A BED of <100 Gy was applied in 27.3% of patients with central tumors vs. 5.4% of patients with peripheral tumors. Patients with central tumors had higher PTV volumes and higher doses to lungs–GTV (mean dose, V5Gy, and V20Gy). Furthermore, we found worse LRC in patients with central tumors (2-year LRC of 64.8% vs. 94.4% in patients with peripheral tumors). When analyzing the outcomes separately for the OAR, we found worse outcomes for the central airways and for the esophagus, but not for the spinal canal.

Our results are in line with previous studies on comparisons of central vs. peripheral tumors in SBRT of early-stage NSCLC. These studies found lower BED (mean 120.2 vs. 143.5 Gy [5]), larger tumor size (as we found larger PTV volumes, with tumors of mean 1.9 vs. 2.5 cm and median 2.6 vs. 3.1 cm in peripheral vs. central location [5,26]), higher lung doses (V5Gy, V20Gy [27]), and worse local control (freedom from local progression,

52% (central) vs. 84% (peripheral) [26]) in central tumors. Additionally, previous studies demonstrated that a BED_{10Gy} of ≥ 100 Gy is associated with higher local control, and that dose escalation increases local control/overall survival and complications [28]. In the presented study, in line with these findings, patients with central lesions received a BED_{10Gy} of <100 Gy in a higher percentage and, consecutively, experienced worse LRC.

In conclusion, in clinical routine, the perception of increased complication risks leads to insufficient doses and reduced outcomes in patients with centrally located tumors [26]. In spite of the perception of high complication risks, previous studies found lower rates of $\geq$grade 3 acute toxicities [5] and low overall rates of toxicities [26] in patients with central tumors. Thus, in clinical routine, balancing dose escalation/tumor control and complication risks (especially concerning the central airways [25]) is very challenging and controversially discussed [29]. In this context, motion management strategies are very important [11]. When active motion management techniques are not available/applicable, safety margins/4D-CT and internal motion have to be considered [11]. However, data on the internal motion of central organs at risk in SBRT of early-stage NSCLC are very rare (e.g., [15]).

When applying the IRV concept (retrospectively, without new optimization), we found maximum differences in the geometric centers of mean 4.2 mm (trachea), 4.3 mm (spinal canal), 5.2 mm (bronchial tree), and 5.5 mm (esophagus). The relative differences in volume (IRV–OAR, mean) were 16.1% (spinal canal), 19.4% (trachea), 40.9% (bronchial tree), and 47.5% (esophagus). The maximum vector of movement for the bronchial tree was greater in males and in tall patients. The volume changes (IRV–OAR) in the esophagus were lower in patients with high BMI.

In the literature, specific data on thoracic organ motion are very rare. When considering our results and the study by Nardone et al. [15], there is evidence that there are relevant volume differences (IRVs–OARs). In detail, the authors reported a difference of 4% (spinal cord), 23% (trachea), and 25% (esophagus) (proximal bronchial tree, absolute difference of 18 vs. 26 cm^3, relative difference not reported, thus, putatively, 44%) [15]. Zhang et al. used the IRV concept for the thoracic and abdominal organs. However, the discussed central OARs (bronchial tree, trachea, esophagus, and spinal canal) were not studied by Zhang et al. [16]. To the authors' knowledge, a putative relationship between patient characteristics and structure movement/volume changes has not been reported. However, an analysis seems reasonable, since previous studies found evidence for increased risks of toxicity associated with SBRT of NSCLC for females (here, for pneumonitis [30]) or obese patients (here, for chest wall pain [31]). After all, our results indicate that organ motion could be more pronounced in males and tall patients, whereas it could be less pronounced in patients with higher BMI. This could have implications for risk-adapted strategies in motion management or toxicity monitoring in these patient groups.

Finally, when comparing OARs and IRVs, we found a relevant increase in dosimetric parameters (D1%, D2%, Dmax) in 12/35 patients (34.3%) with central tumors. Nardone et al. found unacceptable radiotherapy plans in 42% of the patients (here, in 63% of the patients, the tumors were located centrally) [15]. These findings demonstrate that the application of the IRV concept has a relevant impact on dosimetric parameters and radiotherapy plans. In further analysis of the 12 patients in our study, the mean absolute increase in NTCPs was 5.5% (0–22.5%), and the mean relative increase was 54.78% (0–181%). It can be assumed that an absolute increase of $\geq$10% in NTCPs could be clinically relevant. This was documented in three patients for the bronchial tree. In these cases, the distance between the tumor and the bronchial tree was 0.3–1.4 cm.

When considering relevant complications in SBRT for central tumors, larger prospective studies pointed towards a particular relevance of the bronchial tree (e.g., Lindberg et al., 8/10 cases of treatment-related death occurred due to bronchopulmonary hemorrhage [25]). The region of ≤ 2 cm around the proximal bronchial tree is generally considered the "no-fly zone", with an increased risk of relevant toxicities [10,32]. Studies have made efforts to further subclassify this area, e.g., when analyzing tumors located nearer (≤ 1 cm) to the bronchial tree [33]. Recently, Lindberg et al. refined the risk factors for toxicity by considering the dose to further substructures (here, mainstem, intermediate, and lobar bronchi) [34]. However, when applying the IRV concept, our study found an increase of ≥10% in NTCPs in three patients with tumors 0.3–1.4 cm from the bronchial tree. Thus, when it comes to these distinct differences or very small substructures, motion management (as a possibility, using the IRV concept) should come into focus. However, as Noël et al. pointed out in 2022, considering the PRV concept in general—albeit already described in 2006—neither definition, purpose, nor dose constraints exist [14,35]. Studies on the IRV concept in thoracic OARs are very rare but could increase the perception of OAR motion in SBRT, in analogy to Galileo's famous comment, 'and yet it moves' [15,16,36]. Finally, recent developments include the implementation of magnetic resonance imaging (MRI) in linear accelerators with the opportunity of real-time tracking for target volumes (four-dimensional MRI, 4D-MRI) [37]. There is evidence that 4D-MRI is a promising technique for lung tumor delineation and motion assessment with greater robustness against inter-fractional changes than 4D-CT-based radiotherapy [37]. Previous studies have reported results when applying 4D-MRI for target volumes [37], whereas thoracic OARs were studied less frequently [38]. Thus, when considering motion management in SBRT for central lung tumors, 4D-MRI can be considered a promising technology for an optimal balance of toxicities and tumor control [39].

5. Conclusions

The IRV concept might improve toxicity profiles in SBRT for NSCLC [13–15]. We studied (1) clinical aspects in central vs. peripheral tumors, (2) the IRV concept in central tumors, (3) organ motion, and (4) associated NTCPs. We found lower biologically effective doses, larger planning target volume sizes, higher lung doses, and worse locoregional control for central tumors. This emphasizes the need to optimize methods to balance dose escalation with toxicities in central tumors. Organ motion was greater in males and tall patients (both, for the bronchial tree), whereas volume changes were lower in patients with higher BMI (for the esophagus). This could have implications for risk-adapted strategies in motion management or toxicity monitoring in these patient groups. Applying the IRV concept (retrospectively, without new optimization), we found an absolute increase of >10% in NTCPs for the bronchial tree in three patients (distance from the bronchial tree, 0.3–1.4 cm). Recent studies made efforts to further subclassify central tumors in the "no-fly zone", either by exact distance or by substructures (e.g., mainstem, intermediate, and lobar bronchi) [33,34]. Based on the NTCP increase in our study, when it comes to these distinct differences or very small sub-structures, motion management (as a possibility, using the IRV concept) should come into focus.

Supplementary Materials: The following supporting information can be downloaded at: https://www.mdpi.com/article/10.3390/cancers16010231/s1, Figure S1: Absolute dose differences [Gy] between organ at risk and internal organs at risk volumes. The dose differences are shown as a function of the distance of the tumors to the respective structure. Each dot (green, D1%, yellow, D2%, red, Dmax) represents the dose difference for one patient. The dashed line marks the cut-off for a relevant dose increase (please see Section 2.3.2). Table S1: Cox regression analysis, distance of the tumor to organs at risk, and outcomes. HR: hazard ratio. OS: overall survival. PFS: progression-free survival. LPFS: local progression-free survival. LRC: locoregional control. CI: confidence interval. [1] Central organs at risk (OARs): central airway, esophagus, and spinal canal. Table S2: Influence of clinical characteristics on structure movement and volume changes. The Mann–Whitney U test was used to test for an influence of the parameters. P-values are given for each parameter. SBRT: stereotactic body radiation therapy. OAR: organ at risk. IRV: internal organ at risk volumes. AIP: average intensity projection. Table S3: Differences in maximum doses and normal tissue complication probabilities (NTCPs) when comparing organ at risk (OAR) and internal organ at risk volumes (IRV). Patients with relevant increases in dosimetric parameters were preselected (Section 2.3.2, Supplementary Figure S1). For these patients ($n = 12$), we present the distance of the tumor to the structures, the maximum doses, and the NTCPs. The NTCPs for the bronchial tree and the trachea were estimated using the graphs for the maximum dose (in EQD2) for the bronchial tree by Dujim et al. The NTCPs for the esophagus and the spinal canal were calculated using the software, 'RADBIOMOD', with the Lyman–Kutcher–Burman model (please see Section 2.3.2 for further details).

Author Contributions: Conceptualization, F.-N.O.J.H., D.S., A.v.H.-E., S.R. and L.H.D.; data curation, F.-N.O.J.H., M.G., M.L. and L.H.D.; formal analysis, F.-N.O.J.H., M.L. and L.H.D.; investigation, F.-N.O.J.H., D.S., D.A.Z., L.A.F., S.B., O.K., H.T., R.K., S.R. and L.H.D.; methodology, F.-N.O.J.H., D.S., T.F., J.F., M.G., S.B., T.R.O., H.T., A.v.H.-E., S.R. and L.H.D.; project administration, F.-N.O.J.H., D.S. and L.H.D.; resources, S.R.; software, D.S., T.F., J.F. and R.E.S.; supervision, D.S., T.R.O., A.v.H.-E., R.K., R.E.S. and L.H.D.; visualization, F.-N.O.J.H., M.L. and L.H.D.; writing—original draft, F.-N.O.J.H. and L.H.D.; writing—review and editing, F.-N.O.J.H., D.S., T.F., D.A.Z., J.F., L.A.F., M.G., S.B., O.K., T.R.O., H.T., A.v.H.-E., R.K., R.E.S., S.R., M.L. and L.H.D. All authors have read and agreed to the published version of the manuscript.

Funding: This research received no external funding.

Institutional Review Board Statement: The study was conducted according to the guidelines of the Declaration of Helsinki. The study was approved by the ethics committee of the University Medical Center Göttingen (application no. 3/10/20, date of approval: 20 October 2020).

Informed Consent Statement: Due to the retrospective study design, additional informed consent was not required.

Data Availability Statement: The data presented in this study are available on reasonable request from the corresponding author.

Conflicts of Interest: The authors declare no conflict of interest.

References

1. Ceniceros, L.; Aristu, J.; Castañón, E.; Rolfo, C.; Legaspi, J.; Olarte, A.; Valtueña, G.; Moreno, M.; Gil-Bazo, I. Stereotactic body radiotherapy (SBRT) for the treatment of inoperable stage I non-small cell lung cancer patients. *Clin. Transl. Oncol.* **2016**, *18*, 259–268. [CrossRef] [PubMed]
2. Soldà, F.; Lodge, M.; Ashley, S.; Whitington, A.; Goldstraw, P.; Brada, M. Stereotactic radiotherapy (SABR) for the treatment of primary non-small cell lung cancer; Systematic review and comparison with a surgical cohort. *Radiother. Oncol.* **2013**, *109*, 1–7. [CrossRef] [PubMed]
3. Kestin, L.; Grills, I.; Guckenberger, M.; Belderbos, J.; Hope, A.J.; Werner-Wasik, M.; Sonke, J.-J.; Bissonnette, J.-P.; Xiao, Y.; Yan, D. Dose–response relationship with clinical outcome for lung stereotactic body radiotherapy (SBRT) delivered via online image guidance. *Radiother. Oncol.* **2014**, *110*, 499–504. [CrossRef] [PubMed]
4. Guckenberger, M.; Andratschke, N.; Alheit, H.; Holy, R.; Moustakis, C.; Nestle, U.; Sauer, O. Definition of stereotactic body radiotherapy: Principles and practice for the treatment of stage I non-small cell lung cancer. *Strahlenther. Onkol.* **2014**, *190*, 26–33. [CrossRef] [PubMed]
5. Park, H.S.; Harder, E.M.; Mancini, B.R.; Decker, R.H. Central versus Peripheral Tumor Location: Influence on Survival, Local Control, and Toxicity Following Stereotactic Body Radiotherapy for Primary Non–Small-Cell Lung Cancer. *J. Thorac. Oncol.* **2015**, *10*, 832–837. [CrossRef] [PubMed]
6. Hoffman, D.; Dragojević, I.; Hoisak, J.; Hoopes, D.; Manger, R. Lung Stereotactic Body Radiation Therapy (SBRT) dose gradient and PTV volume: A retrospective multi-center analysis. *Radiat. Oncol.* **2019**, *14*, 162. [CrossRef]
7. Kang, K.H.; Okoye, C.C.; Patel, R.B.; Siva, S.; Biswas, T.; Ellis, R.J.; Yao, M.; Machtay, M.; Lo, S.S. Complications from Stereotactic Body Radiotherapy for Lung Cancer. *Cancers* **2015**, *7*, 981–1004. [CrossRef] [PubMed]
8. Wu, A.J.; Williams, E.; Modh, A.; Foster, A.; Yorke, E.; Rimner, A.; Jackson, A. Dosimetric predictors of esophageal toxicity after stereotactic body radiotherapy for central lung tumors. *Radiother. Oncol.* **2014**, *112*, 267–271. [CrossRef]
9. van Hoorn, J.E.; Dahele, M.; Daniels, J.M.A. Late Central Airway Toxicity after High-Dose Radiotherapy: Clinical Outcomes and a Proposed Bronchoscopic Classification. *Cancers* **2021**, *13*, 1313. [CrossRef]
10. Timmerman, R.; McGarry, R.; Yiannoutsos, C.; Papiez, L.; Tudor, K.; DeLuca, J.; Ewing, M.; Abdulrahman, R.; DesRosiers, C.; Williams, M.; et al. Excessive toxicity when treating central tumors in a phase II study of stereotactic body radiation therapy for medically inoperable early-stage lung cancer. *J. Clin. Oncol.* **2006**, *24*, 4833–4839. [CrossRef]
11. Schmitt, D.; Blanck, O.; Gauer, T.; Fix, M.K.; Brunner, T.B.; Fleckenstein, J.; Loutfi-Krauss, B.; Manser, P.; Werner, R.; Wilhelm, M.-L.; et al. Technological quality requirements for stereotactic radiotherapy: Expert review group consensus from the DGMP Working Group for Physics and Technology in Stereotactic Radiotherapy. *Strahlenther. Onkol.* **2020**, *196*, 421–443. [CrossRef] [PubMed]
12. Yeo, S.-G.; Kim, E.S. Efficient approach for determining four-dimensional computed tomography-based internal target volume in stereotactic radiotherapy of lung cancer. *Radiat. Oncol. J.* **2013**, *31*, 247–251. [CrossRef] [PubMed]

13. De Ruysscher, D.; Faivre-Finn, C.; Moeller, D.; Nestle, U.; Hurkmans, C.W.; Le Péchoux, C.; Belderbos, J.; Guckenberger, M.; Senan, S. European Organization for Research and Treatment of Cancer (EORTC) recommendations for planning and delivery of high-dose, high precision radiotherapy for lung cancer. *Radiother. Oncol.* **2017**, *124*, 1–10. [CrossRef] [PubMed]
14. Stroom, J.C.; Heijmen, B.J. Limitations of the planning organ at risk volume (PRV) concept. *Int. J. Radiat. Oncol. Biol. Phys.* **2006**, *66*, 279–286. [CrossRef]
15. Nardone, V.; Giugliano, F.M.; Reginelli, A.; Sangiovanni, A.; Mormile, M.; Iadanza, L.; Cappabianca, S.; Guida, C. 4D CT analysis of organs at risk (OARs) in stereotactic radiotherapy. *Radiother. Oncol.* **2020**, *151*, 10–14. [CrossRef] [PubMed]
16. Zhang, J.; Markova, S.; Garcia, A.; Huang, K.; Nie, X.; Choi, W.; Lu, W.; Wu, A.; Rimner, A.; Li, G. Evaluation of automatic contour propagation in T2-weighted 4DMRI for normal-tissue motion assessment using internal organ-at-risk volume (IRV). *J. Appl. Clin. Med. Phys.* **2018**, *19*, 598–608. [CrossRef] [PubMed]
17. Andruska, N.; Stowe, H.B.; Crockett, C.; Liu, W.; Palma, D.; Faivre-Finn, C.; Badiyan, S.N. Stereotactic Radiation for Lung Cancer: A Practical Approach to Challenging Scenarios. *J. Thorac. Oncol.* **2021**, *16*, 1075–1085. [CrossRef]
18. Habermann, F.-N.O.J.; Schmitt, D.; Failing, T.; Fischer, J.; Ziegler, D.A.; Fischer, L.A.; Alt, N.J.; Muster, J.; Donath, S.; Hille, A.; et al. Patterns of Pretreatment Diagnostic Assessment in Patients Treated with Stereotactic Body Radiation Therapy (SBRT) for Non-Small Cell Lung Cancer (NSCLC): Special Characteristics in the COVID Pandemic and Influence on Outcomes. *Curr. Oncol.* **2022**, *29*, 1080–1092. [CrossRef]
19. Chang, J.Y.; Bezjak, A.; Mornex, F. Stereotactic ablative radiotherapy for centrally located early stage non-small-cell lung cancer: What we have learned. *J. Thorac. Oncol.* **2015**, *10*, 577–585. [CrossRef]
20. Gross, A.; Ziepert, M.; Scholz, M. KMWin—A convenient tool for graphical presentation of results from Kaplan-Meier survival time analysis. *PLoS ONE* **2012**, *7*, e38960. [CrossRef]
21. Kong, F.-M.S.; Quint, L.; Machtay, M.; Bradley, J. Atlases for Organs at Risk (OARs) in Thoracic Radiation Therapy. Available online: https://www.nrgoncology.org/Portals/0/Scientific%20Program/CIRO/Atlases/Lung%20Organs%20at%20Risk.ppt (accessed on 6 August 2021).
22. Chang, J.H.; Gehrke, C.; Prabhakar, R.; Gill, S.; Wada, M.; Joon, D.L.; Khoo, V. RADBIOMOD: A simple program for utilising biological modelling in radiotherapy plan evaluation. *Phys. Medica* **2016**, *32*, 248–254. [CrossRef] [PubMed]
23. Duijm, M. Outcome and Toxicity Modelling after Stereoactic Radiotherapy of Central Lung Tumors. Available online: https://www.google.com/url?sa=t&rct=j&q=&esrc=s&source=web&cd=&ved=2ahUKEwjpi-3Y7MvyAhX2R_EDHUUNAb8QFnoECAQQAQ&url=https://repub.eur.nl/pub/134875/Embargo-version-thesis-M-Duijm.pdf&usg=AOvVaw0yAt8B78bxLWtOomr_zQCw (accessed on 25 August 2021).
24. Murrell, D.H.; Laba, J.M.; Erickson, A.; Millman, B.; Palma, D.A.; Louie, A.V. Stereotactic ablative radiotherapy for ultra-central lung tumors: Prioritize target coverage or organs at risk? *Radiat. Oncol.* **2018**, *13*, 57. [CrossRef] [PubMed]
25. Lindberg, K.; Grozman, V.; Karlsson, K.; Lindberg, S.; Lax, I.; Wersäll, P.; Persson, G.F.; Josipovic, M.; Khalil, A.A.; Moeller, D.S.; et al. The HILUS-Trial—A Prospective Nordic Multicenter Phase 2 Study of Ultracentral Lung Tumors Treated with Stereotactic Body Radiotherapy. *J. Thorac. Oncol.* **2021**, *16*, 1200–1210. [CrossRef] [PubMed]
26. Schanne, D.H.; Nestle, U.; Allgäuer, M.; Andratschke, N.; Appold, S.; Dieckmann, U.; Ernst, I.; Ganswindt, U.; Grosu, A.L.; Holy, R.; et al. Stereotactic body radiotherapy for centrally located stage I NSCLC: A multicenter analysis. *Strahlenther Onkol.* **2015**, *191*, 125–132. [CrossRef] [PubMed]
27. He, J.; Huang, Y.; Shi, S.; Hu, Y.; Zeng, Z. Comparison of Effects Between Central and Peripheral Stage I Lung Cancer Using Image-Guided Stereotactic Body Radiotherapy via Helical Tomotherapy. *Technol. Cancer Res. Treat.* **2015**, *14*, 701–707. [CrossRef] [PubMed]
28. Yu, T.; Shin, I.-S.; Yoon, W.S.; Rim, C.H. Stereotactic Body Radiotherapy for Centrally Located Primary Non–Small-Cell Lung Cancer: A Meta-Analysis. *Clin. Lung Cancer* **2019**, *20*, e452–e462. [CrossRef] [PubMed]
29. Roesch, J.; Panje, C.; Sterzing, F.; Mantel, F.; Nestle, U.; Andratschke, N.; Guckenberger, M. SBRT for centrally localized NSCLC—What is too central? *Radiat. Oncol.* **2016**, *11*, 157. [CrossRef] [PubMed]
30. Takeda, A.; Ohashi, T.; Kunieda, E.; Sanuki, N.; Enomoto, T.; Takeda, T.; Oku, Y.; Shigematsu, N. Comparison of clinical, tumour-related and dosimetric factors in grade 0–1, grade 2 and grade 3 radiation pneumonitis after stereotactic body radiotherapy for lung tumours. *Br. J. Radiol.* **2012**, *85*, 636–642. [CrossRef]
31. Welsh, J.; Thomas, J.; Shah, D.; Allen, P.K.; Wei, X.; Mitchell, K.; Gao, S.; Balter, P.; Komaki, R.; Chang, J.Y. Obesity increases the risk of chest wall pain from thoracic stereotactic body radiation therapy. *Int. J. Radiat. Oncol. Biol. Phys.* **2011**, *81*, 91–96. [CrossRef]
32. Thompson, M.; Rosenzweig, K.E. The evolving toxicity profile of SBRT for lung cancer. *Transl. Lung Cancer Res.* **2019**, *8*, 48–57. [CrossRef]
33. Haseltine, J.M.; Rimner, A.; Gelblum, D.Y.; Modh, A.; Rosenzweig, K.E.; Jackson, A.; Yorke, E.D.; Wu, A.J. Fatal complications after stereotactic body radiation therapy for central lung tumors abutting the proximal bronchial tree. *Pract. Radiat. Oncol.* **2016**, *6*, e27–e33. [CrossRef] [PubMed]
34. Lindberg, S.; Grozman, V.; Karlsson, K.; Onjukka, E.; Lindbäck, E.; Al Jirf, K.; Lax, I.; Wersäll, P.; Persson, G.F.; Josipovic, M.; et al. Expanded HILUS Trial: A Pooled Analysis of Risk Factors for Toxicity from Stereotactic Body Radiation Therapy of Central and Ultracentral Lung Tumors. *Int. J. Radiat. Oncol. Biol. Phys.* **2023**. [CrossRef] [PubMed]
35. Noël, G.; Antoni, D. Organs at risk radiation dose constraints. *Cancer Radiother.* **2022**, *26*, 59–75. [CrossRef] [PubMed]
36. Almeida, P.F. And Yet It Moves. *Biophys. J.* **2017**, *113*, 759–761. [CrossRef]

37. Rabe, M.; Thieke, C.; Düsberg, M.; Neppl, S.; Gerum, S.; Reiner, M.; Nicolay, N.H.; Schlemmer, H.; Debus, J.; Dinkel, J.; et al. Real-time 4DMRI-based internal target volume definition for moving lung tumors. *Med. Phys.* **2020**, *47*, 1431–1442. [CrossRef]
38. Habatsch, M.; Schneider, M.; Requardt, M.; Doussin, S. Movement assessment of breast and organ-at-risks using free-breathing, self-gating 4D magnetic resonance imaging workflow for breast cancer radiation therapy. *Phys. Imaging Radiat. Oncol.* **2022**, *22*, 111–114. [CrossRef]
39. Crockett, C.B.; Samson, P.; Chuter, R.; Dubec, M.; Faivre-Finn, C.; Green, O.L.; Hackett, S.L.; McDonald, F.; Robinson, C.; Shiarli, A.-M.; et al. Initial Clinical Experience of MR-Guided Radiotherapy for Non-Small Cell Lung Cancer. *Front. Oncol.* **2021**, *11*, 617681. [CrossRef]

Disclaimer/Publisher's Note: The statements, opinions and data contained in all publications are solely those of the individual author(s) and contributor(s) and not of MDPI and/or the editor(s). MDPI and/or the editor(s) disclaim responsibility for any injury to people or property resulting from any ideas, methods, instructions or products referred to in the content.

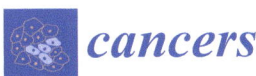

Article

Radiomodulating Properties of Superparamagnetic Iron Oxide Nanoparticle (SPION) Agent Ferumoxytol on Human Monocytes: Implications for MRI-Guided Liver Radiotherapy

Michael R. Shurin [1,*], Vladimir A. Kirichenko [2], Galina V. Shurin [1], Danny Lee [2], Christopher Crane [3] and Alexander V. Kirichenko [2,*]

1. Department of Pathology, University of Pittsburgh Medical Center, Pittsburgh, PA 15213, USA; shuringv@upmc.edu
2. Department of Radiation Oncology, Allegheny Health Network Cancer Institute, Pittsburgh, PA 15224, USA; vak8238@gmail.com (V.A.K.); danny.lee@ahn.org (D.L.)
3. Department of Radiation Oncology, Memorial Sloan Kettering Cancer Center, New York, NY 10065, USA; cranec1@mskcc.org
* Correspondence: shurinmr@upmc.edu (M.R.S.); alexander.kirichenko@ahn.org (A.V.K.)

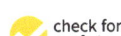

Citation: Shurin, M.R.; Kirichenko, V.A.; Shurin, G.V.; Lee, D.; Crane, C.; Kirichenko, A.V. Radiomodulating Properties of Superparamagnetic Iron Oxide Nanoparticle (SPION) Agent Ferumoxytol on Human Monocytes: Implications for MRI-Guided Liver Radiotherapy. *Cancers* **2024**, *16*, 1318. https://doi.org/10.3390/cancers16071318

Received: 19 February 2024
Revised: 26 March 2024
Accepted: 26 March 2024
Published: 28 March 2024

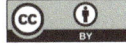

Copyright: © 2024 by the authors. Licensee MDPI, Basel, Switzerland. This article is an open access article distributed under the terms and conditions of the Creative Commons Attribution (CC BY) license (https://creativecommons.org/licenses/by/4.0/).

Simple Summary: Image-guided stereotactic body radiation therapy (SBRT), utilizing biocompatible superparamagnetic iron oxide nanoparticles (SPION), like ferumoxytol, has emerged as a non-invasive, safe, and effective therapy for liver tumors. However, the radiomodulating properties of ferumoxytol on hepatic macrophages have never been directly investigated. We showed that ferumoxytol affected human monocytes increasing their resistance to radiation-induced cell death. These findings provide the basis for mechanism-based optimization of SPION-enhanced image-guided functional treatment planning platform for reducing hepatotoxicity in patients with advanced hepatic cirrhosis undergoing liver SBRT for liver cancer before liver transplant.

Abstract: Superparamagnetic iron oxide nanoparticles (SPION) have attracted great attention not only for therapeutic applications but also as an alternative magnetic resonance imaging (MRI) contrast agent that helps visualize liver tumors during MRI-guided stereotactic body radiotherapy (SBRT). SPION can provide functional imaging of liver parenchyma based upon its uptake by the hepatic resident macrophages or Kupffer cells with a relative enhancement of malignant tumors that lack Kupffer cells. However, the radiomodulating properties of SPION on liver macrophages are not known. Utilizing human monocytic THP-1 undifferentiated and differentiated cells, we characterized the effect of ferumoxytol (Feraheme®), a carbohydrate-coated ultrasmall SPION agent at clinically relevant concentration and therapeutically relevant doses of gamma radiation on cultured cells in vitro. We showed that ferumoxytol affected both monocytes and macrophages, increased the resistance of monocytes to radiation-induced cell death and inhibition of cell activity, and supported the anti-inflammatory phenotype of human macrophages under radiation. Its effect on human cells depended on the duration of SPION uptake and was radiation dose-dependent. The results of this pilot study support a strong mechanism-based optimization of SPION-enhanced MRI-guided liver SBRT for primary and metastatic liver tumors, especially in patients with liver cirrhosis awaiting a liver transplant.

Keywords: magnetic iron oxide nanoparticles; monocytes; macrophages; liver cancer; biomedical application

1. Introduction

Hepatocellular carcinoma (HCC) is the sixth most common cancer and the third leading cause of cancer-related death worldwide [1,2]. Liver cirrhosis predisposes the development of HCC, with 80–90% of HCC cases occurring in cirrhotic livers. In the USA, chronic hepatitis C, alcohol abuse, and non-alcoholic steatohepatitis are the leading causes of hepatic cirrhosis leading to HCC [3,4]. The high prevalence of hepatic cirrhosis and portal hypertension in patients with HCC markedly limits the choice of curative liver resection: only 15–30% of HCC patients with cirrhosis are eligible for curative partial hepatectomy [5,6]. Selective internal radiation therapy (SIRT) or radioembolization is one of the targeted treatments for unresectable liver tumors where radioactive microspheres are infused via the hepatic artery for internal tumor irradiation. Although it is generally considered efficacious in patients with unresectable HCC and unresectable hepatic metastatic disease, practical guidance on personalized dosimetry performance is still in progress.

Therefore, the most appropriate therapy for patients with HCC is liver transplantation, which addresses both the underlying cirrhosis and the HCC with a five-year survival rate of up to 85%, however, only 10% of patients are eligible [7].

Patients with HCC and liver cirrhosis face major challenges, as cancer must be under control, while patients remain on a waiting list for liver transplantation. During this waiting time, the progression of the tumor is unpredictable, resulting in an average dropout rate of ~25% [8] or as high as ~40% in 12 months [9,10]. Therefore, extended control of HCC is even more important for patients on the transplant waiting list to successfully reach liver transplants. Given the above, local therapy for HCC has been investigated as a bridge to liver transplant with the aim of decreasing tumor progression and reducing the risk of dropout rate from the waiting list.

Over the past decade, stereotactic body radiation therapy (SBRT) has emerged as a non-invasive, safe, and effective therapy for liver tumors providing local control and prolonging survival for many HCC patients who were not eligible for standard local regional treatment [11–13]. Image-guided SBRT for unresectable HCC sustained local control rates ranging from 75 to 100% in prospective phase I/II clinical trials [12,14]. Several prospective studies have shown SBRT as a highly effective ablative therapy for primary liver tumors and used as a bridge to liver transplant for inoperable patients with HCC [12,14,15]. Combined with appropriate diagnostic imaging, SBRT delivers the ablative radiation dose to liver tumor with conformal avoidance of residual functionally active hepatic parenchyma thus minimizing the risk of developing radiation-induced liver disease in patients with liver cirrhosis [13,16,17]. In this regard, biocompatible superparamagnetic iron oxide nanoparticles (SPION) have attracted a great deal of interest as contrast agents for magnetic resonance imaging (MRI) providing differential contrast enhancement imaging for functionally active, macrophage-infiltrated hepatic parenchyma and liver tumors for treatment planning of liver SBRT on MRI-Linac in patients with hepatic cirrhosis [18,19].

Ferumoxytol (Feraheme®) is a carbohydrate-coated ultrasmall SPION agent that is FDA-approved for the treatment of iron deficiency anemia. Because of its clearance through the reticuloendothelial system, ferumoxytol has been recently adopted for off-label clinical use as an MRI contrast agent for clinical imaging of liver parenchyma involving contrast uptake by hepatic macrophages (Kupffer cells) [20,21]. Once intravascularly injected, ferumoxytol nanoparticles stay trapped within hepatic Kupffer cells for several weeks causing T2-weighted signal loss within functionally active liver parenchyma [22]. Malignant tumors lacking Kupffer cells exhibit no signal change resulting in increased tumor-to-liver contrast difference allowing diagnostic quality MR imaging with contouring of liver tumors for precision targeting and functional hepatic parenchyma for guided avoidance during liver SBRT planning.

However, the radiomodulating properties of Feraheme on hepatic macrophages have never been directly investigated. Moreover, patients with primary and metastatic hepatic malignancies often present with iron-deficiency anemia due to chronic blood loss and require therapeutic Feraheme injections, raising the same question on the potential radiosensitizing effect of Feraheme on hepatic parenchyma when the liver is irradiated simultaneously with Feraheme injections. Although radiation-induced damage of Kupffer cells is well described [23], published results focusing on macrophage polarization after SPION treatment are highly inconsistent. For instance, previous studies reported that SPION polarizes macrophages into M1-phenotype [24,25], has no M1 polarization effect [26], or increases the production of anti-inflammatory IL-10 (i.p., M2 polarization) [27,28]. Furthermore, ferumoxytol upregulated macrophage polarization associated with pro-inflammatory Th1-type responses [29]. In vivo, ferumoxytol could inhibit tumor growth in mice, which was accompanied by tumor infiltration with pro-inflammatory M1 macrophages [29]. Finally, ferumoxytol might also cause tumor cell ferroptosis, an iron-dependent cell death, by triggering the transformation of infiltrating macrophages to the M1 phenotype [30]. However, the effect of ferumoxytol on macrophage polarization, cytokine release, and apoptosis under irradiation has never been investigated.

This study aimed to develop, optimize, and characterize the pre-clinical model allowing the determination of functional and phenotypic alterations of human macrophages treated with SPION at therapeutically relevant doses of ionizing radiation in vitro. Our results revealed that iron loading significantly improved monocyte and macrophage survival under low-dose irradiation. We also demonstrated that SPION supports the anti-inflammatory phenotype of human macrophages under radiation and that the effects of SPION depended on the duration of iron particle uptake and were radiation dose-dependent. Our data help to understand mechanisms of radiation-induced liver damage and provide the basis for the safe administration of Feraheme as an MRI contrast agent during SPION-enhanced MRI-guided liver SBRT to HCC in patients with hepatic cirrhosis awaiting a liver transplant.

2. Materials and Methods

2.1. Cell Cultures

THP-1 cells, a spontaneously immortalized monocyte-like cell line derived from the peripheral blood of a childhood case of acute monocytic leukemia (M5 subtype) [31] were purchased from ATCC (TIB-202). Cells were cultured in RPMI-1640 medium (Thermo Fisher Scientific, Waltham, MA, USA) supplemented with 0.2 mM of L-glutamine, 50 µ/mL of penicillin, 50 µg/mL of streptomycin, 10 mM HEPES (Invitrogen Life Technologies, Waltham, MA, USA), and 10% heat-inactivated fetal bovine serum (FBS, Gemini Bio-Products, West Sacramento, CA, USA) (complete RPMI-1640 medium) and maintained at 37 °C, 5% CO_2 in a humidified tissue culture incubator. For macrophage differentiation, 1×10^6 THP-1 cells/mL were cultured in a complete RPMI-1640 medium supplemented with 20 ng/mL recombinant human M-CSF (Peprotech Inc., Rocky Hill, NJ, USA) for five days. All cells were authenticated, mycoplasma tested, were contaminant-free, and used at low passage. For macrophage harvesting, trypsin was added to flasks until cells became detached and RPMI medium +10% FCS was added to neutralize the effects of the enzyme. The cell suspension was centrifuged at $400 \times g$ for 5 min and re-suspended in a lower volume of media. Cell number was determined using the hemocytometer and Trypan Blue staining (Sigma, Burlington, MA, USA).

2.2. Cell Proliferation Assay

To examine the cell proliferative activity of treated and control cells, 1×10^4 cells per well were seeded in 96-well plates in a culture medium. Following appropriate treatments, 1 mg/mL MTT reagent (Sigma, Burlington, MA, USA) was added to each well for 4 h at 37 °C. The cells were then suspended in dimethyl sulfoxide for 3 h at 37 °C and detected using multimode microplate readers (BioRad, Hercules, CA, USA) at a wavelength of 540 nm. Quadruplicates were used in each experiment. The MTT (3-[4,5-dimethylthiazol-2-yl]-2,5 diphenyl tetrazolium bromide) assay is based on the conversion of MTT into formazan crystals by living cells, which determines mitochondrial activity and reflects cell proliferative activity.

2.3. Annexin V/PI Apoptosis Assay

Cells were collected, pelleted, and washed twice in PBS. The resulting pellets were resuspended in 100 µL of 1X Annexin V binding buffer and stained with 5 µL Annexin

V-FITC and 10 µL propidium iodide (PI) (BioLegend, San Diego, CA, USA). Samples were kept at room temperature for 15 min and protected from light. After the incubation period, 400 µL of Annexin V binding buffer was added to each tube. Samples were analyzed immediately by flow cytometry (BD LSR II, Franklin Lakes, NJ, USA). Data were analyzed using FlowJo software V9 (FlowJo LLC., Ashland, OR, USA).

2.4. Flow Cytometry

After experimental and control treatments, cells were collected by gentle enzymatic detachment, resuspended, counted, and resuspended in flow cytometry staining buffer (PBS supplemented with 2% BSA) at 1×10^6 cells/mL. Aliquots of cells were stained for 30 min at room temperature and protected from light with fluorescently conjugated antibodies (HLA-DR-FITC, CD86-PerCp-Cy5.5, CD11b-PE, CD14-APC from Biolegend) according to the concentrations indicated by the suppliers. Flow cytometric acquisition was performed on a Becton Dickinson LSR II instrument. Data were analyzed using FlowJo software V9 (FlowJo LLC.). A minimum of 10,000 events were acquired for each sample and the experiments were repeated three times independently.

2.5. Cytokine Secretion

Cell culture supernatants from M-CSF-differentiated macrophages were collected at the end of the polarization period and appropriate treatments. Secretion of cytokines was quantified using a multi-cytokine–chemokine panel 27plex assay, according to the manufacturer's instructions (Bio-Rad, Hercules, CA, USA). The results were normalized to the total protein concentration in the cell culture supernatant samples. Data are derived from two independent experiments performed in triplicate.

2.6. Experimental Design

Monocytes or macrophages (200,000 cells/mL) were stabilized in cell cultures, harvested in fresh medium, and treated with ferumoxytol (510 mg/17 mL vial at a neutral pH, AMAG Pharmaceuticals, Inc., Waltham, MA, USA)—30 µg Fe/mL, 2 or 24 h, 37 °C. Ferumoxytol is a superparamagnetic iron oxide nanoparticle, 17–31 nm in diameter (topological polar surface area 74.6 $Å^2$), coated with a low molecular weight semi-synthetic carbohydrate (polyglucose sorbitol and carboxymethyl ether shell) and having ~2000 magnetite iron (Fe_3O_4) molecules in the core with the relaxometric properties at 1.5 Tesla and 37 °C of $r_1 = 15$ and $r_2 = 89$ $mM^{-1}s^{-1}$ [20,32]. The coating material is about 1.7 nm thick (10 kDa in molecular weight) and provides ferumoxytol with a neutrally charged surface [30]. The concentration of ferumoxytol for our studies was selected based on previous in vitro data investigating the dose-dependent effects of SPION on monocytes and macrophages [24,33–35] and in vivo data on ferumoxytol pharmacodynamics and pharmacokinetics [12,36,37]. Uptake of iron oxide nanoparticles by macrophages has been well documented previously [22,32,35,38,39]. After iron uptake, cells were washed twice and treated with therapeutically relevant doses of gamma radiation (300, 500, 1000, or 3000 rad) (Gamma Cell 1000 Elite, Nordion International Inc., Ottawa, ON, Canada). Next, cells were cultured again in 96-well plates (MTT assay and cytokine expression) or 6-well plates (phenotyping and apoptosis assay) for 24 or 48 h and analyzed in different assays as indicated in individual result sections.

2.7. Statistical Analysis

For a single comparison of two groups, the Student *t*-test was used after the evaluation of normality. If data distribution was not normal, the Mann–Whitney rank-sum test was performed. For the comparison of multiple groups, ANOVA was applied. SigmaStat Software V4.0 was used for data analysis (SyStat Software, Inc., Chicago, IL, USA). For all statistical analyses, $p < 0.05$ was considered significant. All experiments were repeated at least two times. Data are presented as the mean ± standard error of the mean (SEM).

3. Results

3.1. Ferumoxytol Decreases Radiation-Induced Cell Death of Human Monocytes In Vitro

First, we tested how the uptake of iron by human monocytes affects their sensitivity to radiation-induced cell death. Figure 1 demonstrates that preincubation of cells with ferumoxytol for either two or 24 h before irradiation significantly increases their survival measured by Annexin V/PI staining for all tested doses of irradiation after 24 h. For instance, the level of cell death in monocytes incubated loaded with SPION for 24 h and irradiated by 500 rad decreased from 11.9 ± 2.1% to 7.7 ± 1.2% (Figure 1B, $p < 0.05$). We also revealed that 3000 rad killed more than 50% of cultured cells and this dose of radiation was omitted from further experiments.

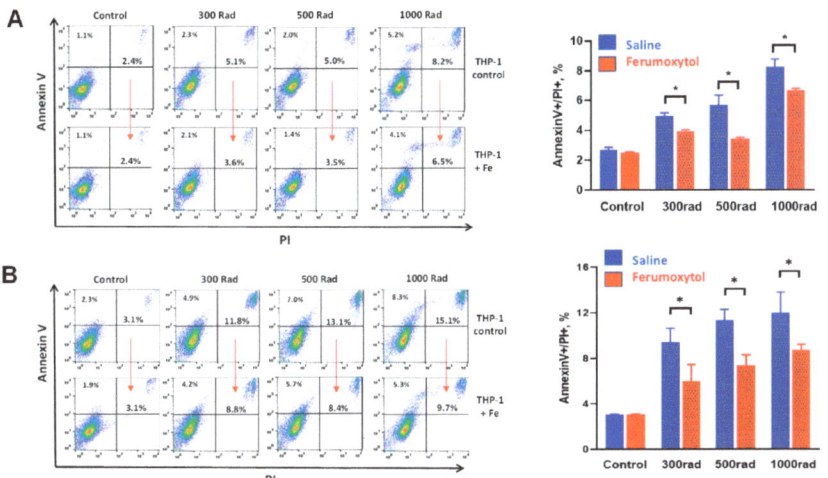

Figure 1. Ferumoxytol decreases radiation-induced apoptosis of human monocytes in vitro. THP-1 monocytes were treated with SPION (30 μg Fe/mL) for two (**A**) and 24 (**B**) hours, washed, irradiated by 300–1000 rad, and analyzed in Annexin V/PI assay 24 h later as described in M&M. Both Annexin V+/PI− (early apoptosis) and Annexin V+/PI+ (all dead) cells were analyzed. Treatment with saline served as a control. All samples were tested in triplicates in each experiment. The left panels represent the results of representative experiments, while the right panels summarize the results of 3–4 independent experiments. Error bars indicate ±SEM of 3–4 independent replicates. *, $p < 0.05$ (Student *t*-test, $n = 3$–4).

To verify these results, all experiments were repeated with a prolonged time of cell culture after irradiation—cell death was assessed 48 h after cell irradiation (300–1000 rad). The results are demonstrated in Figure 2. Short (2 h, Figure 2A) loading of THP-1 cells with iron nanoparticles did not protect cells from higher doses of irradiation (500 and 1000 rad), while the protective effect was still detected at 300 rad: cells death significantly decreased from 5.5 ± 0.6% to 3.9 ± 0.3% ($p < 0.05$). Importantly, preincubation of cells with SPION for 24 h (Figure 2B) significantly decreased cell death induced by all tested doses of radiation. For instance, the level of cell death in monocytes incubated loaded with SPION for 24 h and irradiated by 500 rad decreased from 23.9 ± 4.2% to 14.8 ± 2.2% ($p < 0.05$).

Thus, these data suggest that human monocytes loaded with iron nanoparticles demonstrate increased resistance to radiation-induced cell death. This raises the next question about how iron uptake can alter the functional and phenotypic characteristics of human monocytes and macrophages.

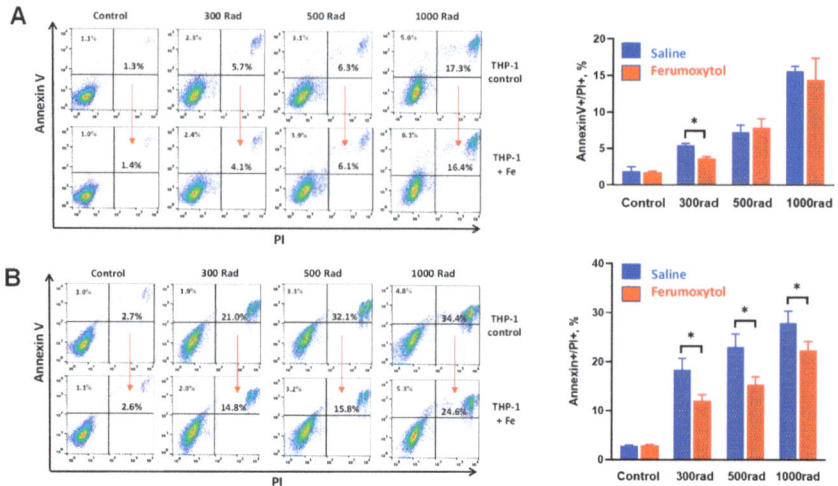

Figure 2. Ferumoxytol decreases radiation-induced apoptosis of human monocytes in vitro. THP-1 monocytes were treated with SPION (30 μg Fe/mL) for 2 (**A**) and 24 (**B**) hours, washed, irradiated by 300–1000 rad, and analyzed in Annexin V/PI assay 48 h later as described in M&M. Both Annexin V+/PI− (early apoptosis) and Annexin V+/PI+ (all dead) cells were analyzed. Treatment with saline served as a control. All samples were tested in triplicates in each experiment. The left panels represent the results of representative experiments, while the right panels summarize the results of 3–4 independent experiments. Error bars indicate ±SEM of 3–4 independent replicates. *, $p < 0.05$ (Student t-test, n = 3–4).

3.2. Ferumoxytol Prevents Radiation-Induced Inhibition of Monocyte Proliferative Activity In Vitro

To determine how the uptake of iron particles alters monocyte proliferation after irradiation, cells were incubated with SPION for 2 and 24 h, irradiated (300, 500, and 1000 rad), and their proliferation was assessed 24 and 48 h later in an MTT assay. Figure 3 demonstrates that radiation dose-dependently inhibits the proliferative activity of human monocytes. Preincubation of cells with SPION for 2 h significantly abrogated this inhibitory effect of all tested doses of radiation seen after 24 h, although the protective effect persisted only for 300 rad if assessed 48 h after irradiation (Figure 3, upper panels). Importantly, significant iron-mediated protection was revealed for both early (24 h) and late (48 h) detection if monocytes were pre-treated with SPION for 24 h (Figure 3, lower panels). For instance, 0.55 ± 0.03 OD versus 0.61 ± 0.06 OD ($p < 0.05$) and 0.62 ± 0.07 OD versus 0.79 ± 0.05 OD ($p < 0.05$) for 500 rad detected in 24 and 48 h, respectively.

Thus, these data suggest that iron nanoparticles significantly inhibit the antiproliferative effect of radiation on human monocytes and that this effect was markedly stronger if cells were pre-treated with SPION for a prolonged time.

3.3. Modulation of Cytokine Production in Monocytes and Macrophages by SPION and Irradiation

Using the THP-1 monocytic cell line, it was reported that gamma radiation triggers monocyte differentiation toward the macrophage phenotype with increased expression of type I interferons and both pro- and anti-inflammatory macrophage phenotyping markers [40]. Therefore, we tested how SPION uptake can alter cytokine production by monocytes and macrophages upon irradiation. Undifferentiated and M-CSF-differentiated THP-1 cells were treated with SPION for 24 h (based on the results above), irradiated with 500 and 1000 rad, and cell-free supernatants were harvested 48 h later for determination of cytokine levels. Figure 4 shows cytokine production by control and treated monocytes. These results revealed that ferumoxytol uptake by human monocytes downregulates expression of pro-inflammatory chemokines MIP-1α (macrophage inflammatory protein 1α), MIP-1β (CCL4), and RANTES (CCL5) but does not significantly alter cytokine expression under radiation conditions. Only radiation (500 rad) induced upregulation of monocyte chemoattractant protein-1 (MCP-1/CCL2), one of the key chemokines that regulate migration and infiltration of monocytes/macrophages, was abrogated by SPION, but this finding should be further investigated. Of note, IL-2, IL-4, IL-5, IL-6, IL-7, IFN-γ, IL-10, IL-12 (p70), IL-13, IL-1β, G-CSF, FGF-2, GM-CSF and PDGF levels were less than 1 ng/mL.

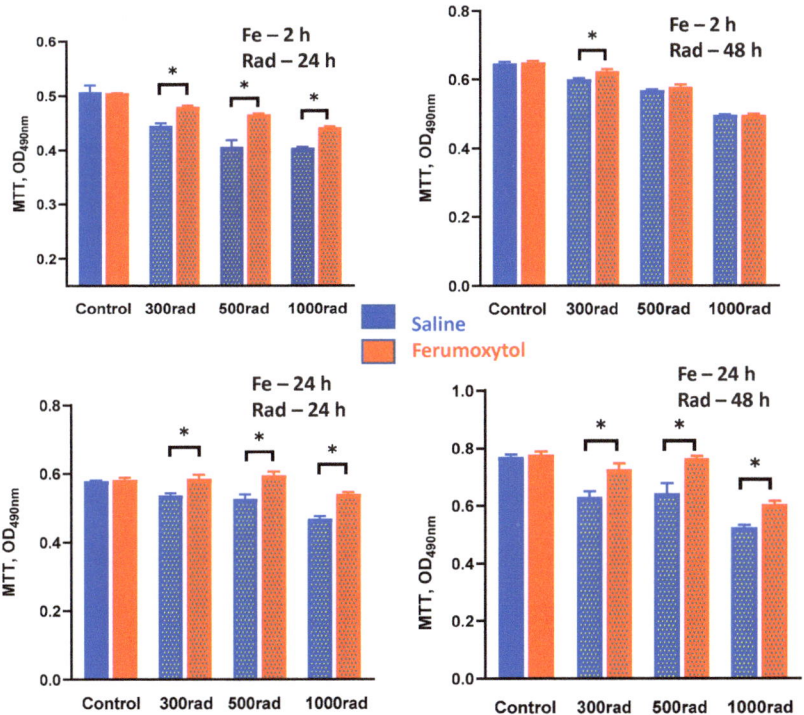

Figure 3. Ferumoxytol prevents radiation-induced inhibition of human monocyte proliferative activity in vitro. THP-1 monocytes were treated with SPION (30 μg Fe/mL) for 2 (**upper panels**) and 24 (**lower panels**) hours, washed, irradiated by 300–1000 rad, and analyzed in MTT assay 24 h (**left panels**) and 48 h (**right panels**) later as described in M&M. Treatment with saline served as a control. All samples were tested in triplicates in each experiment. Error bars indicate ±SEM of four independent replicates. *, $p < 0.05$ (Student t-test, $n = 4$).

Next, using a similar experimental design, we tested cytokine expression in macrophages differentiated from THP-1 cells and treated with SPION and irradiation. Results in Figure 5 show that macrophages produce significantly higher levels of cytokines, when compared with monocytes, and are much more sensitive to iron uptake and radiation treatment. For instance, ferumoxytol uptake by macrophages significantly upregulated the expression of MCP-1 (CCL2) in control and irradiated cells ($p < 0.05$). SPION also reversed the effect of radiation (500 rad) on the expression of IL-1RA, IL-8, VEGF, CCL5, and TNF-α. Interestingly, if irradiation upregulated cytokine expression (IL-1RA, TNF-α, CCL5), iron particles downregulated their expression. However, if irradiation decreased cytokine release from macrophages (IL-8, VEGF), iron increased cytokine production. Furthermore, strong stimulation of MCP-1, MIP-1α, and MIP-1β expression in macrophages by ferumoxytol upon cell irradiation should be further investigated. Also, expression of

IL-2, IL-4, IL-5, IL-6, IL-7, IFN-γ, IL-10, IL-12 (p70), IL-13, IL-1β, G-CSF, FGF-2, GM-CSF and PDGF was not observed.

Together, these results suggest that iron uptake by human monocytes and macrophages may alter their sensitivity to irradiation-induced cytokine expression.

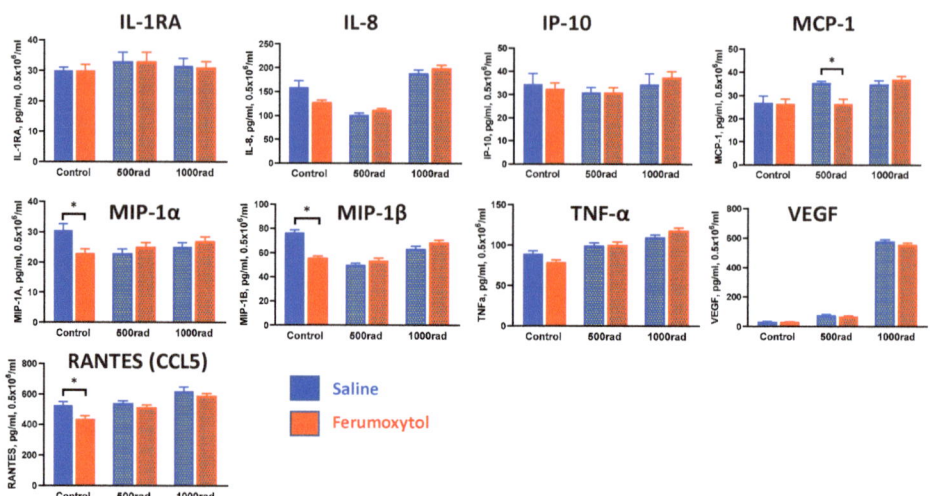

Figure 4. Ferumoxytol and radiation modulate cytokine expression in human monocytes in vitro. THP-1 monocytes were treated with SPION (30 μg Fe/mL) for 24 h, washed, irradiated by 500 or 1000 rad, and cultured for an additional 48 h before supernatants were collected for cytokine assessment as described in M&M. Treatment with saline served as a control. All samples were tested in triplicates in each experiment. Results are shown as mean ± SEM. *, $p < 0.05$ (Student t-test, $n = 3$).

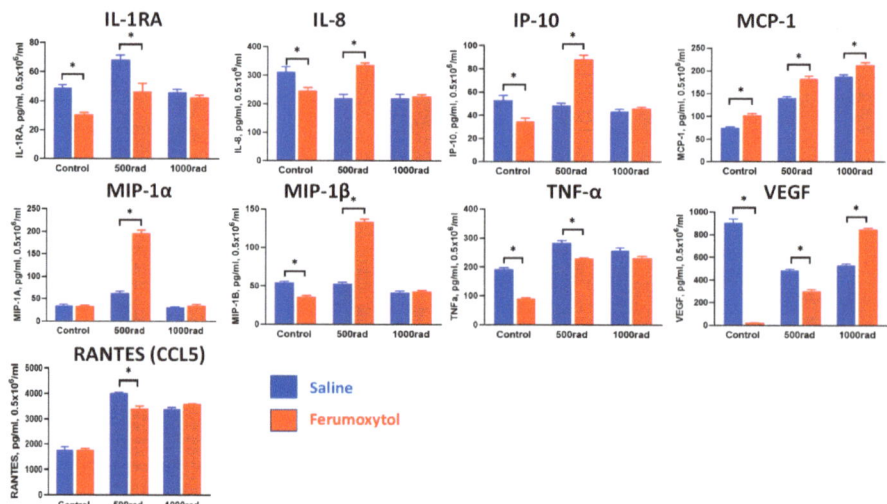

Figure 5. Ferumoxytol and radiation modulate cytokine expression in human macrophages in vitro. THP-1 monocytes were treated with M-CSF (20 ng/mL) for five days, then loaded with SPION (30 μg Fe/mL) for 24 h, washed, irradiated by 500 or 1000 rad and cultured for an additional 48 h with M-CSF (10 ng/mL) before supernatants were collected for cytokine assessment as described in M&M. Treatment with saline instead of SPION served as a control. All samples were tested in triplicates in each experiment. Results are shown as mean ± SEM. *, $p < 0.05$ (Student t-test, $n = 3$).

3.4. Ferumoxytol Changes the Phenotype of Monocytes/Macrophages Altered by Radiation

Finally, we asked whether iron nanoparticles could alter monocyte and macrophage phenotype in response to gamma irradiation. First, we showed that 1000 rad treatment of THP-1 cells decreased the percentage of CD11b$^+$ CD14$^+$ cells from 92.3 ± 5.0% to 65.2 ± 6.2% ($p < 0.05$) 48 h after irradiation but the preincubation with SPION for 24 h before irradiation kept the percentage of double-positive cells at 82.6 ± 7.3% level. Furthermore, while 1000 rad increased CD11b^{neg} CD14^{neg} cells from 2.3 ± 0.1% to 21.7 ± 4.6% ($p < 0.05$), SPION reversed this effect to 7.1 ± 1.1% ($p < 0.05$). Importantly, a similar anti-radiation effect of SPION was also seen in macrophage cultures: while 1000 rad significantly upregulated CD11b$^+$CD14$^+$ cells from 56.7 ± 7.4% to 75.5 ± 8.2%, iron nanoparticles prevented this increase to 62.3 ± 6.3% level ($p < 0.05$). As an example, Figure 6 demonstrates that expression of HLA-DR in human macrophages decreased under irradiation and, interestingly, uptake of iron particles before cell irradiation decreased even more: 94.1 ± 7.2% versus 75.4 ± 9.1% ($p < 0.05$). Furthermore, radiation upregulated the expression of CD86 in macrophages, and SPION augmented it further: 3.9 ± 0.2% versus 18.5 ± 2.2% ($p < 0.05$) (Figure 6). As a control, Figure 6 shows that SPION does not change the expression of HLA-DR and CD86 on preloaded macrophages in control non-irradiated cultures.

Thus, these data suggest that SPION can attenuate polarization of macrophages induced by radiation, although the effect depends on the dose of radiation and phenotypic markers.

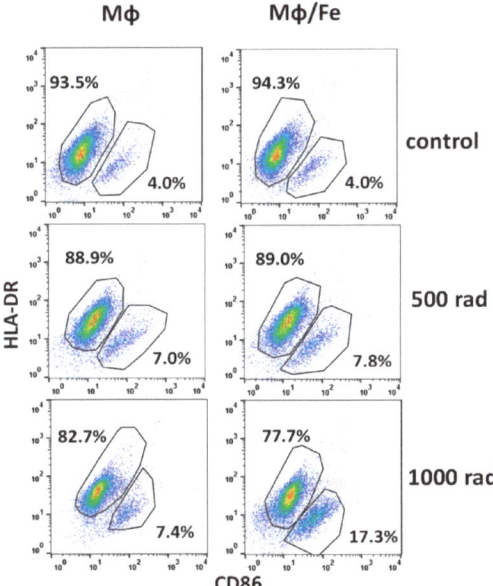

Figure 6. Ferumoxytol changed phenotypic alterations of monocytes and macrophages induced by radiation in vitro. Undifferentiated and macrophage-differentiated (M-CSF, 20 ng/mL, five days) THP-1 cells were treated with medium (control) or ferumoxytol (30 µg Fe/mL, 24 h) and irradiated by 500 and 1000 rad. Cells were then cultured for an additional 48 h with medium (monocytes) or M-CSF, 10 ng/mL (macrophages) before their phenotype was assessed by flow cytometry as described in M&M. Results from a representative experiment are shown. Mϕ, macrophages.

4. Discussion

MRI-guided radiotherapy on a hybrid MR-Linac (a magnetic resonance-guided linear accelerator) is a rapidly evolving new technology allowing superior soft tissue imaging for liver SBRT compared with conventional CT-guided radiotherapy. Reliable identification of liver tumors and functional hepatic parenchyma on MR-Linac has a direct impact on the quality of radiotherapy planning and treatment outcomes. However, using repeated MRI with conventional IV contrast, such as gadolinium chloride for daily image-guided radiotherapy carries the potential risk of toxicity and is contraindicated in patients with impaired kidney function.

Ferumoxytol (Feraheme®), as a SPION-based contrast agent with unique pharmacological, metabolic, and imaging properties, may play a crucial role in the future MR liver imaging [30,39] with important safety features: (a) it can be safely administered in the population of patients with impaired renal function in whom gadolinium-based MRI contrast agents are contraindicated; (b) the use of ferumoxytol is not associated with concerns of a long-term accumulation from repeated applications, such as is the case with brain deposition of gadolinium-containing agents [40,41].

Ferumoxytol is eventually taken up by tissue-resident macrophages/the reticuloendothelial system in the liver, spleen, bone marrow, and lymph nodes, and this uptake mechanism is being extensively explored for the enhanced MR imaging approach for tumors, vascular lesions, and lymph nodes [20]. For instance, the utilization of ferumoxytol as an off-label contrast agent has been recently reported to increase the detection rate of colorectal cancer liver metastases and may aid in preoperative decision-making [41].

Lately, superparamagnetic iron oxide nanoparticles have been used to diagnose focal liver lesions and the progression of fibrosis in steatohepatitis by the analysis of iron nanoparticles in liver Kupffer cells. It was reported that alteration of Kupffer cell phagocytic function evaluated with SPION-MRI correlated with the severity of non-alcoholic steatohepatitis [42]. Furthermore, analysis of the diagnostic value of SPION/MR imaging for the characterization of focal liver lesions, both primary and metastatic, in patients with cancer and hepatic cirrhosis revealed a diagnostic incremental value of using iron oxide particles [43]. The usefulness of SPION was based on the high uptake of the SPION by the Kupffer cells: a shortage of T2W signal was seen in the volumes of functional hepatic parenchyma diffusely infiltrated by Kupffer cells, with no signal changes in hepatic lesions lacking Kupffer cells [44].

As the use of ferumoxytol, a novel ultrasmall SPION formulation, as a contrast agent for MRI is constantly increasing, it is critical to understand its radiomodulating effects on liver parenchyma infiltrated by hepatic resident macrophages in a setting of SPION-enhanced MRI-guided SBRT to primary and metastatic liver tumors.

Iron oxide nanoparticles have been reported to augment a "pro-inflammatory" immune cell phenotype in macrophages and their antitumor potential [29,45,46]. For instance, the growth of breast adenocarcinomas in mice was markedly repressed by ferumoxytol, which was associated with the alteration of pro-inflammatory M1 macrophages in the tumor tissues [29]. In addition to stimulating macrophages, ferumoxytol can reduce the immunosuppressive function of myeloid-derived suppressor cells (MDSC) known to play a key role in the formation of immunosuppressive tumor microenvironment and resistance to anti-cancer therapy [47].

The radiosensitizing potential of SPION is intensively investigated revealing the diversity of results among the multiple research groups [48]. Even though radiation-induced modulation of monocytes and macrophages has been described [40,49,50] to the best of our knowledge, there are no data describing the effect of ferumoxytol on human monocytes and macrophages under clinically relevant doses of radiation.

Here we demonstrated that preloading of human monocyte cell line with ferumoxytol significantly decreased radiation-induced cell death of human monocytes in vitro. The effect was revealed using doses of gamma radiation within the liver SBRT clinical dose range. Although Wu et al. demonstrated that Fe_3O_4 nanoparticles could reduce macrophage viability via activation of ferroptosis after 48 h through the upregulation of p53 [51] we did not observe the effect of ferumoxytol on THP-1 cell death in vitro. However, as expected, we observed radiation-induced cell death, which was significantly attenuated by cell preincubation with iron oxide nanoparticles. Our data were further confirmed by the demonstration that ferumoxytol prevented radiation-induced inhibition of monocyte proliferative activity in vitro. The inhibitory effect of gamma radiation on primary macrophages has been described [52], but our data demonstrated for the first time that monocytes preloaded with ferumoxytol displayed increased resistance to the anti-proliferative effect of radiation on human monocytes. Interestingly, Teresa Pinto et al. reported that irradiated (200 rad/fraction/day for a week) human monocyte-derived macrophages remained viable and metabolically active, and increased Bcl-xL expression evidenced the promotion of pro-survival activity [49]. It would be interesting to assess the potential role of SPION in macrophage longevity in this experimental model.

Furthermore, we investigated the cytokine production by human monocytes and macrophages treated with ferumoxytol and radiation. The pattern of altered cytokine expression did not allow for a conclusion about a definite pro- or anti-inflammatory phenotypic polarization of treated cells, which was not a surprising finding based on previously published contradicting data. Our observation of the absence of strong pro-inflammatory polarization of monocytes loaded with iron nanoparticles agrees with Raynal et al. who reported that uptake of even high concentrations of SPION (ferumoxide or ferumoxtran-10) by activated THP-1 cells caused a very low IL-1 expression [53]. However, Laskar et al. reported that SPION induced a phenotypic shift in THP-1-derived M2 macrophages towards a high CD86+ and high TNF-α+ macrophage subtype [25]. Nonetheless, irradiation of human monocyte-derived macrophages with 200, 600, or 1000 rad has been reported to result in reduced expression of anti-inflammatory genes [49]. Because of the visual increase in pro-inflammatory macrophage markers CD80, CD86, and HLA-DR, but not TNF-α and IL-1β after 1000 rad cumulative doses, with downregulated anti-inflammatory markers and IL-10 expression, the authors concluded about the modulation towards a more pro-inflammatory phenotype. Interestingly, we observed that preloading of THP-1-derived macrophages with ferumoxytol downregulated the expression of HLA-DR and upregulated the expression of CD86. The most interesting observation is that radiation may augment both of these pathways.

Here It is important to understand that multiple controversies between published data can be explained by other results demonstrating that different types of SPION particles display differential effects on macrophages due to their size, polarity, cover layers, and cytotoxic properties [48,54,55]. Next, the uptake and effect of SPION particles also depend on the subset of monocytes and macrophages used for evaluation, including their state of activation and polarization, culture conditions, source, and species [25,27,28,56]. Similarly, the alteration of monocytes and macrophages under irradiation conditions also depends on the type of radiation, accumulative dose, radiation schedule, and type of cells used for the assay [49,52,57,58]. Additional evaluation of ferumoxytol and radiation combination on primary human monocytes and macrophages harvested from healthy donors and patients with different diseases is needed to confirm our initial experience.

In conclusion, we have demonstrated that ferumoxytol, in addition to being an FDA-approved iron oxide nanoparticle agent for the treatment of iron-deficiency anemia, possesses unique radiomodulating effects on human monocytes and macrophages irradiated within therapeutically relevant doses of gamma radiation. Ferumoxytol affected both human monocytes and macrophages, increased the resistance of monocytes to radiation-induced cell death, alleviated inhibition of cell activity, and supported the anti-inflammatory phenotype of human macrophages under clinically relevant doses of radiation. Its effect on human monocytes depended on the duration of iron particle uptake and was radiation dose-dependent. In future studies, we expect to investigate the radiomodulating effects of ferumoxytol on primary human monocytes and Kupffer cells, focusing on the analysis of how SPION-preloaded macrophages regulate the viability and function of primary human hepatocytes within the normal liver, in the presence of tumors, and under cirrhotic microenvironments in vitro and in vivo. These studies will further investigate the diagnostic and therapeutic properties of ferumoxytol and provide new insight into the limitations and emerging applications of SPIONs in biomedicine.

Author Contributions: M.R.S., G.V.S. and A.V.K. designed the study. G.V.S. and V.A.K. performed all experiments. G.V.S. and M.R.S. analyzed experimental data and designed the figures. D.L., A.V.K. and M.R.S. developed the theoretical framework. M.R.S., G.V.S. and C.C. drafted the manuscript with input from all authors. C.C., V.A.K. and D.L. edited the initial and final version of the manuscript. M.R.S. supervised the project and oversaw overall direction and planning. All authors provided critical feedback and helped shape the research, analysis, and manuscript preparation. All authors have read and agreed to the published version of the manuscript.

Funding: This work was supported by the Elekta Research Grant, Department of Pathology, University of Pittsburgh Medical Center, and Allegheny-Singer Research Institute, Pittsburgh, PA, USA.

Institutional Review Board Statement: Not applicable.

Informed Consent Statement: Not applicable.

Data Availability Statement: The original contributions presented in the study are included in the article, further inquiries can be directed to the corresponding author(s).

Conflicts of Interest: The authors declare that the research was conducted in the absence of any commercial or financial relationships that could be construed as a potential conflict of interest. The authors are accountable for all aspects of the work in ensuring that questions related to the accuracy or integrity of any part of the work are appropriately investigated and resolved.

References

1. El-Serag, H.B.; Rudolph, K.L. Hepatocellular carcinoma: Epidemiology and molecular carcinogenesis. *Gastroenterology* **2007**, *132*, 2557–2576. [CrossRef] [PubMed]
2. Siegel, R.L.; Miller, K.D.; Wagle, N.S.; Jemal, A. Cancer statistics, 2023. *CA Cancer J. Clin.* **2023**, *73*, 17–48. [CrossRef]
3. O'Leary, J.G.; Landaverde, C.; Jennings, L.; Goldstein, R.M.; Davis, G.L. Patients with NASH and cryptogenic cirrhosis are less likely than those with hepatitis C to receive liver transplants. *Clin. Gastroenterol. Hepatol.* **2011**, *9*, 700–704.e1. [CrossRef] [PubMed]
4. Ascha, M.S.; Hanouneh, I.A.; Lopez, R.; Tamimi, T.A.; Feldstein, A.F.; Zein, N.N. The incidence and risk factors of hepatocellular carcinoma in patients with nonalcoholic steatohepatitis. *Hepatology* **2010**, *51*, 1972–1978. [CrossRef] [PubMed]
5. Minagawa, M.; Ikai, I.; Matsuyama, Y.; Yamaoka, Y.; Makuuchi, M. Staging of hepatocellular carcinoma: Assessment of the Japanese TNM and AJCC/UICC TNM systems in a cohort of 13,772 patients in Japan. *Ann. Surg.* **2007**, *245*, 909–922. [CrossRef]
6. Makuuchi, M.; Sano, K. The surgical approach to HCC: Our progress and results in Japan. *Liver Transplant.* **2004**, *10*, S46–S52. [CrossRef]
7. Fortune, B.E.; Umman, V.; Gilliland, T.; Emre, S. Liver transplantation for hepatocellular carcinoma: A surgical perspective. *J. Clin. Gastroenterol.* **2013**, *47*, S37–S42. [CrossRef]
8. Yao, F.Y.; Bass, N.M.; Nikolai, B.; Davern, T.J.; Kerlan, R.; Wu, V.; Ascher, N.L.; Roberts, J.P. Liver transplantation for hepatocellular carcinoma: Analysis of survival according to the intention-to-treat principle and dropout from the waiting list. *Liver Transplant.* **2002**, *8*, 873–883. [CrossRef]
9. Maddala, Y.K.; Stadheim, L.; Andrews, J.C.; Burgart, L.J.; Rosen, C.B.; Kremers, W.K.; Gores, G. Drop-out rates of patients with hepatocellular cancer listed for liver transplantation: Outcome with chemoembolization. *Liver Transplant.* **2004**, *10*, 449–455. [CrossRef]
10. Decaens, T.; Roudot-Thoraval, F.; Hadni-Bresson, S.; Meyer, C.; Gugenheim, J.; Durand, F.; Bernard, P.H.; Boillot, O.; Sulpice, L.; Calmus, Y.; et al. Impact of UCSF criteria according to pre- and post-OLT tumor features: Analysis of 479 patients listed for HCC with a short waiting time. *Liver Transplant.* **2006**, *12*, 1761–1769. [CrossRef]
11. Rusthoven, K.E.; Kavanagh, B.D.; Cardenes, H.; Stieber, V.W.; Burri, S.H.; Feigenberg, S.J.; Chidel, M.A.; Pugh, T.J.; Franklin, W.; Kane, M.; et al. Multi-institutional phase I/II trial of stereotactic body radiation therapy for liver metastases. *J. Clin. Oncol.* **2009**, *27*, 1572–1578. [CrossRef] [PubMed]
12. Safavi, A.H.; Dawson, L.A.; Mesci, A. Do We Have a Winner? Advocating for SBRT in HCC Management. *Clin. Transl. Radiat. Oncol.* **2024**, *45*, 100740. [CrossRef] [PubMed]
13. Kirichenko, A.; Gayou, O.; Parda, D.; Kudithipudi, V.; Tom, K.; Khan, A.; Abrams, P.; Szramowski, M.; Oliva, J.; Monga, D.; et al. Stereotactic body radiotherapy (SBRT) with or without surgery for primary and metastatic liver tumors. *HPB* **2016**, *18*, 88–97. [CrossRef] [PubMed]
14. Cardenes, H.R.; Price, T.R.; Perkins, S.M.; Maluccio, M.; Kwo, P.; Breen, T.E.; Henderson, M.A.; Schefter, T.E.; Tudor, K.; Deluca, J.; et al. Phase I feasibility trial of stereotactic body radiation therapy for primary hepatocellular carcinoma. *Clin. Transl. Oncol.* **2010**, *12*, 218–225. [CrossRef] [PubMed]
15. Uemura, N.; Yagi, H.; Uemura, M.T.; Hatanaka, Y.; Yamakado, H.; Takahashi, R. Inoculation of alpha-synuclein preformed fibrils into the mouse gastrointestinal tract induces Lewy body-like aggregates in the brainstem via the vagus nerve. *Mol. Neurodegener.* **2018**, *13*, 21. [CrossRef] [PubMed]

16. Gayou, O.; Day, E.; Mohammadi, S.; Kirichenko, A. A method for registration of single photon emission computed tomography (SPECT) and computed tomography (CT) images for liver stereotactic radiotherapy (SRT). *Med. Phys.* **2012**, *39*, 7398–7401. [CrossRef]
17. Rodríguez, M.R.; Chen-Zhao, X.; Hernando, O.; Flamarique, S.; Fernández-Letón, P.; Campo, M.; López, M.; Zucca, D.; Martínez, D.; Sánchez-Saugar, E.; et al. SBRT-SG-01: Final results of a prospective multicenter study on stereotactic body radiotherapy for liver metastases. *Clin. Transl. Oncol.* **2024**, *Online ahead of print*. [CrossRef] [PubMed]
18. Si, G.; Du, Y.; Tang, P.; Ma, G.; Jia, Z.; Zhou, X.; Mu, D.; Shen, Y.; Lu, Y.; Mao, Y.; et al. Unveiling the next generation of MRI contrast agents: Current insights and perspectives on ferumoxytol-enhanced MRI. *Natl. Sci. Rev.* **2024**, *2024*, nwae057. [CrossRef]
19. Bae, S.H.; Chun, S.-J.; Chung, J.-H.; Kim, E.; Kang, J.-K.; Jang, W.I.; Moon, J.E.; Roquette, I.; Mirabel, X.; Kimura, T.; et al. Stereotactic Body Radiation Therapy for Hepatocellular Carcinoma: Meta-Analysis and International Stereotactic Radiosurgery Society Practice Guidelines. *Int. J. Radiat. Oncol. Biol. Phys.* **2024**, *118*, 337–351. [CrossRef]
20. Smith, L.; Byrne, H.L.; Waddington, D.; Kuncic, Z. Nanoparticles for MRI-guided radiation therapy: A review. *Cancer Nano* **2022**, *13*, 38. [CrossRef]
21. Long, M.; Li, Y.; He, H.; Gu, N. The Story of Ferumoxytol: Synthesis Production, Current Clinical Applications, and Therapeutic Potential. *Adv. Healthc. Mater.* **2023**, *13*, e2302773. [CrossRef] [PubMed]
22. Daldrup-Link, H.E. Ten Things You Might Not Know about Iron Oxide Nanoparticles. *Radiology* **2017**, *284*, 616–629. [CrossRef]
23. Takamatsu, S.; Kozaka, K.; Kobayashi, S.; Yoneda, N.; Yoshida, K.; Inoue, D.; Kitao, A.; Ogi, T.; Minami, T.; Kouda, W.; et al. Pathology and images of radiation-induced hepatitis: A review article. *Jpn. J. Radiol.* **2018**, *36*, 241–256. [CrossRef]
24. Zhang, W.; Cao, S.; Liang, S.; Tan, C.H.; Luo, B.; Xu, X.; Saw, P.E. Differently Charged Super-Paramagnetic Iron Oxide Nanoparticles Preferentially Induced M1-Like Phenotype of Macrophages. *Front. Bioeng. Biotechnol.* **2020**, *8*, 537. [CrossRef]
25. Laskar, A.; Eilertsen, J.; Li, W.; Yuan, X.M. SPION primes THP1 derived M2 macrophages towards M1-like macrophages. *Biochem. Biophys. Res. Commun.* **2013**, *441*, 737–742. [CrossRef]
26. Sharkey, J.; Starkey Lewis, P.J.; Barrow, M.; Alwahsh, S.M.; Noble, J.; Livingstone, E.; Lennen, R.J.; Jansen, M.A.; Carrion, J.G.; Liptrott, N.; et al. Functionalized superparamagnetic iron oxide nanoparticles provide highly efficient iron-labeling in macrophages for magnetic resonance-based detection in vivo. *Cytotherapy* **2017**, *19*, 555–569. [CrossRef]
27. Rojas, J.M.; Sanz-Ortega, L.; Mulens-Arias, V.; Gutiérrez, L.; Pérez-Yagüe, S.; Barber, D.F. Superparamagnetic iron oxide nanoparticle uptake alters M2 macrophage phenotype, iron metabolism, migration and invasion. *Nanomed. Nanotechnol. Biol. Med.* **2016**, *12*, 1127–1138. [CrossRef]
28. Xu, Y.; Li, Y.; Liu, X.; Pan, Y.; Sun, Z.; Xue, Y.; Wang, T.; Dou, H.; Hou, Y. SPIONs enhances IL-10-producing macrophages to relieve sepsis via Cav1-Notch1/HES1-mediated autophagy. *Int. J. Nanomed.* **2019**, *14*, 6779–6797. [CrossRef]
29. Zanganeh, S.; Hutter, G.; Spitler, R.; Lenkov, O.; Mahmoudi, M.; Shaw, A.; Pajarinen, J.S.; Nejadnik, H.; Goodman, S.; Moseley, M.; et al. Iron oxide nanoparticles inhibit tumour growth by inducing pro-inflammatory macrophage polarization in tumour tissues. *Nat. Nanotechnol.* **2016**, *11*, 986–994. [CrossRef]
30. Huang, Y.; Hsu, J.C.; Koo, H.; Cormode, D.P. Repurposing ferumoxytol: Diagnostic and therapeutic applications of an FDA-approved nanoparticle. *Theranostics* **2022**, *12*, 796–816. [CrossRef]
31. Tsuchiya, S.; Yamabe, M.; Yamaguchi, Y.; Kobayashi, Y.; Konno, T.; Tada, K. Establishment and characterization of a human acute monocytic leukemia cell line (THP-1). *Int. J. Cancer* **1980**, *26*, 171–176. [CrossRef] [PubMed]
32. Corot, C.; Robert, P.; Idée, J.-M.; Port, M. Recent advances in iron oxide nanocrystal technology for medical imaging. *Adv. Drug Deliv. Rev.* **2006**, *58*, 1471–1504. [CrossRef] [PubMed]
33. Zhao, J.; Zhang, Z.; Xue, Y.; Wang, G.; Cheng, Y.; Pan, Y.; Zhao, S.; Hou, Y. Anti-tumor macrophages activated by ferumoxytol combined or surface-functionalized with the TLR3 agonist poly (I: C) promote melanoma regression. *Theranostics* **2018**, *8*, 6307–6321. [CrossRef] [PubMed]
34. Ariza de Schellenberger, A.; Poller, W.C.; Stangl, V.; Landmesser, U.; Schellenberger, E. Macrophage uptake switches on OCT contrast of superparamagnetic nanoparticles for imaging of atherosclerotic plaques. *Int. J. Nanomed.* **2018**, *13*, 7905–7913. [CrossRef] [PubMed]
35. Wang, G.; Serkova, N.J.; Groman, E.V.; Scheinman, R.I.; Simberg, D. Feraheme (Ferumoxytol) Is Recognized by Proinflammatory and Anti-inflammatory Macrophages via Scavenger Receptor Type AI/II. *Mol. Pharm.* **2019**, *16*, 4274–4281. [CrossRef] [PubMed]
36. Sakashita, M.; Nangaku, M. Ferumoxytol: An emerging therapeutic for iron deficiency anemia. *Expert Opin. Pharmacother.* **2023**, *24*, 171–175. [CrossRef] [PubMed]
37. Ding, Y.; Zhu, X.; Li, X.; Zhang, H.; Wu, M.; Liu, J.; Palmen, M.; Roubert, B.; Li, C. Pharmacokinetic, Pharmacodynamic, and Safety Profiles of Ferric Carboxymaltose in Chinese Patients with Iron-deficiency Anemia. *Clin. Ther.* **2020**, *42*, 276–285. [CrossRef] [PubMed]
38. Alam, S.R.; Stirrat, C.; Richards, J.; Mirsadraee, S.; Semple, S.I.; Tse, G.; Henriksen, P.; Newby, D.E. Vascular and plaque imaging with ultrasmall superparamagnetic particles of iron oxide. *J. Cardiovasc. Magn. Reson.* **2015**, *17*, 83. [CrossRef]
39. Toth, G.B.; Varallyay, C.G.; Horvath, A.; Bashir, M.R.; Choyke, P.L.; Daldrup-Link, H.E.; Dosa, E.; Finn, J.P.; Gahramanov, S.; Harisinghani, M.; et al. Current and potential imaging applications of ferumoxytol for magnetic resonance imaging. *Kidney Int.* **2017**, *92*, 47–66. [CrossRef]

40. Mikhalkevich, N.; O'Carroll, I.P.; Tkavc, R.; Lund, K.; Sukumar, G.; Dalgard, C.L.; Johnson, K.R.; Li, W.; Wang, T.; Nath, A.; et al. Response of human macrophages to gamma radiation is mediated via expression of endogenous retroviruses. *PLoS Pathog.* **2021**, *17*, e1009305. [CrossRef]
41. Carney, B.W.; Gholami, S.; Fananapazir, G.; Sekhon, S.; Lamba, R.; Loehfelm, T.W.; Wilson, M.D.; Corwin, M.T. Utility of combined gadoxetic acid and ferumoxytol-enhanced liver MRI for preoperative detection of colorectal cancer liver metastases: A pilot study. *Acta Radiol.* **2023**, *64*, 1357–1362. [CrossRef] [PubMed]
42. Tonan, T.; Fujimoto, K.; Qayyum, A.; Morita, Y.; Nakashima, O.; Ono, N.; Kawahara, A.; Kage, M.; Hayabuchi, N.; Ueno, T. CD14 expression and Kupffer cell dysfunction in non-alcoholic steatohepatitis: Superparamagnetic iron oxide-magnetic resonance image and pathologic correlation. *J. Gastroenterol. Hepatol.* **2012**, *27*, 789–796. [CrossRef] [PubMed]
43. Maurea, S.; Mainenti, P.P.; Tambasco, A.; Imbriaco, M.; Mollica, C.; Laccetti, E.; Camera, L.; Liuzzi, R.; Salvatore, M. Diagnostic accuracy of MR imaging to identify and characterize focal liver lesions: Comparison between gadolinium and superparamagnetic iron oxide contrast media. *Quant. Imaging Med. Surg.* **2014**, *4*, 181–189. [CrossRef] [PubMed]
44. Serkova, N.J. Nanoparticle-Based Magnetic Resonance Imaging on Tumor-Associated Macrophages and Inflammation. *Front. Immunol.* **2017**, *8*, 590. [CrossRef] [PubMed]
45. Li, K.; Lu, L.; Xue, C.; Liu, J.; He, Y.; Zhou, J.; Xia, Z.; Dai, L.; Luo, Z.; Mao, Y.; et al. Polarization of tumor-associated macrophage phenotype via porous hollow iron nanoparticles for tumor immunotherapy in vivo. *Nanoscale* **2020**, *12*, 130–144. [CrossRef] [PubMed]
46. Korangath, P.; Barnett, J.D.; Sharma, A.; Henderson, E.T.; Stewart, J.; Yu, S.H.; Kandala, S.K.; Yang, C.T.; Caserto, J.S.; Hedayati, M.; et al. Nanoparticle interactions with immune cells dominate tumor retention and induce T cell-mediated tumor suppression in models of breast cancer. *Sci. Adv.* **2020**, *6*, eaay1601. [CrossRef] [PubMed]
47. Xue, Y.; Xu, Y.; Liu, X.; Sun, Z.; Pan, Y.; Lu, X.; Liang, H.; Dou, H.; Hou, Y. Ferumoxytol Attenuates the Function of MDSCs to Ameliorate LPS-Induced Immunosuppression in Sepsis. *Nanoscale Res. Lett.* **2019**, *14*, 379. [CrossRef] [PubMed]
48. Vangijzegem, T.; Lecomte, V.; Ternad, I.; Van Leuven, L.; Muller, R.N.; Stanicki, D.; Laurent, S. Superparamagnetic Iron Oxide Nanoparticles (SPION): From Fundamentals to State-of-the-Art Innovative Applications for Cancer Therapy. *Pharmaceutics* **2023**, *15*, 236. [CrossRef]
49. Teresa Pinto, A.; Laranjeiro Pinto, M.; Patrícia Cardoso, A.; Monteiro, C.; Teixeira Pinto, M.; Filipe Maia, A.; Castro, P.; Figueira, R.; Monteiro, A.; Marques, M.; et al. Ionizing radiation modulates human macrophages towards a pro-inflammatory phenotype preserving their pro-invasive and pro-angiogenic capacities. *Sci. Rep.* **2016**, *6*, 18765. [CrossRef]
50. Beach, C.; MacLean, D.; Majorova, D.; Arnold, J.N.; Olcina, M.M. The effects of radiation therapy on the macrophage response in cancer. *Front. Oncol.* **2022**, *12*, 1020606. [CrossRef]
51. Wu, C.; Shen, Z.; Lu, Y.; Sun, F.; Shi, H. p53 Promotes Ferroptosis in Macrophages Treated with Fe(3)O(4) Nanoparticles. *ACS Appl. Mater. Interfaces* **2022**, *14*, 42791–42803. [CrossRef] [PubMed]
52. Sadhu, S.; Decker, C.; Sansbury, B.E.; Marinello, M.; Seyfried, A.; Howard, J.; Mori, M.; Hosseini, Z.; Arunachalam, T.; Finn, A.V.; et al. Radiation-Induced Macrophage Senescence Impairs Resolution Programs and Drives Cardiovascular Inflammation. *J. Immunol.* **2021**, *207*, 1812–1823. [CrossRef] [PubMed]
53. Raynal, I.; Prigent, P.; Peyramaure, S.; Najid, A.; Rebuzzi, C.; Corot, C. Macrophage endocytosis of superparamagnetic iron oxide nanoparticles: Mechanisms and comparison of ferumoxides and ferumoxtran-10. *Investig. Radiol.* **2004**, *39*, 56–63. [CrossRef] [PubMed]
54. Dulińska-Litewka, J.; Łazarczyk, A.; Hałubiec, P.; Szafrański, O.; Karnas, K.; Karewicz, A. Superparamagnetic Iron Oxide Nanoparticles-Current and Prospective Medical Applications. *Materials* **2019**, *12*, 617. [CrossRef] [PubMed]
55. Friedrich, B.; Auger, J.P.; Dutz, S.; Cicha, I.; Schreiber, E.; Band, J.; Boccacccini, A.R.; Krönke, G.; Alexiou, C.; Tietze, R. Hydroxyapatite-Coated SPIONs and Their Influence on Cytokine Release. *Int. J. Mol. Sci.* **2021**, *22*, 4143. [CrossRef]
56. Su, L.; Dong, Y.; Wang, Y.; Wang, Y.; Guan, B.; Lu, Y.; Wu, J.; Wang, X.; Li, D.; Meng, A.; et al. Potential role of senescent macrophages in radiation-induced pulmonary fibrosis. *Cell Death Dis.* **2021**, *12*, 527. [CrossRef] [PubMed]
57. Heylmann, D.; Rödel, F.; Kindler, T.; Kaina, B. Radiation sensitivity of human and murine peripheral blood lymphocytes, stem and progenitor cells. *Biochim. Biophys. Acta* **2014**, *1846*, 121–129. [CrossRef]
58. Zhou, Y.J.; Tang, Y.; Liu, S.J.; Zeng, P.H.; Qu, L.; Jing, Q.C.; Yin, W.J. Radiation-induced liver disease: Beyond DNA damage. *Cell Cycle* **2022**, *22*, 506–526. [CrossRef]

Disclaimer/Publisher's Note: The statements, opinions and data contained in all publications are solely those of the individual author(s) and contributor(s) and not of MDPI and/or the editor(s). MDPI and/or the editor(s) disclaim responsibility for any injury to people or property resulting from any ideas, methods, instructions or products referred to in the content.

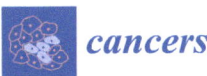

Article

Daily Diagnostic Quality Computed Tomography-on-Rails (CTOR) Image Guidance for Abdominal Stereotactic Body Radiation Therapy (SBRT)

Rachael M. Martin-Paulpeter [1,*], P. James Jensen [1], Luis A. Perles [1], Gabriel O. Sawakuchi [1], Prajnan Das [2], Eugene J. Koay [2], Albert C. Koong [2], Ethan B. Ludmir [2], Joshua S. Niedzielski [1] and Sam Beddar [1,*]

[1] Department of Radiation Physics, The University of Texas MD Anderson Cancer Center, Houston, TX 77030, USA; laperles@mdanderson.org (L.A.P.)
[2] Department of Gastrointestinal Radiation Oncology, The University of Texas MD Anderson Cancer Center, Houston, TX 77030, USA
* Correspondence: rmmartin@mdanderson.org (R.M.M.-P.); abeddar@mdanderson.org (S.B.); Tel.: +1-346-228-5339 (R.M.M.-P.); +1-832-794-3349 (S.B.)

Simple Summary: Radiation therapy is becoming increasingly important in the treatment of liver and pancreatic tumors, particularly in situations where high doses of radiation can be delivered safely. However, there are several challenges to treating tumors in the abdomen, including poor visibility of the tumor and movements due to breathing and digestion. The typical imaging available at the time of treatment makes it difficult to see both the tumor and nearby portions of the digestive tract, which is particularly sensitive to radiation damage. This paper describes the workflow involved when using high-quality computed tomography imaging at the time of treatment, to ensure that the tumor is accurately targeted and normal tissues are avoided. This study shows that by using these images and the planned dose distribution, the dose to normal structures can be maintained below specified targets. With this technology and workflow, more patients can benefit from high-dose radiation treatment to the liver and pancreas.

Abstract: Background/Objectives: Stereotactic body radiation therapy (SBRT) for abdominal targets faces a variety of challenges, including motion caused by the respiration and digestion and a relatively poor level of contrast between the tumor and the surrounding tissues. Breath-hold treatments with computed tomography-on-rails (CTOR) image guidance is one way of addressing these challenges, allowing for both the tumor and normal tissues to be well-visualized. Using isodose lines (IDLs) from CT simulations as a guide, the anatomical information can be used to shift the alignment or trigger a replan, such that normal tissues receive acceptable doses of radiation. Methods: This study aims to describe the workflow involved when using CTOR for pancreas and liver SBRT and demonstrates its effectiveness through several case studies. Results: In these case studies, using the anatomical information gained through diagnostic-quality CT guidance to make slight adjustments to the alignment, resulted in reductions in the maximum dose to the stomach. Conclusions: High-quality imaging, such as CTOR, and the use of IDLs to estimate the doses to OARs, enable the safe delivery of SBRT, without the added complexity and resource commitment required by daily online adaptive planning.

Keywords: SBRT; liver; pancreas; CT; image guidance; motion management; CT-on-rails system

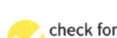

Citation: Martin-Paulpeter, R.M.; Jensen, P.J.; Perles, L.A.; Sawakuchi, G.O.; Das, P.; Koay, E.J.; Koong, A.C.; Ludmir, E.B.; Niedzielski, J.S.; Beddar, S. Daily Diagnostic Quality Computed Tomography-on-Rails (CTOR) Image Guidance for Abdominal Stereotactic Body Radiation Therapy (SBRT). *Cancers* **2024**, *16*, 3770. https://doi.org/10.3390/cancers16223770

Academic Editor: Dania Cioni

Received: 14 October 2024
Accepted: 6 November 2024
Published: 8 November 2024

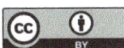

Copyright: © 2024 by the authors. Licensee MDPI, Basel, Switzerland. This article is an open access article distributed under the terms and conditions of the Creative Commons Attribution (CC BY) license (https://creativecommons.org/licenses/by/4.0/).

1. Introduction

Liver and pancreatic cancers are both challenging to treat, with poor overall prognoses. The overall survival benefit of radiation for pancreatic cancer [1–13] has been the subject of debate, partially due to the prevalence of distant failures and the use of less advanced radiation techniques in some studies. However, local control benefits have been observed, particularly with sufficient dose escalation. Additionally, radiation allows some patients with borderline resectable disease to become candidates for surgery. The role of radiation in liver cancer [14–19] is similarly the subject of debate, with local control benefits being observed, especially with dose escalation. The local control offered by radiation therapy in regard to both cancers becomes more relevant as improvements are made to systemic treatments. With sufficient care in avoiding organs at risk (OARs), stereotactic and other hypofractionated dose regimes that allow for dose escalation have become important tools for treating these diseases.

There are a number of challenges facing liver and pancreatic stereotactic body radiation therapy (SBRT) that can limit the ability to safely escalate the radiation dose if they are not addressed properly [20]. The first is intra-fraction motion, due to respiration and motility of gastrointestinal (GI) organs [21–25]. A number of strategies exist to address respiratory motion, including the breath-hold (BH) technique, abdominal compression, free breathing gating, and four-dimensional computed tomography (4DCT)-based motion margins [22,24,26,27]. Another type of motion that should be addressed is inter-fraction motion, caused by changes in the stomach and bowel related to stomach filling and intestinal gas [28]. These changes could cause sensitive GI structures to move closer to the treatment field than they were during simulation, either through organ or tumor motion, potentially resulting in unanticipated damage if not properly accounted for.

Another challenge in regard to the abdomen is the limited soft-tissue contrast, especially between the tumor and the surrounding normal tissue. Iodinated contrast media can be used during simulation to define the gross tumor volume (GTV) [29], but daily contrast injections during treatment require the dilution of the contrast agent and adds time and complexity to the treatment process [30]. Gas within the abdomen can cause streak artifacts in cone-beam computed tomography (CBCT) images, further compounding the visibility challenges. These artifacts are more pronounced in free-breathing CBCT images, but are often still present in breath-hold images. Advanced imaging, such as diagnostic-quality CT or MRI, can allow for sufficient gross tumor volume (GTV) and normal tissue visualization to ensure proper alignment with the target and avoidance of OARs [31–33]. Without advanced imaging, the treatment margins may need to be increased or fiducials put in place to ensure target coverage [34,35] and the prescriptions may need to be adjusted to ensure that OARs do not exceed the dose tolerance thresholds [36]. A comparison is shown in Figure 1 between diagnostic-quality CT used for alignment and CBCT. This article will focus on the technical aspects of the use of a CT-on-rails (CTOR) system [37–41], utilizing BH gating to address the challenges to delivering a high dose of radiation to the abdomen, allowing a safe level of dose escalation that ensures the dose constraints in regard to radiosensitive GI organs are met. This study aims to describe the workflow involved and demonstrate the benefits and potential pitfalls related to the use of this technology through several case studies.

Daily online adaptive planning has been shown to allow for improved target coverage, while maintaining normal tissue constraints [36,42–55]. However, online adaptive systems can be time consuming and resource intensive, generally requiring extensive medical physics and physician involvement during treatment [56,57]. Such systems can also add complexity, as they often require a separate treatment planning system (TPS) and may face challenges relating to interfacing with outside records and systems verification. While online adaptive planning is generally ideal when dealing with the abdomen, it may not be feasible to implement in all treatment centers or for all patient populations. Offline adaptation can be used, but may cause treatment delays and add complexity and require more personnel resources. Additionally, further changes to the patient's anatomy could again lead to OARs receiving higher doses of SBRT than expected. Offline adaptation is best employed when consistent changes in the anatomy are observed. Another strategy is to lower the prescription dose, such that the OARs will not receive a dose above the stipulated tolerance regardless of any anatomical changes. This decrease in treatment efficacy may be needed when OARs are not visible in the daily alignment images, due to image quality limitations. An intermediate solution is to use isodose line (IDL) contours, derived from the planning CT displayed on the daily image to identify and avoid any excessive doses to normal tissues. This strategy will be explored in this paper. A comparison of these strategies is presented in Table 1.

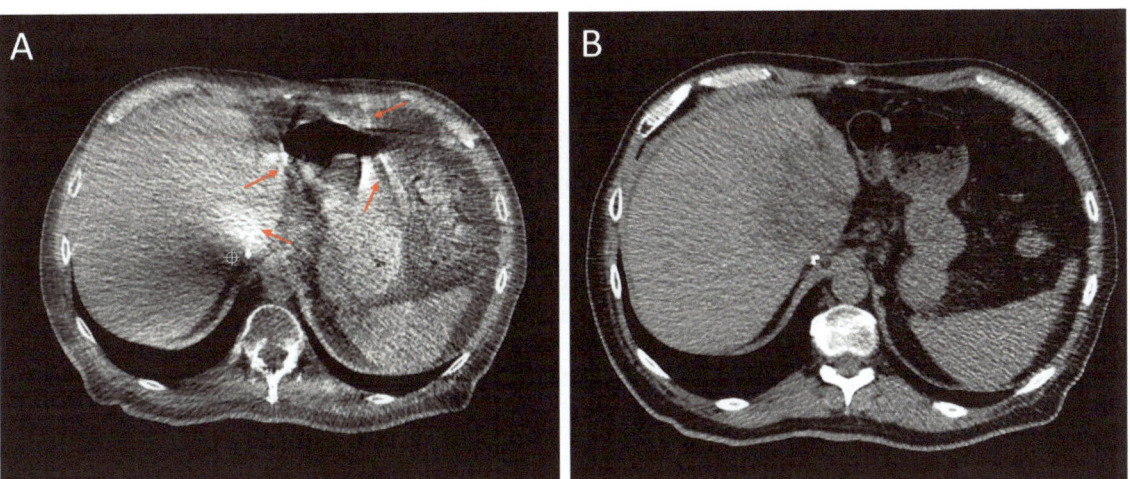

Figure 1. A comparison between (**A**) a BH CBCT image and (**B**) a BH CT-on-rails image of the same patient and anatomical location. Note the artifacts (red arrows) near the gas and high-density object in the CBCT image, which are not shown in the CTOR image. The boundaries of the stomach and bowel are also more clearly visualized in the CTOR image, compared to the CBCT image. Also visible in the CTOR image, are features within the liver itself.

Table 1. Relative comparison of methods used to avoid exceeding GI organ-at-risk (OAR) tolerance during the delivery of SBRT to the abdomen.

Approach	Risk to OARs	Treatment Efficacy	Complexity of Treatment	Physician Time Requirement	Requires High Quality Imaging
Lower prescription dose	low	low	low	low	no
Use IDLs to avoid OARs	med	med	low	med	yes
Offline adaptation	med	med	med	high	yes
Online adaptation	low	high	high	high	yes

Overall, this paper aims to demonstrate the workflow involved when using CTOR-based daily imaging and planning CT-based isodose contours to improve target alignment and normal tissue avoidance, during abdominal SBRT and hypofractionated treatments. After a description of the workflow steps, three case studies are presented to demonstrate the alignment improvements that are possible when using the daily CTOR system.

2. Methods and Materials

The protocol described in this section was approved by the University of Texas MD Anderson Cancer Center institutional review board (PA14-0646). MD Anderson Cancer Center has two CTOR treatment rooms, with beam-matched linacs and matched CTs. The vast majority of liver and pancreatic SBRT and hypofractionated treatments at our institution are conducted using these machines, while standard fractionated treatments generally use CBCT alignment. The patients presenting here were simulated using breath-hold (BH) image gating and CTOR image guidance. For patients receiving abdominal SBRT at our institution, BH is preferred for patients that can tolerate it. With this motion management technique, the motion of both the OARs and the tumor can be controlled, allowing for a larger portion of the tumor to be safely treated with a high dose. Inhalation BH is typically used, as it is generally easier for patients to understand the instructions, but exhalation BH is considered when it is dosimetrically favorable. For patients that cannot tolerate holding their breath repeatedly, 4DCT is used and an internal GTV (IGTV) is created. A compression belt is considered for patients who cannot hold their breath, but have large tumor motion.

2.1. Simulation

Patients are scanned using a Philips Big Bore CT scanner (Philips, Andover, MA, USA). To improve consistency in terms of the stomach-filling and bowel position, patients are instructed prior to the simulation not to eat or drink anything ("nil per os", abbreviated to NPO) for three hours before arriving and are given instructions on the appropriate diet and/or medications to manage gas. These preparations are maintained during the treatment to improve consistency. Patients are positioned in a long stereotactic cradle over a wingboard, with their hands above their heads, holding a T-bar. A Varian Medical Systems (Varian, Palo Alto, CA, USA) real-time position management (RPM) box is placed on the patient's abdomen and they are instructed to hold a comfortable breath multiple times, before a gating window is set centered on their natural breath-hold position. After establishing the baseline breath window, visual feedback goggles are used to assist the patient in consistently reproducing this breath-hold level. After a free-breathing scan, at least one breath-hold scan without contrast is acquired, followed by 3 or 4 scans with the use of iodinated intravenous (IV) contrast media. The contrast scans are started 30 s after contrast media injection and are acquired back-to-back to capture different contrast phases. A planning image is chosen based on the breath-hold position and contrast phase with the best tumor visualization.

If prior non-contrast imaging suggests that there will not be an anatomical landmark to align with, then fiducials may be implanted near the tumor prior to simulation [58–60]. However, generally the tumor itself or a surrogate structure can be visualized on daily non-contrast CT images, so the added risk involving implantation into the patient is avoided. Potential surrogate structures include blood vessels, fissures within the liver, cysts, or the edge of the liver.

2.2. Treatment Planning

To account for variations in the breath-hold position, an IGTV is contoured that includes the tumor position across all the breath-hold scans. A simultaneous integrated boost (SIB) approach is often utilized to allow for partial dose escalation, while protecting normal tissues [61,62]. The approach used at our institution is detailed in the work by Koay et al. [61] and is briefly described here. A PRV (planning OAR volume) expansion of 5 mm is added around all GI luminal structures and the heart. The high-dose planning target volume (PTV) is created as a margin around the IGTV subtracting the PRV and a lower dose PTV fills in the areas that have been carved out. Figure 2 demonstrates this technique in a patient, where their stomach and large bowel were close to the IGTV. Treatment planning is completed in RayStation, using the collapsed cone dose calculation algorithm. For OARs that have a maximum dose constraint, IDL contours are created and exported to be used during the alignment. The prescription dose levels are also exported as IDL contours.

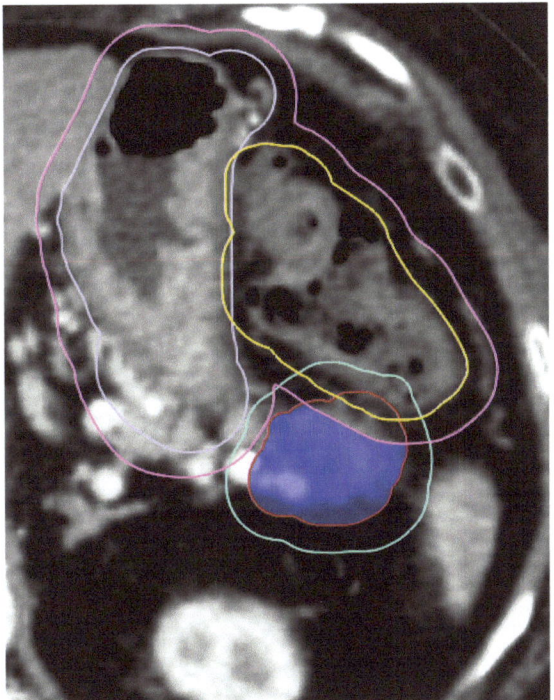

Figure 2. Example of an SIB approach to account for nearby radiosensitive OARs. In this case, the large bowel (orange) overlaps with the GTV (red) and the stomach (purple) is also close by. A GI PRV (pink) is created as an expansion of the GI luminal structures and is carved out from the high-dose PTV (shaded blue). An expanded low-dose PTV (teal) includes portions of the GTV that are not covered by the high-dose PTV.

2.3. Description of the CT-on-Rails System and Workflow

The CT-on-rails delivery system consists of a GE CT scanner on rails, a Varian Clinac 21EX linac, and a couch that can rotate 180 degrees between the linac position and the CT scanning position (Figure 3). The overall workflow used for SBRT in patients treated with CTOR alignment is shown in Figure 4. The SBRT patients are treated during 40 min time slots, with an extra 10 min added on the first day. The patient is initially set up with the couch in the linac position. After the patient's position within the cradle and rotation are verified in terms of free breathing, the patient is shifted to the final isocenter position. A gating window is set up, using the same window parameters as at the simulation (distance from normal breathing exhale to the bottom of the gating window and window width) and the patient is given feedback goggles to assist them in reaching the correct BH level. An RPM camera, attached to the end of the couch, is used so the camera is in the same position relative to the patient in both the linac and CT configurations. Radiopaque ball bearings (BBs) are placed on the patient when they are in the final isocenter position, while they are holding their breath, and are verified with a repeat BH. Since the CT and linac systems are separate systems, the BBs serve as the reference position in the CT scan to relate the coordinates back to the linac position. The initial couch coordinates are recorded and the patient is rotated into the CT position. A BH CT scan is then acquired with our GE LightSpeed 16 scanner (GE, Chicago, IL, USA), with a 0.98 × 0.98 mm^2 pixel size, a 2.5 mm slice thickness, a 0.5 s rotation time, a 50 cm field-of-view, 120 kVp, and 250–350 mA (depending on the patient's habitus and tumor contrast). Daily CT-on-rails images are aligned to the reference planning CT images using in-house software [63] (see next section), which calculates the final couch position from the inputted BB-aligned couch position. A rigid registration without rotation is performed, since the specialized rotating couch is not capable of 6 degrees-of-freedom motion. After image registration, the patient is rotated back to the treatment position and aligned to the BBs during a breath hold. The couch coordinates are compared to those initially recorded. A difference of 3 mm or more indicates that the patient has moved, which necessitates a repeat CT scan using the new BB position. Once the BB position is verified, the patient is shifted to the final couch position. Care is taken to verify the couch positions for multiple steps, since the manual entry of numbers is involved.

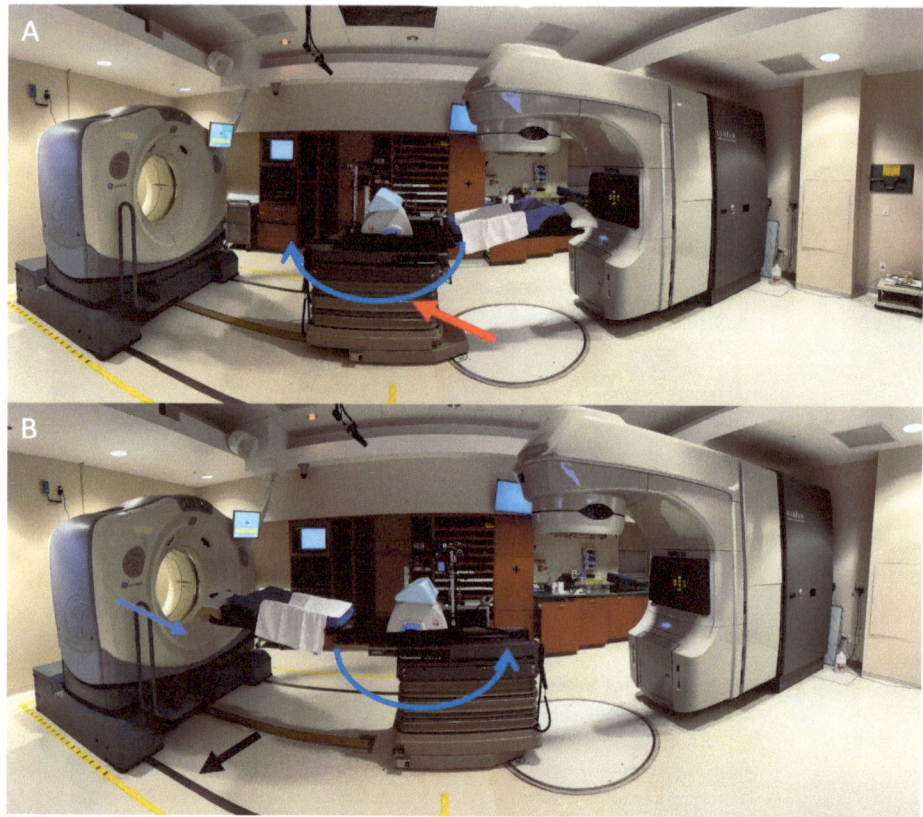

Figure 3. Photos of the CTOR–linac set up. First the patient is set up in the treatment position, with the couch positioned in the linac position (**A**) and BBs are placed in the laser positions. The base of the couch (red arrow) is then rotated 180° (curved blue arrows), according to the CT scanner position (**B**). The CT scanner moves along the rails on the floor (black arrow) in the direction of the straight blue arrow to take a scan. After image alignment, the patient is rotated back to the linac position and the lasers are aligned with the BBs. Final couch shifts are made from this position.

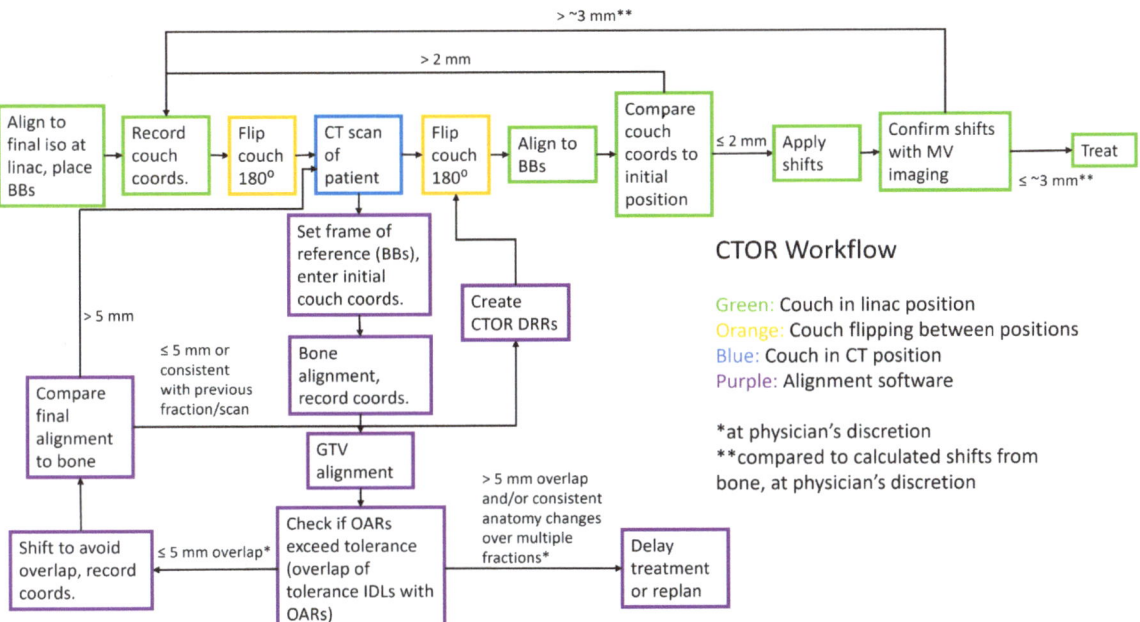

Figure 4. Flowchart of overall CTOR workflow (Section 2.3), including CTOR-based alignment and evaluation (Section 2.4) and verification imaging (Section 2.5).

2.4. CT-on-Rails-Based Alignment

Daily CTOR images are aligned to the reference planning CT images, using the in-house software. First, a reference point is set at the location of the BBs in the CT scan. The longitudinal and vertical position are determined using one or both lateral BBs and the lateral position is determined using the anterior BB. Next, an alignment to the vertebral bodies near the GTV is performed, as a reference for how the internal anatomy has changed relative to bone. Then, the GTV is aligned to the planning CT. Any shifts away from GTV alignment to avoid OARs exceeding the tolerance dose (discussed in more detail below) are now made, resulting in what will be called GTV* alignment for clarity. A comparison is then made between bone and the GTV* alignment, in the spirit of creating action levels for large anatomical variations, as suggested by AAPM's task group 101 on SBRT [64], and to help to detect outlier breath holds. If the difference between bone and the GTV* alignment is greater than 5 mm and the alignment is not consistent with previous fractions, subsequent CTOR images are acquired, until the GTV* position is consistent with the previous scan. If the patient's positioning is demonstrated to be inconsistent by four CTOR images, the treatment will be aborted for the day and possibly replanned. An example of the CTOR alignment workflow is shown in Figure 5.

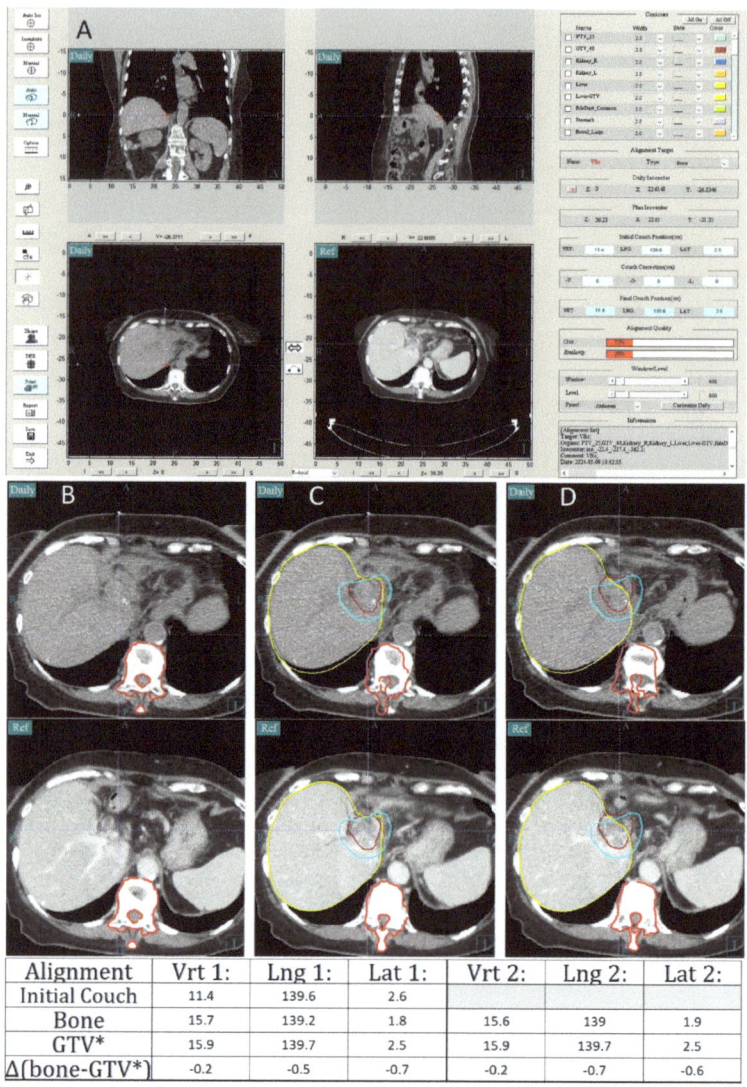

Figure 5. Example demonstrating the alignment workflow using in-house software for CTOR. A screenshot of the alignment software is shown in (**A**). As seen in (**A**), first the user aligns with the BBs to set the reference point and enters the initial couch positions, when the lasers were aligned to the BBs in the treatment position. Next, they align to the vertebral bodies (VBs) near the GTV, as shown in (**B**), with the daily CTOR image above and the CT simulation reference image below (red contour). Then, (**C**) they align to the GTV (dark red contour) and check that the desired IDL (teal contour) does not overlap with the relevant OARs. In this example, the difference between the bone alignment and GTV alignment is greater than 5 mm, as seen in alignment 1 in the chart at the bottom, so a second CTOR image is acquired. Again, the BB position is set and VB alignment is conducted, followed by GTV* alignment (**D**). The chart at the bottom of the figure shows the recorded couch positions (in cm) and differences between the bone and GTV* alignment for both scans. Since the differences between the bone and GTV* were within a few millimeters between the two scans, the couch positions from the second alignment were used as the treatment isocenter.

Despite a lack of contrast agents for daily imaging, the GTV or a surrogate can generally be visualized in the CTOR image. Fiducial markers can be inserted in more difficult cases, but are not generally needed with CTOR. For tumors of the pancreas, surrogates such as blood vessels and the pancreas shape can be used when the tumor itself is difficult to visualize (Figure 6). For tumors of the liver, surrogates such as the nearby liver shape, blood vessels, fissures, or cysts can be used, when there is not enough contrast to visualize the tumor (Figure 7). Changing the CT image's window and level can also help with visualizing the tumor itself (Figure 7). A window/level of 400/800 Hounsfield units (HU) is used for the visualization of organs at risk and 180/950 HU is used to visualize tumors and blood vessels in the liver. Prior to simulation, the physician should consider whether the tumor or a sufficient surrogate will be visible on non-contrast CT scans or whether fiducial markers should be inserted, using prior diagnostic non-contrast CT scans as a guide as to what should be visible when needed.

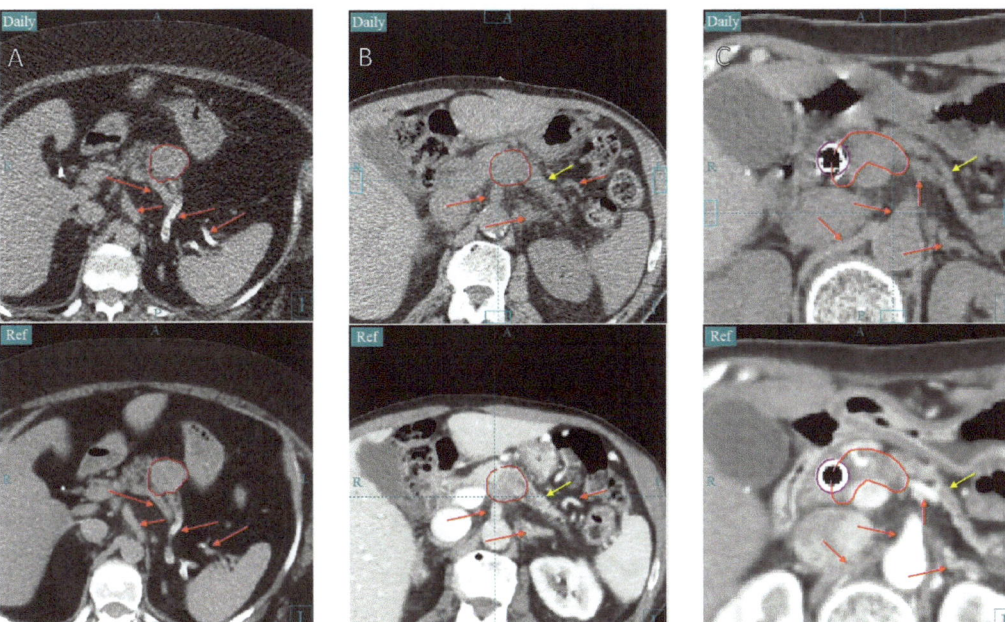

Figure 6. This figure demonstrates the ability to visualize with CTOR images the pancreas and the surrounding anatomy necessary to align with the GTV (red contour). The top row is the CTOR images and the bottom is the planning CT images. Comparing nearby blood vessels (red arrows) and the pancreas shape (yellow arrows) between the two images can be used to achieve good alignment in the superior–inferior direction, which is often the hardest, and can aide in the alignment in other directions as well. Calcifications within blood vessels (as seen in (**A,B**)) can also be a useful tool. Stents (purple contour in (**C**)) can be used to assist with alignment, but should be used with caution, as they may move relative to the tumor. The window/level for all the images is 400/800 HU.

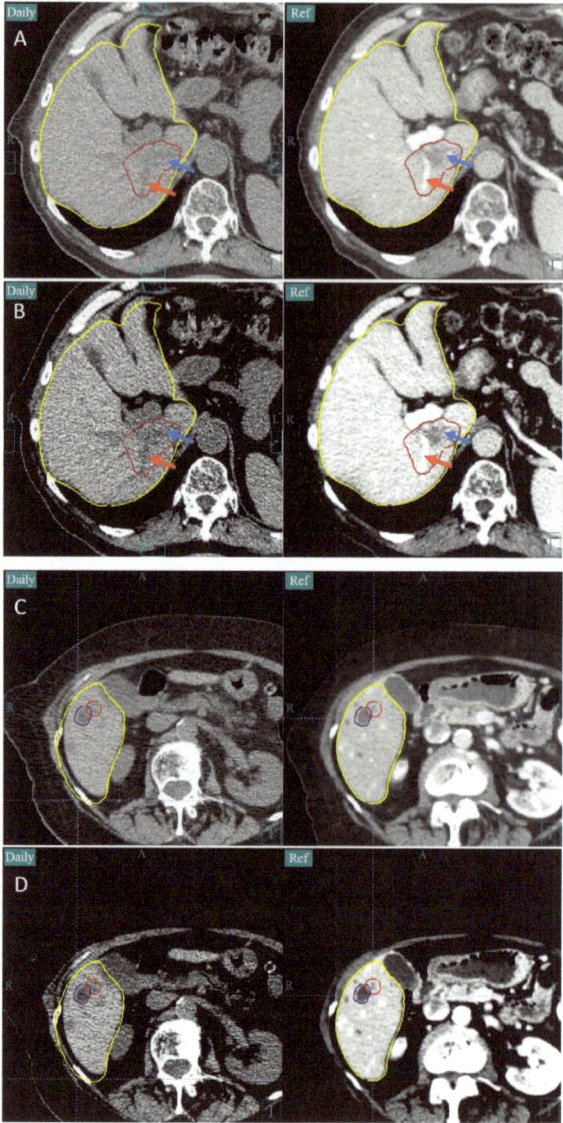

Figure 7. This figure demonstrates the ability to visualize the CTOR features within the liver necessary to accurately align with the GTV. In the left column are the CTOR images and in the right are the planning CT images. For the patient in (**A**), the liver shape (yellow contour), blood vessels, liver fissures in the vicinity of the tumor can be used to align to the GTV (red contour). Additionally, the tumor itself is somewhat visible (blue arrow), along with a blood vessel within the liver (red arrow). Using a different window and level (**B**) can improve the visualization of the tumor and interior blood vessel. In (**C**), the tumor itself is difficult to distinguish from normal liver, but a cyst (purple contour) right next to the tumor (red contour), along with the inferior liver shape, can be used to achieve accurate alignment. With a different window and level (**D**), the cyst becomes easier to distinguish and there is some distinction between the tumor and normal liver. In (**A**,**C**), a window level of 400/800 HU is used and, in (**B**,**D**), a window level of 180/950 HU is used.

To assist with alignment evaluation, isodose lines are created in the TPS on the planning CT and transferred to the alignment software. Isodose lines for the maximum dose constraints of the structures near the GTV are displayed after GTV alignment; the daily image is then checked for overlaps between the maximum dose constraint isodose contours and the associated OARs. Typically for SBRT (5 fractions), the goal is for less than 1 cm^3 of a given GI luminal structure to receive 35 Gy or higher, with a maximum of less than 40 Gy. However, these goals may vary depending on patient-specific factors, clinical trial enrollment, and anatomic consistency, among other factors. For slight overlaps (on the order of the PTV margin or smaller), the alignment can be shifted, such that the GTV contour is slightly misaligned in regard to the daily GTV position, but the IDL no longer overlaps the OAR. After slight GTV misalignment or for cases where the GTV is rotated or deformed relative to the simulation, sufficient GTV coverage can be evaluated using the prescription dose IDL. For larger overlaps, the treatment should be aborted and reattempted later in the day or the following day. For patients with repeated large overlaps, an adaptive plan could be created offline, using the daily CTOR image. Note that for the purpose of comparing bone to GTV alignment as described above, the final alignment (shifted slightly off GTV if needed for OAR sparing) is what is used (GTV*).

To demonstrate the appropriateness of using IDLs that were calculated on the planning CT and then transferred to the daily CT, the dose was recalculated in regard to the daily CTOR images for several patients and compared to the IDLs from the planning CT. Additionally, to demonstrate the appropriateness of shifting away from the GTV to satisfy maximum dose constraints related to the bowel, the dose was recalculated in regard to the daily CTOR images with and without this shift to compare GTV coverage and OAR doses. The results of these comparisons are detailed in Sections 3.2 and 3.3.

2.5. Verification Imaging

Prior to each treatment, orthogonal digitally reconstructed radiographs (DRRs) from the CTOR image are calculated as a reference for the expected bony anatomy position relative to the daily treatment isocenter. To verify that the patient has not moved and that shifts have been applied correctly, orthogonal MV images are acquired. Both the MV images and CTOR-derived DRRs are compared to the DRRs from the planning CT. The MV images are expected to have the same shifts (within a few millimeters at the physician's discretion) away from the bony anatomy alignment as is observed in the CTOR DRRs, which should numerically agree with the shifts between the bone and GTV alignment that were recorded during the alignment process. Any discrepancies warrant further investigation and likely a repeat of the CTOR scan in order to repeat the workflow.

3. Results

3.1. Case Study 1

The first case study focuses on the effects of changes in bowel gas between the simulation and treatment. This patient with adenocarcinoma of the pancreas received SBRT to the pancreas, with a dose of 40 Gy in five fractions. They had a sizeable gas bubble close to the GTV in their stomach during the simulation, which resolved itself for part of their treatment. The fraction with the most dramatic difference in terms of the gas is illustrated in Figure 8. When the dose is recalculated in regard to the daily CTOR image without the gas, a decrease in the target coverage is observed. The dose volume histogram (DVH) for the GTV is shifted to the left by 36 cGy for the single fraction, which would extrapolate out to a 180 cGy shift if the dose distribution was the same for all the fractions (as shown in Figure 8D). This example illustrates the importance of managing bowel gas and paying attention to large changes in gas between the simulation and treatment. Since previous treatments of this patient had involved gas levels that were similar to those that occurred during the simulation, this deviation was deemed acceptable. However, consistent changes in gas or a more dramatic change could warrant requiring the patient to return later to try again or for the application of a verification plan. In addition to unexpected loss of target coverage, the accuracy of the IDL contours used to evaluate OAR avoidance during alignment is of potential concern in similar cases. Large changes in gas near the tumor could result in changes to the IDL shape, which could result in unnecessary shifts away from GTV or higher than anticipated doses to the OARs. In this patient, the difference in the shapes of the lower dose IDLs was very small, so the OAR avoidance strategy was not changed. Noticeable unanticipated differences in doses to the targets and OARs can generally be avoided by being observant enough to notice changes in gas distribution during alignment, noting patterns in gas filling over multiple fractions when larger fractional changes are observed, and being aware of the limitations of using IDLs calculated from the simulation CT in these situations. Other solutions for mitigating the effects of gas include dietary restrictions and gas medications; overriding large, unexpected areas of gas in the planning CT with water; and delaying the treatment and recalculating the dose in regard to the daily CTOR image for verification. The amount of gas and the number of fractions affected was deemed small enough that overriding the gas and dose recalculation were not used in this case.

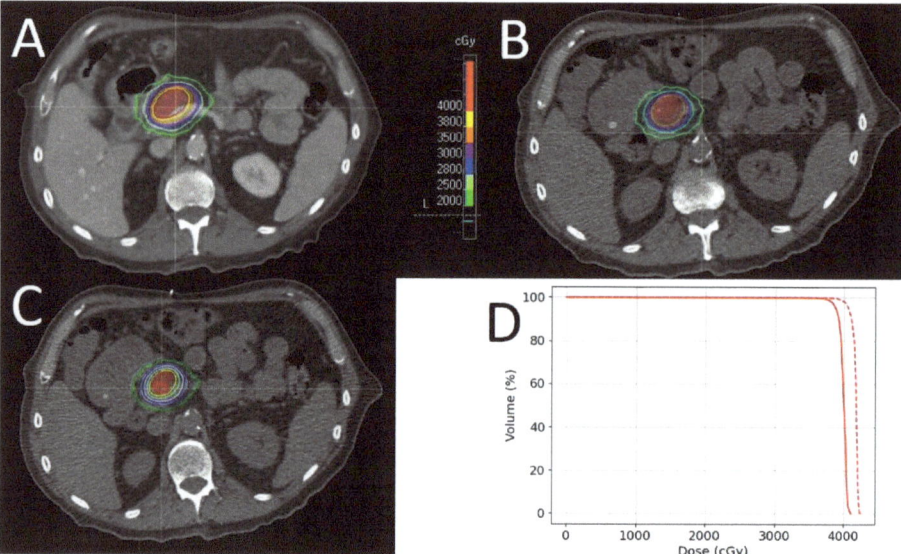

Figure 8. An example of the effect of gas bubbles on the planned vs. actual dose distribution. (**A**) Shows the treatment plan according to the simulation, with the GTV in red and various isodose levels shown; here, a large gas bubble is very close to the GTV. (**B**) Shows the day-of CTOR image with the original dose distribution, while (**C**) shows the day-of CTOR image with the dose recalculated to account for the now-absent gas bubble, showing a decrease in target coverage. (**D**) Shows the planned (dashed) vs. actual (solid) DVHs for the GTV for this fraction, extrapolated to five fractions, assuming the same dose is delivered to each fraction.

3.2. Case Study 2

The second case study examines pancreatic SBRT treatment, where anatomy changes near the target are present. This patient with adenocarcinoma of the pancreas received an SIB prescription of 50 Gy in five fractions, with a low-dose PTV prescription of 30 Gy in five fractions. The clinical goal for the duodenum (blue contour) and stomach (green contour) in regard to this treatment was V33 Gy < 0.5 cm^3. To ensure this goal was met, a 33 Gy IDL (orange contour) was sent to the alignment software from the treatment planning system. For three out of the five fractions, a small overlap between the 33 Gy IDL and the stomach or duodenum was noted. To meet the clinical goal for these OARs, the alignment was shifted away from perfect GTV alignment, until the IDL just skimmed the edge of the OAR. Figure 9 shows the fraction with the largest difference in the anatomy (black arrow) between the simulation (Figure 9A) and treatment (Figure 9B,C) CT scan. Using the GTV to align the simulation CT to the daily CT without accounting for the OARs would have resulted in a portion of the stomach receiving 33 Gy, as seen in Figure 8B. If this strategy were to be repeated for all the fractions, the total maximum dose to the stomach would have been 39.4 Gy, with 0.15 cm^3 receiving 33 Gy or higher (Figure 9D). However, by shifting the isocenter 3 mm laterally and 1 mm posteriorly, the 33 Gy IDL no longer overlaps with the stomach (Figure 9C). Using this strategy, the maximum dose to the stomach would be 37.7 Gy, with 0.13 cm^3 receiving 33 Gy or higher, with a modest, but clinically acceptable, drop in GTV coverage (D95% = 97.6%).

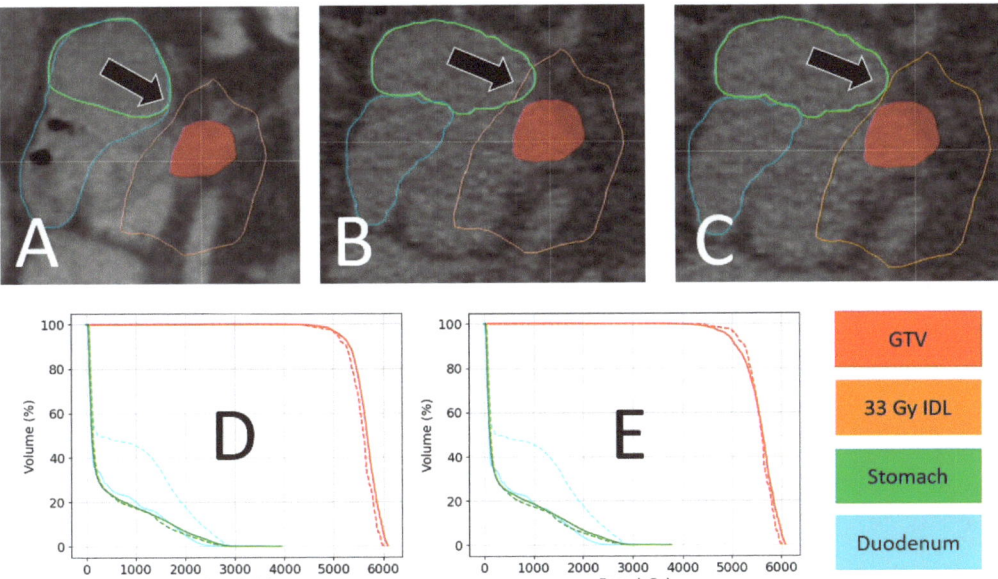

Figure 9. An example of pre-treatment shifting via CTOR. (**A**) Shows the treatment plan according to the simulation, with the GTV in red, stomach in green, duodenum in blue, and the 33 Gy isodose line in orange. Here, the plan was designed to stop 33 Gy from being received by the stomach and duodenum (acceptable within 0.5 cm^3). (**B**) Shows the day-of CTOR image, which indicates that the stomach would partially receive 33 Gy near the black arrow if nothing is done. (**C**) Shows the results of manually shifting the isocenter by 3 mm laterally and 1 mm posteriorly, causing the 33 Gy isodose line to stay away from the stomach. (**D**) Compares the DVHs of the planned and day-of GTV-aligned dose distributions as a sum of all the fractions (unshifted daily dose in solid lines, planned dose in dashed lines), while (**E**) compares the planned and day-of manually shifted dose distributions as a sum of all the fractions (shifted daily dose in solid lines, planned dose in dashed lines).

3.3. Case Study 3

The third case study looks at an example of a patient with a more dramatic difference in their anatomy between the simulation (Figure 10A) and treatment (Figure 10B,C) CT scans. This patient with adenocarcinoma of the pancreas received SBRT to the pancreas with a prescription of 36 Gy in five fractions, with a clinical goal being for the stomach and duodenum to be subject to a V33 Gy < 0.5 cm^3. For this patient, four out of five fractions required an isocenter shift to avoid the 33 Gy IDL overlapping the stomach. Aligning to the GTV and ignoring the IDL overlaps with the bowel would have resulted in total doses (Figure 10D) of 22.0 Gy and 35.7 Gy as the maximum dose and 0.0 cc and 0.41 cc > 33 Gy for the duodenum and stomach, respectively. Shifting the IDL away from the stomach, as in Figure 10C, results in total doses (Figure 10E) of 19.9 Gy and 34.9 Gy as the maximum dose and 0.0 cm^3 and 0.25 cm^3 > 33 Gy for the duodenum and stomach, respectively. The target coverage (D95%) in this case was reduced from 100 to 96.6%.

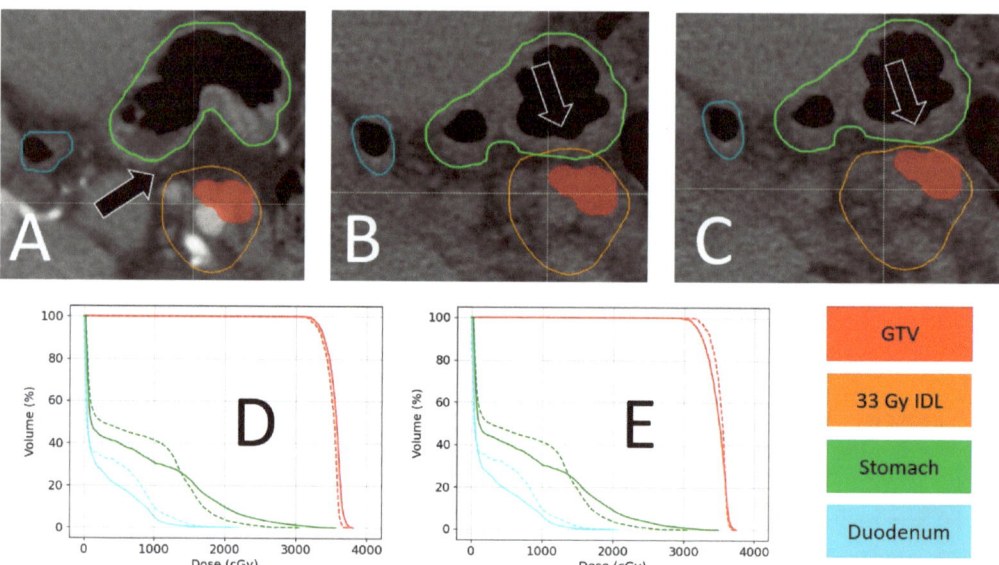

Figure 10. Example of pre-treatment shifting via CTOR. (**A**) Shows the treatment plan according to the simulation, with the GTV in red, stomach in green, duodenum in blue, and the 33 Gy isodose line in orange. Here, the plan was designed to stop 33 Gy from being received by the stomach and duodenum (acceptable within 0.5 cm^3). (**B**) Shows the day-of CTOR image, which indicates that the stomach partially receives 33 Gy near the black arrow. (**C**) Shows the results of manually shifting the isocenter by 0.3 cm laterally, 0.2 cm superiorly, and 0.4 cm posteriorly, causing the 33 Gy isodose line to stay away from the stomach. (**D**) Compares the DVHs of the planned and day-of GTV-aligned dose distributions as a sum of all the fractions (unshifted daily dose in solid lines, planned dose in dashed lines), while (**E**) compares the planned and day-of manually shifted dose distributions as a sum of all the fractions (shifted daily dose in solid lines, planned dose in dashed lines).

4. Discussion

This paper has described one approach to addressing the many challenges to safely delivering high doses of radiation to the abdomen and has demonstrated its validity in three patients. The high contrast and relatively low noise imaging of CT-based alignment allows for accurate GTV alignment and the evaluation of the OAR dose, based on planning CT IDLs. Slight adjustments to the alignment to avoid high doses of SBRT to OARs enable safe dose escalation, without the added complexity of daily adaptive treatments. In each of the patients examined, changes in their anatomy could lead to unexpectedly low target coverage (case 1) or unexpectedly high OAR doses (cases 2 and 3), if one were to rely solely on GTV alignment. These examples, as well as a number of more extensive studies, illustrate the consequences of treatment strategies that do not account for changing anatomy in the abdomen. With standard CBCT, it is not always possible to accurately evaluate the OAR positions due to image quality limitations, which emphasizes the importance of high-quality imaging, such as CTOR.

As is often the case in the abdomen, a balance must be struck between avoiding normal tissue toxicity and maximizing the dose to the tumor. It should be noted that the strategy discussed in this paper is conservative in terms of ensuring normal tissue sparing at the potential cost of GTV coverage. For each fraction, the assumption is that the fractional dose distribution will be the total dose distribution, even though on other days the OAR in question may be further away. It should be noted that in case studies 2 and 3, the total doses to the stomach and duodenum with GTV only alignment, while higher than with shifts away from the OARs, were still within the tolerance thresholds. However, without knowing the cumulative dose at the time of treatment, caution is warranted to ensure the tolerance thresholds are met. In the work by Niedzielski et. al., the author retrospectively calculated the cumulative dose in regard to CTOR images with simulated fiducial-only alignment, and three out of eleven patients had at least one OAR that exceeded the tolerance level [36]. While this strategy is necessarily conservative in sparing normal tissues, due to the seriousness of potential toxicity, clinical judgement should be used to ensure the proper balance is being met. Further study on the effects of alignment adjustments based on IDLs would be beneficial to better understand this tradeoff, as only two cases were examined closely in this study.

While a dosimetrically ideal solution would be to use daily online adaptive planning, the strategy demonstrated here involving the use of IDLs to shift away from OARs shows improved OAR doses with clinically acceptable overall decreases in the GTV dose compared to simply aligning with the GTV. Note that the patient case studies discussed here represent some of the larger changes seen in a patient's anatomy that were still treatable without adaptation, and that typically smaller shifts away from the GTV are observed. Online adaptive planning is time consuming and personnel resource intensive, decreasing the overall throughput and leaving less time for physicists and physicians to work on other tasks. In regard to this workflow, physicians are only required to review images (5 to 10 min), whereas with an online adaptive workflow, they would be required to perform or approve the contouring and revised plan as well. The added time between imaging and treatment with an online adaptive workflow increases the likelihood that the patient's internal anatomy will have shifted. Overall, the strategy presented here represents a good middle ground that can reduce the chances of overdosing OARs, without the added time required and complexity of online adaptive planning.

A limitation of using IDLs that are derived from simulation CT scans is that changes in the patient's anatomy could affect the dose distribution. Changes are particularly likely when large differences in the amount of gas are present, as in case 1. Caution should be used when these differences are observed and strategies, such as NPO instructions and gas reduction medications, should be employed to lessen the probability of them occurring. However, note that even in the patient with a noticeable difference in the amount of gas in their system and in the target coverage area, the lower dose IDLs were very similar to the simulation and were unlikely to impact the quality of the treatment if relied on. A more extensive study would be necessary to more quantitatively study this effect.

A key aspect of safely delivering high doses of SBRT to tumors that are close to GI luminal structures is sufficient image quality to be able to visualize both the GTV and the surrounding OARs, particularly at their borders. As can be seen from the CTOR images in this paper, this treatment modality has sufficient image quality to visualize both the targets (or nearby surrogates) and the OARs. Traditionally, artifacts and relatively poor contrast have made such visualization difficult in CBCT images, especially in larger patients or patients with implanted metal or excessive gas. However, improvements in CBCT imaging are closing the gap between diagnostic-quality CT and CBCT, potentially allowing for similar strategies to be applied to CBCT-based SBRT [65–69]. While the specialized technology described in this paper is of limited availability, the strategies acquired from our institution's extensive experience with CTOR and the methods described in this paper can help to lower the human expertise gap in implementing these commercially available products.

The motion management in terms of inhale BH gating with RPM-based motion tracking that is described in this paper should be understood as one of several valid options for dealing with respiratory motion. Other strategies include exhale BH, compression belts, gating, or 4DCT-based ITV. However, the user should use caution when opting for free-breathing strategies that use CTOR (or fast CBCT) to avoid aligning to the tumor when it is in the extreme inhale or exhale phase.

A limitation of this study is that the low number of patients examined does not allow for definitive conclusions about the dose distributions resulting from shifting away from OARs and how these compare to CBCT-based alignment. A full quantitative analysis of this strategy is an area in need of future work. However, evidence exists for the exceedance of OAR tolerances in the abdomen when the alignment focus is only on the GTV [36]. In both our work and the work by Niedzielski et al., the assumption in comparing to CBCT-based alignment is that CBCT alignment is solely based on fiducial markers. This oversimplification ignores the fact that OARs can been seen on CBCT images in some patients and, thus, be avoided. Another area of future work is to review patient outcomes from this treatment approach and compare them to standard-of-care methods to better understand the clinical benefits of this technique.

5. Conclusions

High-quality daily imaging for abdominal SBRT allows the adequate visualization of both the tumor and organs at risk (OARs). A clear OAR delineation allows for the use of isodose line contours to shift high-dose regions away from OARs. Accurate target localization and OAR avoidance enables safe dose escalation, which can help to more effectively treat challenging tumors.

Author Contributions: Conceptualization, R.M.M.-P., S.B. and J.S.N.; methodology, R.M.M.-P., P.J.J., L.A.P., G.O.S., P.D., E.J.K., A.C.K., E.B.L., J.S.N. and S.B.; software, R.M.M.-P. and P.J.J.; validation, R.M.M.-P., P.J.J. and S.B.; formal analysis, R.M.M.-P.; investigation, R.M.M.-P.; resources, R.M.M.-P., P.J.J., L.A.P., G.O.S., P.D., E.J.K., A.C.K., E.B.L., J.S.N. and S.B.; data curation, R.M.M.-P. and P.J.J.; writing—original draft preparation, R.M.M.-P. and P.J.J.; writing—review and editing, R.M.M.-P., P.J.J., L.A.P., G.O.S., P.D., E.J.K., A.C.K., E.B.L., J.S.N. and S.B.; visualization, R.M.M.-P. and P.J.J.; project administration, S.B. and E.J.K. All authors have read and agreed to the published version of the manuscript.

Funding: This research received no external funding.

Institutional Review Board Statement: The study was conducted in accordance with the Declaration of Helsinki, and approved by the Institutional Review Board of The University of Texas MD Anderson Cancer Center (PA14-0646) with latest approval on 4 October 2022.

Informed Consent Statement: Patient consent was waived by the IRB due to the study being retrospective and involving standard of care treatments.

Data Availability Statement: The raw data supporting the conclusions of this article will be made available by the authors on request.

Conflicts of Interest: The authors declare no conflict of interest.

References

1. Bouchart, C.; Navez, J.; Closset, J.; Hendlisz, A.; Van Gestel, D.; Moretti, L.; Van Laethem, J.-L. Novel strategies using modern radiotherapy to improve pancreatic cancer outcomes: Toward a new standard? *Ther. Adv. Med. Oncol.* **2020**, *12*, 175883592093609. [CrossRef] [PubMed]
2. Arcelli, A.; Guido, A.; Buwenge, M.; Simoni, N.; Mazzarotto, R.; Macchia, G.; Deodato, F.; Cilla, S.; Bonomo, P.; Scotti, V.; et al. Higher Biologically Effective Dose Predicts Survival in SBRT of Pancreatic Cancer: A Multicentric Analysis (PAULA-1). *Anticancer Res.* **2020**, *40*, 465–472. [CrossRef] [PubMed]
3. Cellini, F.; Arcelli, A.; Simoni, N.; Caravatta, L.; Buwenge, M.; Calabrese, A.; Brunetti, O.; Genovesi, D.; Mazzarotto, R.; Deodato, F.; et al. Basics and Frontiers on Pancreatic Cancer for Radiation Oncology: Target Delineation, SBRT, SIB Technique, MRgRT, Particle Therapy, Immunotherapy and Clinical Guidelines. *Cancers* **2020**, *12*, 1729. [CrossRef]
4. Chang, D.T.; Schellenberg, D.; Shen, J.; Kim, J.; Goodman, K.A.; Fisher, G.A.; Ford, J.M.; Desser, T.; Quon, A.; Koong, A.C. Stereotactic radiotherapy for unresectable adenocarcinoma of the pancreas. *Cancer* **2009**, *115*, 665–672. [CrossRef]
5. Chen-Zhao, X.; Hernando, O.; López, M.; Sánchez, E.; Montero, A.; García-Aranda, M.; Ciérvide, R.; Valero, J.; Alonso, R.; Cárdenas-Rebollo, J.M.; et al. A prospective observational study of the clinical and pathological impact of stereotactic body

radiotherapy (SBRT) as a neoadjuvant strategy of chemoradiation in pancreatic cancer. *Clin. Transl. Oncol.* **2020**, *22*, 1499–1505. [CrossRef]
6. Dalwadi, S.M.; Herman, J.M.; Das, P.; Holliday, E.B. Novel Radiotherapy Technologies in the Treatment of Gastrointestinal Malignancies. *Hematol. Oncol. Clin. N. Am.* **2020**, *34*, 29–43. [CrossRef]
7. Mahadevan, A.; Jain, S.; Goldstein, M.; Miksad, R.; Pleskow, D.; Sawhney, M.; Brennan, D.; Callery, M.; Vollmer, C. Stereotactic Body Radiotherapy and Gemcitabine for Locally Advanced Pancreatic Cancer. *Int. J. Radiat. Oncol.* **2010**, *78*, 735–742. [CrossRef]
8. Mellon, E.A.; Hoffe, S.E.; Springett, G.M.; Frakes, J.M.; Strom, T.J.; Hodul, P.J.; Malafa, M.P.; Chuong, M.D.; Shridhar, R. Long-term outcomes of induction chemotherapy and neoadjuvant stereotactic body radiotherapy for borderline resectable and locally advanced pancreatic adenocarcinoma. *Acta Oncol.* **2015**, *54*, 979–985. [CrossRef]
9. Petrelli, F.; Comito, T.; Ghidini, A.; Torri, V.; Scorsetti, M.; Barni, S. Stereotactic Body Radiation Therapy for Locally Advanced Pancreatic Cancer: A Systematic Review and Pooled Analysis of 19 Trials. *Int. J. Radiat. Oncol.* **2017**, *97*, 313–322. [CrossRef]
10. Reyngold, M.; Parikh, P.; Crane, C.H. Ablative radiation therapy for locally advanced pancreatic cancer: Techniques and results. *Radiat. Oncol.* **2019**, *14*, 95. [CrossRef]
11. Zhong, J.; Patel, K.; Switchenko, J.; Cassidy, R.J.; Hall, W.A.; Gillespie, T.; Patel, P.R.; Kooby, D.; Landry, J. Outcomes for patients with locally advanced pancreatic adenocarcinoma treated with stereotactic body radiation therapy versus conventionally fractionated radiation. *Cancer* **2017**, *123*, 3486–3493. [CrossRef] [PubMed]
12. Palta, M.; Godfrey, D.; Goodman, K.A.; Hoffe, S.; Dawson, L.A.; Dessert, D.; Hall, W.A.; Herman, J.M.; Khorana, A.A.; Merchant, N.; et al. Radiation Therapy for Pancreatic Cancer: Executive Summary of an ASTRO Clinical Practice Guideline. *Pract. Radiat. Oncol.* **2019**, *9*, 322–332. [CrossRef] [PubMed]
13. Herman, J.M.; Chang, D.T.; Goodman, K.A.; Dholakia, A.S.; Raman, S.P.; Hacker-Prietz, A.; Iacobuzio-Donahue, C.A.; Griffith, M.E.; Pawlik, T.M.; Pai, J.S.; et al. Phase 2 multi-institutional trial evaluating gemcitabine and stereotactic body radiotherapy for patients with locally advanced unresectable pancreatic adenocarcinoma. *Cancer* **2015**, *121*, 1128–1137. [CrossRef] [PubMed]
14. Poon, R.T.-P.; Fan, S.-T.; Lo, C.-M.; Ng, I.O.-L.; Liu, C.-L.; Lam, C.-M.; Wong, J. Improving Survival Results After Resection of Hepatocellular Carcinoma: A Prospective Study of 377 Patients Over 10 Years. *Ann. Surg.* **2001**, *234*, 63–70. [CrossRef]
15. Mornex, F.; Girard, N.; Beziat, C.; Kubas, A.; Khodri, M.; Trepo, C.; Merle, P. Feasibility and efficacy of high-dose three-dimensional-conformal radiotherapy in cirrhotic patients with small-size hepatocellular carcinoma non-eligible for curative therapies—Mature results of the French Phase II RTF-1 trial. *Int. J. Radiat. Oncol.* **2006**, *66*, 1152–1158. [CrossRef]
16. Ben-Josef, E.; Normolle, D.; Ensminger, W.D.; Walker, S.; Tatro, D.; Ten Haken, R.K.; Knol, J.; Dawson, L.A.; Pan, C.; Lawrence, T.S. Phase II Trial of High-Dose Conformal Radiation Therapy With Concurrent Hepatic Artery Floxuridine for Unresectable Intrahepatic Malignancies. *J. Clin. Oncol.* **2005**, *23*, 8739–8747. [CrossRef]
17. Skinner, H.D.; Sharp, H.J.; Kaseb, A.O.; Javle, M.M.; Vauthey, J.N.; Abdalla, E.K.; Delclos, M.E.; Das, P.; Crane, C.H.; Krishnan, S. Radiation treatment outcomes for unresectable hepatocellular carcinoma. *Acta Oncol.* **2011**, *50*, 1191–1198. [CrossRef]
18. Tao, R.; Krishnan, S.; Bhosale, P.R.; Javle, M.M.; Aloia, T.A.; Shroff, R.T.; Kaseb, A.O.; Bishop, A.J.; Swanick, C.W.; Koay, E.J.; et al. Ablative Radiotherapy Doses Lead to a Substantial Prolongation of Survival in Patients With Inoperable Intrahepatic Cholangiocarcinoma: A Retrospective Dose Response Analysis. *J. Clin. Oncol.* **2016**, *34*, 219–226. [CrossRef]
19. McPartlin, A.; Swaminath, A.; Wang, R.; Pintilie, M.; Brierley, J.; Kim, J.; Ringash, J.; Wong, R.; Dinniwell, R.; Craig, T.; et al. Long-Term Outcomes of Phase 1 and 2 Studies of SBRT for Hepatic Colorectal Metastases. *Int. J. Radiat. Oncol.* **2017**, *99*, 388–395. [CrossRef]
20. Chang, B.K.; Timmerman, R.D. Stereotactic Body Radiation Therapy: A Comprehensive Review. *Am. J. Clin. Oncol.* **2007**, *30*, 637–644. [CrossRef]
21. Grimbergen, G.; Eijkelenkamp, H.; Heerkens, H.D.; Raaymakers, B.W.; Intven, M.P.W.; Meijer, G.J. Intrafraction pancreatic tumor motion patterns during ungated magnetic resonance guided radiotherapy with an abdominal corset. *Phys. Imaging Radiat. Oncol.* **2022**, *21*, 1–5. [CrossRef] [PubMed]
22. Ge, J.; Santanam, L.; Noel, C.; Parikh, P.J. Planning 4-Dimensional Computed Tomography (4DCT) Cannot Adequately Represent Daily Intrafractional Motion of Abdominal Tumors. *Int. J. Radiat. Oncol.* **2013**, *85*, 999–1005. [CrossRef] [PubMed]
23. Marchant, T.E.; Amer, A.M.; Moore, C.J. Measurement of inter and intra fraction organ motion in radiotherapy using cone beam CT projection images. *Phys. Med. Biol.* **2008**, *53*, 1087–1098. [CrossRef] [PubMed]
24. Minn, A.Y.; Schellenberg, D.; Maxim, P.; Suh, Y.; McKenna, S.; Cox, B.; Dieterich, S.; Xing, L.; Graves, E.; Goodman, K.A.; et al. Pancreatic Tumor Motion on a Single Planning 4D-CT Does Not Correlate With Intrafraction Tumor Motion During Treatment. *Am. J. Clin. Oncol.* **2009**, *32*, 364–368. [CrossRef]
25. Rusu, D.N.; Cunningham, J.M.; Arch, J.V.; Chetty, I.J.; Parikh, P.J.; Dolan, J.L. Impact of intrafraction motion in pancreatic cancer treatments with MR-guided adaptive radiation therapy. *Front. Oncol.* **2023**, *13*, 1298099. [CrossRef]
26. Hooshangnejad, H.; Miles, D.; Hill, C.; Narang, A.; Ding, K.; Han-Oh, S. Inter-Breath-Hold Geometric and Dosimetric Variations in Organs at Risk during Pancreatic Stereotactic Body Radiotherapy: Implications for Adaptive Radiation Therapy. *Cancers* **2023**, *15*, 4332. [CrossRef]
27. Keall, P.J. The management of respiratory motion in radiation oncology report of AAPM Task Group 76a. *Med. Phys.* **2006**, *33*, 3874–3900. [CrossRef]
28. Young, T.; Lee, M.; Johnston, M.; Nguyen, T.; Ko, R.; Arumugam, S. Assessment of interfraction dose variation in pancreas SBRT using daily simulation MR images. *Phys. Eng. Sci. Med.* **2023**, *46*, 1619–1627. [CrossRef]

29. Beddar, A.S.; Briere, T.M.; Balter, P.; Pan, T.; Tolani, N.; Ng, C.; Szklaruk, J.; Krishnan, S. 4D-CT imaging with synchronized intravenous contrast injection to improve delineation of liver tumors for treatment planning. *Radiother. Oncol.* 2008, 87, 445–448. [CrossRef]
30. Eccles, C.L.; Tse, R.V.; Hawkins, M.A.; Lee, M.T.; Moseley, D.J.; Dawson, L.A. Intravenous contrast-enhanced cone beam computed tomography (IVCBCT) of intrahepatic tumors and vessels. *Adv. Radiat. Oncol.* 2016, 1, 43–50. [CrossRef]
31. Daamen, L.A.; Parikh, P.J.; Hall, W.A. The Use of MR-Guided Radiation Therapy for Pancreatic Cancer. *Semin. Radiat. Oncol.* 2024, 34, 23–35. [CrossRef] [PubMed]
32. Gough, J.; Hall, W.; Good, J.; Nash, A.; Aitken, K. Technical Radiotherapy Advances—The Role of Magnetic Resonance Imaging-Guided Radiation in the Delivery of Hypofractionation. *Clin. Oncol.* 2022, 34, 301–312. [CrossRef] [PubMed]
33. Prime, S.; Schiff, J.P.; Hosni, A.; Stanescu, T.; Dawson, L.A.; Henke, L.E. The Use of MR-Guided Radiation Therapy for Liver Cancer. *Semin. Radiat. Oncol.* 2024, 34, 36–44. [CrossRef] [PubMed]
34. Breazeale, A.; Rahmani, R.; Gallagher, K.; Nabavizadeh, N. Liver stereotactic body radiation therapy without fiducial or retained ethiodized oil guidance warrants greater than 5 mm planning target volumes. *J. Med. Radiat. Sci.* 2024, 71, 110–113. [CrossRef] [PubMed]
35. Moskalenko, M.; Jones, B.L.; Mueller, A.; Lewis, S.; Shiao, J.C.; Zakem, S.J.; Robin, T.P.; Goodman, K.A. Fiducial Markers Allow Accurate and Reproducible Delivery of Liver Stereotactic Body Radiation Therapy. *Curr. Oncol.* 2023, 30, 5054–5061. [CrossRef]
36. Niedzielski, J.S.; Liu, Y.; Ng, S.S.W.; Martin, R.M.; Perles, L.A.; Beddar, S.; Rebueno, N.; Koay, E.J.; Taniguchi, C.; Holliday, E.B.; et al. Dosimetric Uncertainties Resulting From Interfractional Anatomic Variations for Patients Receiving Pancreas Stereotactic Body Radiation Therapy and Cone Beam Computed Tomography Image Guidance. *Int. J. Radiat. Oncol.* 2021, 111, 1298–1309. [CrossRef]
37. Hammers, J.; Lindsay, D.; Narayanasamy, G.; Sud, S.; Tan, X.; Dooley, J.; Marks, L.B.; Chen, R.C.; Das, S.K.; Mavroidis, P. Evaluation of the clinical impact of the differences between planned and delivered dose in prostate cancer radiotherapy based on CT-on-rails IGRT and patient-reported outcome scores. *J. Appl. Clin. Med. Phys.* 2023, 24, e13780. [CrossRef]
38. Li, X.; Quan, E.M.; Li, Y.; Pan, X.; Zhou, Y.; Wang, X.; Du, W.; Kudchadker, R.J.; Johnson, J.L.; Kuban, D.A.; et al. A Fully Automated Method for CT-on-Rails-Guided Online Adaptive Planning for Prostate Cancer Intensity Modulated Radiation Therapy. *Int. J. Radiat. Oncol.* 2013, 86, 835–841. [CrossRef]
39. Ma, C.-M.C.; Paskalev, K. In-room CT techniques for image-guided radiation therapy. *Med. Dosim.* 2006, 31, 30–39. [CrossRef]
40. Owen, R.; Kron, T.; Foroudi, F.; Milner, A.; Cox, J.; Duchesne, G.; Cleeve, L.; Zhu, L.; Cramb, J.; Sparks, L.; et al. Comparison of CT on Rails With Electronic Portal Imaging for Positioning of Prostate Cancer Patients With Implanted Fiducial Markers. *Int. J. Radiat. Oncol.* 2009, 74, 906–912. [CrossRef]
41. Yang, Z.; Chang, Y.; Brock, K.K.; Cazoulat, G.; Koay, E.J.; Koong, A.C.; Herman, J.M.; Park, P.C.; Poenisch, F.; Li, Q.; et al. Effect of setup and inter-fraction anatomical changes on the accumulated dose in CT-guided breath-hold intensity modulated proton therapy of liver malignancies. *Radiother. Oncol.* 2019, 134, 101–109. [CrossRef] [PubMed]
42. Bohoudi, O.; Bruynzeel, A.M.E.; Meijerink, M.R.; Senan, S.; Slotman, B.J.; Palacios, M.A.; Lagerwaard, F.J. Identification of patients with locally advanced pancreatic cancer benefitting from plan adaptation in MR-guided radiation therapy. *Radiother. Oncol.* 2019, 132, 16–22. [CrossRef] [PubMed]
43. Chuong, M.D.; Bryant, J.; Mittauer, K.E.; Hall, M.; Kotecha, R.; Alvarez, D.; Romaguera, T.; Rubens, M.; Adamson, S.; Godley, A.; et al. Ablative 5-Fraction Stereotactic Magnetic Resonance–Guided Radiation Therapy With On-Table Adaptive Replanning and Elective Nodal Irradiation for Inoperable Pancreas Cancer. *Pract. Radiat. Oncol.* 2021, 11, 134–147. [CrossRef] [PubMed]
44. Doty, D.G.; Chuong, M.D.; Gomez, A.G.; Bryant, J.; Contreras, J.; Romaguera, T.; Alvarez, D.; Kotecha, R.; Mehta, M.P.; Gutierrez, A.N.; et al. Stereotactic MR-guided online adaptive radiotherapy reirradiation (SMART reRT) for locally recurrent pancreatic adenocarcinoma: A case report. *Med. Dosim.* 2021, 46, 384–388. [CrossRef] [PubMed]
45. Ermongkonchai, T.; Khor, R.; Muralidharan, V.; Tebbutt, N.; Lim, K.; Kutaiba, N.; Ng, S.P. Stereotactic radiotherapy and the potential role of magnetic resonance-guided adaptive techniques for pancreatic cancer. *World J. Gastroenterol.* 2022, 28, 745–754. [CrossRef]
46. Hawranko, R.; Sohn, J.J.; Neiderer, K.; Bump, E.; Harris, T.; Fields, E.C.; Weiss, E.; Song, W.Y. Investigation of Isotoxic Dose Escalation and Plan Quality with TDABC Analysis on a 0.35 T MR-Linac (MRL) System in Ablative 5-Fraction Stereotactic Magnetic Resonance-Guided Radiation Therapy (MRgRT) for Primary Pancreatic Cancer. *J. Clin. Med.* 2022, 11, 2584. [CrossRef]
47. Herr, D.J.; Wang, C.; Mendiratta-Lala, M.; Matuszak, M.; Mayo, C.S.; Cao, Y.; Parikh, N.D.; Ten Haken, R.; Owen, D.; Evans, J.R.; et al. A Phase II Study of Optimized Individualized Adaptive Radiotherapy for Hepatocellular Carcinoma. *Clin. Cancer Res.* 2023, 29, 3852–3858. [CrossRef]
48. Hill, C.S.; Han-Oh, S.; Cheng, Z.; Wang, K.K.-H.; Meyer, J.J.; Herman, J.M.; Narang, A.K. Fiducial-based image-guided SBRT for pancreatic adenocarcinoma: Does inter-and intra-fraction treatment variation warrant adaptive therapy? *Radiat. Oncol.* 2021, 16, 53. [CrossRef]
49. Lee, D.; Renz, P.; Oh, S.; Hwang, M.-S.; Pavord, D.; Yun, K.L.; Collura, C.; McCauley, M.; Colonias, A.; Trombetta, M.; et al. Online Adaptive MRI-Guided Stereotactic Body Radiotherapy for Pancreatic and Other Intra-Abdominal Cancers. *Cancers* 2023, 15, 5272. [CrossRef]

50. Magallon-Baro, A.; Granton, P.V.; Milder, M.T.W.; Loi, M.; Zolnay, A.G.; Nuyttens, J.J.; Hoogeman, M.S. A model-based patient selection tool to identify who may be at risk of exceeding dose tolerances during pancreatic SBRT. *Radiother. Oncol.* **2019**, *141*, 116–122. [CrossRef]
51. Mittauer, K.E.; Yarlagadda, S.; Bryant, J.M.; Bassiri, N.; Romaguera, T.; Gomez, A.G.; Herrera, R.; Kotecha, R.; Mehta, M.P.; Gutierrez, A.N.; et al. Online adaptive radiotherapy: Assessment of planning technique and its impact on longitudinal plan quality robustness in pancreatic cancer. *Radiother. Oncol.* **2023**, *188*, 109869. [CrossRef] [PubMed]
52. Rhee, D.J.; Beddar, S.; Jaoude, J.A.; Sawakuchi, G.; Martin, R.; Perles, L.; Yu, C.; He, Y.; Court, L.E.; Ludmir, E.B.; et al. Dose Escalation for Pancreas SBRT: Potential and Limitations of using Daily Online Adaptive Radiation Therapy and an Iterative Isotoxicity Automated Planning Approach. *Adv. Radiat. Oncol.* **2023**, *8*, 101264. [CrossRef] [PubMed]
53. Prasad Venkatesulu, B.; Ness, E.; Ross, D.; Saripalli, A.L.; Abood, G.; Badami, A.; Cotler, S.; Dhanarajan, A.; Knab, L.M.; Lee, B.; et al. MRI-guided Real-time Online Gated Stereotactic Body Radiation Therapy for Liver Tumors. *Am. J. Clin. Oncol.* **2023**, *46*, 530–536. [CrossRef] [PubMed]
54. Weykamp, F.; Katsigiannopulos, E.; Piskorski, L.; Regnery, S.; Hoegen, P.; Ristau, J.; Renkamp, C.K.; Liermann, J.; Forster, T.; Lang, K.; et al. Dosimetric Benefit of Adaptive Magnetic Resonance-Guided Stereotactic Body Radiotherapy of Liver Metastases. *Cancers* **2022**, *14*, 6041. [CrossRef]
55. Wu, T.C.; Yoon, S.M.; Cao, M.; Raldow, A.C.; Xiang, M. Identifying predictors of on-table adaptation for pancreas stereotactic body radiotherapy (SBRT). *Clin. Transl. Radiat. Oncol.* **2023**, *40*, 100603. [CrossRef]
56. Chuong, M.D.; Clark, M.A.; Henke, L.E.; Kishan, A.U.; Portelance, L.; Parikh, P.J.; Bassetti, M.F.; Nagar, H.; Rosenberg, S.A.; Mehta, M.P.; et al. Patterns of utilization and clinical adoption of 0.35 Tesla MR-guided radiation therapy in the United States—Understanding the transition to adaptive, ultra-hypofractionated treatments. *Clin. Transl. Radiat. Oncol.* **2023**, *38*, 161–168. [CrossRef]
57. Garcia Schüler, H.I.; Pavic, M.; Mayinger, M.; Weitkamp, N.; Chamberlain, M.; Reiner, C.; Linsenmeier, C.; Balermpas, P.; Krayenbühl, J.; Guckenberger, M.; et al. Operating procedures, risk management and challenges during implementation of adaptive and non-adaptive MR-guided radiotherapy: 1-year single-center experience. *Radiat. Oncol.* **2021**, *16*, 217. [CrossRef]
58. Sanders, M.K.; Moser, A.J.; Khalid, A.; Fasanella, K.E.; Zeh, H.J.; Burton, S.; McGrath, K. EUS-guided fiducial placement for stereotactic body radiotherapy in locally advanced and recurrent pancreatic cancer. *Gastrointest. Endosc.* **2010**, *71*, 1178–1184. [CrossRef]
59. Krishnan, S.; Briere, T.M.; Dong, L.; Murthy, R.; Ng, C.; Balter, P.; Mohan, R.; Gillin, M.T.; Beddar, A.S. Daily targeting of liver tumors: Screening patients with a mock treatment and using a combination of internal and external fiducials for image-guided respiratory-gated radiotherapya. *Med. Phys.* **2007**, *34*, 4591–4593. [CrossRef]
60. Slagowski, J.M.; Colbert, L.E.; Cazacu, I.M.; Singh, B.S.; Martin, R.; Koay, E.J.; Taniguchi, C.M.; Koong, A.C.; Bhutani, M.S.; Herman, J.M.; et al. Evaluation of the Visibility and Artifacts of 11 Common Fiducial Markers for Image Guided Stereotactic Body Radiation Therapy in the Abdomen. *Pract. Radiat. Oncol.* **2020**, *10*, 434–442. [CrossRef]
61. Koay, E.J.; Hania, A.N.; Hall, W.A.; Taniguchi, C.M.; Rebueno, N.; Myrehaug, S.; Aitken, K.L.; Dawson, L.A.; Crane, C.H.; Herman, J.M.; et al. Dose-Escalated Radiation Therapy for Pancreatic Cancer: A Simultaneous Integrated Boost Approach. *Pract. Radiat. Oncol.* **2020**, *10*, e495–e507. [CrossRef] [PubMed]
62. Simoni, N.; Micera, R.; Paiella, S.; Guariglia, S.; Zivelonghi, E.; Malleo, G.; Rossi, G.; Addari, L.; Giuliani, T.; Pollini, T.; et al. Hypofractionated Stereotactic Body Radiation Therapy with Simultaneous Integrated Boost and Simultaneous Integrated Protection in Pancreatic Ductal Adenocarcinoma. *Clin. Oncol.* **2021**, *33*, e31–e38. [CrossRef] [PubMed]
63. Zhang, L.; Dong, L.; Court, L.; Wang, H.; Gillin, M.; Mohan, R. TU-EE-A4-05: Validation of CT-Assisted Targeting (CAT) Software for Soft Tissue and Bony Target Localization. *Med. Phys.* **2005**, *32*, 2106. [CrossRef]
64. Benedict, S.H.; Yenice, K.M.; Followill, D.; Galvin, J.M.; Hinson, W.; Kavanagh, B.; Keall, P.; Lovelock, M.; Meeks, S.; Papiez, L.; et al. Stereotactic body radiation therapy: The report of AAPM Task Group 101. *Med. Phys.* **2010**, *37*, 4078–4101. [CrossRef]
65. Robar, J.L.; Cherpak, A.; MacDonald, R.L.; Yashayaeva, A.; McAloney, D.; McMaster, N.; Zhan, K.; Cwajna, S.; Patil, N.; Dahn, H. Novel Technology Allowing Cone Beam Computed Tomography in 6 Seconds: A Patient Study of Comparative Image Quality. *Pract. Radiat. Oncol.* **2024**, *14*, 277–286. [CrossRef]
66. Zhang, Q.; Hu, Y.; Liu, F.; Goodman, K.; Rosenzweig, K.E.; Mageras, G.S. Correction of motion artifacts in cone-beam CT using a patient-specific respiratory motion model. *Med. Phys.* **2010**, *37*, 2901–2909. [CrossRef]
67. Dai, X.; Lei, Y.; Wynne, J.; Janopaul-Naylor, J.; Wang, T.; Roper, J.; Curran, W.J.; Liu, T.; Patel, P.; Yang, X. Synthetic CT-aided multiorgan segmentation for CBCT-guided adaptive pancreatic radiotherapy. *Med. Phys.* **2021**, *48*, 7063–7073. [CrossRef]
68. Gao, L.; Xie, K.; Sun, J.; Lin, T.; Sui, J.; Yang, G.; Ni, X. Streaking artifact reduction for CBCT-based synthetic CT generation in adaptive radiotherapy. *Med. Phys.* **2023**, *50*, 879–893. [CrossRef]
69. Hrinivich, W.T.; Chernavsky, N.E.; Morcos, M.; Li, T.; Wu, P.; Wong, J.; Siewerdsen, J.H. Effect of subject motion and gantry rotation speed on image quality and dose delivery in CT-guided radiotherapy. *Med. Phys.* **2022**, *49*, 6840–6855. [CrossRef]

Disclaimer/Publisher's Note: The statements, opinions and data contained in all publications are solely those of the individual author(s) and contributor(s) and not of MDPI and/or the editor(s). MDPI and/or the editor(s) disclaim responsibility for any injury to people or property resulting from any ideas, methods, instructions or products referred to in the content.

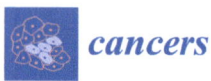 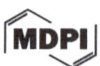

Article

Upper Urinary Tract Stereotactic Body Radiotherapy Using a 1.5 Tesla Magnetic Resonance Imaging-Guided Linear Accelerator: Workflow and Physics Considerations

Yao Zhao [1,†], Adrian Cozma [2,†], Yao Ding [1], Luis Augusto Perles [1], Reza Reiazi [1], Xinru Chen [1,3], Anthony Kang [1,3], Surendra Prajapati [1], Henry Yu [1], Ergys David Subashi [1], Kristy Brock [1,3,4], Jihong Wang [1], Sam Beddar [1], Belinda Lee [1], Mustefa Mohammedsaid [2], Sian Cooper [5], Rosalyne Westley [5], Alison Tree [5], Osama Mohamad [2], Comron Hassanzadeh [2], Henry Mok [2], Seungtaek Choi [2], Chad Tang [2,*,‡] and Jinzhong Yang [1,3,*,‡]

[1] Department of Radiation Physics, The University of Texas MD Anderson Cancer Center, Houston, TX 77030, USA; yzhao15@mdandrson.org (Y.Z.); yding1@mdanderson.org (Y.D.); laperles@mdanderson.org (L.A.P.); rreiazi@mdanderson.org (R.R.); xchen20@mdanderson.org (X.C.); anthony.m.kang@uth.tmc.edu (A.K.); sprajapati1@mdanderson.org (S.P.); zyu1@mdanderson.org (H.Y.); edsubashi@mdanderson.org (E.D.S.); kkbrock@mdanderson.org (K.B.); jihong.wang@mdanderson.org (J.W.); abeddar@mdanderson.org (S.B.); blee5@mdanderson.org (B.L.)

[2] Department of Radiation Oncology, The University of Texas MD Anderson Cancer Center, Houston, TX 77030, USA; adrian.i.cozma@gmail.com (A.C.); mmsaid@mdanderson.org (M.M.); omohamad@mdanderson.org (O.M.); cjhassanzadeh@mdanderson.org (C.H.); hmok@mdanderson.org (H.M.); stchoi@mdanderson.org (S.C.)

[3] The University of Texas MD Anderson Cancer Center UTHealth Houston Graduate School of Biomedical Sciences, Houston, TX 77030, USA

[4] Department of Imaging Physics, The University of Texas MD Anderson Cancer Center, Houston, TX 77030, USA

[5] The Royal Marsden Hospital, Institute of Cancer Research, London SW3 6JJ, UK; sian.cooper@rmh.nhs.uk (S.C.); rosalyne.westley@rmh.nhs.uk (R.W.); alison.tree@icr.ac.uk (A.T.)

* Correspondence: ctang1@mdanderson.org (C.T.); jyang4@mdanderson.org (J.Y.)

† These authors contributed equally to this work.

‡ These authors contributed equally to this work as joint senior authors.

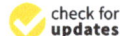

Citation: Zhao, Y.; Cozma, A.; Ding, Y.; Perles, L.A.; Reiazi, R.; Chen, X.; Kang, A.; Prajapati, S.; Yu, H.; Subashi, E.D.; et al. Upper Urinary Tract Stereotactic Body Radiotherapy Using a 1.5 Tesla Magnetic Resonance Imaging-Guided Linear Accelerator: Workflow and Physics Considerations. *Cancers* **2024**, *16*, 3987. https://doi.org/10.3390/cancers16233987

Academic Editor: Hideya Yamazaki

Received: 24 October 2024
Revised: 25 November 2024
Accepted: 26 November 2024
Published: 27 November 2024

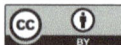

Copyright: © 2024 by the authors. Licensee MDPI, Basel, Switzerland. This article is an open access article distributed under the terms and conditions of the Creative Commons Attribution (CC BY) license (https:// creativecommons.org/licenses/by/ 4.0/).

Simple Summary: The MR-Linac (or MRL) is a powerful new device that integrates high-resolution magnetic resonance imaging (MRI) within a linear accelerator to enhance the precision of radiation treatment delivery beyond the predominantly CT-guided standard of care. Our institution was one of the seven founding members of the consortium that tested and refined the 1.5 Tesla MR-Linac in preparation for the first-in-human clinical trials, resulting in several years of early clinical experience. Its application in delivering ablative doses (stereotactic ablative radiation therapy; SBRT) to renal cell carcinoma (RCC) or upper tract urothelial carcinomas (UTUC) has been of particular interest out of clinical necessity and technical challenge. We present a retrospective analysis of our multi-year experience using MRL-SBRT, with emphasis on our evolving treatment setup and early clinical outcomes. Our aim is to contribute to and support the development and innovation of further programs using one of the largest worldwide single-institution cohorts.

Abstract: Background/Objectives: Advancements in radiotherapy technology now enable the delivery of ablative doses to targets in the upper urinary tract, including primary renal cell carcinoma (RCC) or upper tract urothelial carcinomas (UTUC), and secondary involvement by other histologies. Magnetic resonance imaging-guided linear accelerators (MR-Linacs) have shown promise to further improve the precision and adaptability of stereotactic body radiotherapy (SBRT). **Methods:** This single-institution retrospective study analyzed 34 patients (31 with upper urinary tract non-metastatic primaries [RCC or UTUC] and 3 with metastases of non-genitourinary histology) who received SBRT from August 2020 through September 2024 using a 1.5 Tesla MR-Linac system. Treatment plans were adjusted by using [online settings] for "adapt-to-position" (ATP) and "adapt-to-shape" (ATS) strategies for anatomic changes that developed during treatment; compression belts were used for motion management. **Results:** The median duration of treatment was 56 min overall and was significantly shorter using the adapt-to-position (ATP) (median 54 min, range 38–97 min) in comparison with adapt-to-shape (ATS) option (median 80, range 53–235 min). Most patients (77%) experienced self-resolving grade 1–2 acute radiation-induced toxicity; none had grade ≥ 3. Three participants (9%) experienced late grade 1–2 toxicity, potentially attributable to SBRT, with one (3%) experiencing grade 3. **Conclusions:** We conclude that MR-Linac-based SBRT, supported by online plan adaptation, is a feasible, safe, and highly precise treatment modality for the definitive management of select upper urinary tract lesions.

Keywords: MR-Linac; MRgRT; kidney; SBRT; RCC; UTUC

1. Introduction

Delivering ablative doses of radiation therapy to upper urinary tract targets is a complex endeavor [1–3]. It involves the accurate tracking and treatment of a critical and mobile retroperitoneal organ in close proximity to visceral structures [4]. Nonetheless, these significant technical challenges must be addressed, as a substantial proportion of patients cannot undergo gold-standard surgical resection due to medical comorbidities and/or risk of treatment-induced renal insufficiency [5].

The integration of magnetic resonance imaging with linear accelerators (MR-Linacs) into the treatment planning and delivery process has shown great promise [6–8]. This technology leverages the superior soft tissue contrast and temporal resolution of MRI to enable direct tumor visualization and real-time monitoring of motion throughout the respiratory phases [9]. Such capabilities facilitate daily adaptation and optimization of the treatment plan, ensuring precise targeting of the tumor while sparing surrounding organs at risk (OARs) [10]. Clinical experience with a 0.35-Tesla (T) MR-Linac system has shown encouraging locoregional control and preservation of renal function in the setting of RCC, highlighting the potential of MR-guided SBRT for the effective management of upper urinary tract malignancies (including primary RCC, UTUC, and secondary involvement by other histologies) [11,12]. However, treatment protocols involving daily online plan adaptation and the use of the more advanced 1.5 T MR-Linac system are underdeveloped, and the outcomes from such treatments have yet to be systematically reported. We describe our retrospective, single-institution experience with 1.5 T MR-Linac guided upper urinary tract SBRT, with a focus on key workflow and physics considerations.

2. Materials and Methods

2.1. Patient Selection

Eligibility for MR-Linac-guided SBRT was jointly determined by a multidisciplinary genitourinary tumor board, on the basis of expected benefit from consolidative radiotherapy for biopsy-proven disease (or in cases with high clinical and/or radiographic suspicion and perceived high risk for biopsies owing to medical comorbidities, although all patients in this analysis had biopsy-confirmed disease prior to treatment), and target movement of ≤ 10 mm on a 4D-CT scan while the patient was immobilized with a Vac-Lok cushion and a compression belt (described further below). Additional considerations included whether patients could fit within the MR-Linac body coil, could maintain a consistent position for extended periods, and had no contraindications to MRI (e.g., implanted ferromagnetic materials or pacemakers). This retrospective study was approved by the institutional review board (IRB 2022-0521), and due to the retrospective nature of the research, informed consent was not required.

2.2. Simulation

Treatment simulation was performed with both MRI and CT on the same day to facilitate precise rigid registration. Patients were positioned head-first supine, with arms up and legs on a knee support. For patients who had difficulty holding both arms up, the arm on the contralateral side was positioned down alongside the body. Patients were immobilized with a Vac-Lok cushion. The field of view of the CT scan was set at 600 mm to ensure that the entire body was visible. The default image matrix size was configured to 512 pixels, and the standard slice thickness for all scans was maintained at 3 mm, with a slice spacing of 2.5 mm. A pneumatic compression belt, modified in-house for adaptability, was used to minimize respiratory motion. Its pressure was adjusted for each patient for comfort, without compromising the effectiveness of the immobilization during simulation.

MR images were obtained with a Unity MR-Linac system (Elekta AB, Stockholm, Sweden) [13], which is based on a Philips 1.5 T Marlin MRI and includes a four-element anterior coil and a built-in four-element posterior coil to provide coverage of the abdominal region. Motion evaluations were performed with cine-mode MRI imaging (a 2D balanced turbo fast echo [TFE] dynamic MR scan; details in Table 1) during the MR simulation to quantify cranial–caudal tumor motion both, with and without use of the compression belt. Initially, MR images were captured without a compression belt, and then patients were fitted with a compression belt to apply a tolerable level of pressure. The cine MR image was aligned to the center of the target in both scenarios, and cine image acquisition lasted approximately 1 min. The motion range of the target was measured by using Philips image tools from the console, along with the cine images. After that, a T2-weighted 3D sequence and a T1-weighted 3D VANE mDixon sequence with fat suppression were acquired for the treatment planning system (Table 1). The 4D CT scans were then obtained with the belt in place to verify the motion consistency and to establish the final motion range.

Table 1. Parameters and acquisition techniques for MR imaging during MR simulation and treatment sessions.

Sequence	T2w 3D	T1w 3D VANE mDixon	Cine MRI for Simulation	Cine MRI for Daily Treatment
Scan Technique	Spin echo	Gradient echo	Gradient echo	Gradient echo
Imaging Mode	Turbo SE	Radial FFE	Balanced TFE	Balanced TFE
Imaging Orientation	Axial	Axial	Sagittal, Coronal	Axial, Sagittal, Coronal
Acquisition Type	3D	3D	2D	2D
Image Contrast	T2	T1	T2/T1	T2/T1
Repetition Time (ms)	1300	6.3	4.3	3.8
Echo Time (ms)	87	1.9/3.6	2.2	1.9
Flip Angle (°)	90	10	40	40
Pixel Bandwidth (Hz)	693	857	478	1085
Echo Train Length (ETL)	90	2	68	48
Radial Oversampling	NA	225	NA	NA
Field of View (cm^3)	48 × 48 × 25	45 × 45 × 24	51 × 51 × 0.6	44 × 44 × 0.5
Voxel Size (mm^3)	0.83 × 0.83 × 1	0.78 × 0.78 × 1.5	0.96 × 0.96 × 6	1.3 × 1.3 × 5
Sense Factor	4	1.3	3	3
Fat Saturation	None	Dixon	None	None
Number of Averages	2	1	1	1
Dynamic Times	1	1	100	>1500
Scan Time (minutes)	4:00	4:30	1:04	>15:00

To assess motion reduction and its consistency from simulation to daily treatment sessions, daily cine MR images, with the same MR sequence used in simulation, were captured and analyzed for each treatment fraction.

2.3. Treatment Planning

The Monaco treatment planning system (Elekta, Inc. Maryland Heights, MO, USA) was used to create reference radiotherapy plans based on the primary CT scan, according to planning directives established by the Genitourinary Radiation Oncology Service at MD Anderson Cancer Center. The GTV was drawn from the maximum intensity projection (MIP) of the 4D-CT scans as volume encompassing the entire tumor, with a subsequent 5 mm isometric expansion of the GTV used to derive the planning target volume (PTV). The clinical goals were to provide at least 100% coverage of the GTV and 95% coverage of the PTV by using prescribed doses of 36 Gy (7 patients; 21%), 39 Gy (1 patient; 3%), or 42 Gy (26 patients; 76%), given in three fractions, every other day. The OAR constraints are summarized in Table 2. Before treatment was delivered, we performed a secondary monitor unit (MU) check by using RadCalc (Version 6.3, Lifeline Software Inc., Austin, TX, USA) and an intensity-modulated radiation therapy (IMRT) QA measurement using ArcCheck MR (Sun Nuclear Corporation, Melbourne, FL, USA) to ensure the accuracy and deliverability of the generated plan.

Table 2. Dose constraints for organs at risk for kidney stereotactic body radiotherapy in three fractions.

	36–42 Gy Plans
Liver	$D700 \text{ cm}^3 \leq 15 \text{ Gy}$
	$Dmean \leq 16 \text{ Gy}$
Spinal Cord	$Dmax \leq 18 \text{ Gy}$
	$D10 \text{ cm}^3 \leq 15 \text{ Gy}$
Contralateral Kidney	$V10 \text{ Gy} \leq 10\%$
Small Bowel	$Dmax \leq 28 \text{ Gy}$
	$V12.5 \text{ Gy} \leq 30 \text{ cm}^3$
Large Bowel	$Dmax \leq 38 \text{ Gy}$
	$V35 \text{ Gy} \leq 1 \text{ cm}^3$
	$V30 \text{ Gy} \leq 10 \text{ cm}^3$
Duodenum	$Dmax \leq 28 \text{ Gy}$
Stomach	$V22.5 \text{ Gy} \leq 4 \text{ cm}^3$
	$Dmax \leq 28 \text{ Gy}$
Target Kidney-GTV	$V10 \text{ Gy} \leq 50\%$ (Optional)
Chest Wall	$D30 \text{ cm}^3 \leq 30 \text{ Gy}$ (Optional)

2.4. Online Plan Adaptation and Treatment Delivery

Patients were positioned on the MR-Linac couch using a pre-established index value from the simulation that guided their longitudinal placement. Because the MR-Linac lacks external lasers, therapists used an internal sagittal laser and leveling markers on each patient's skin to ascertain lateral positioning and to mitigate any potential body rotations. After setup, a T1 3D mDixon (water phase) MRI scan was obtained and subsequently fused with the reference plan image for plan adaptation. Plans could be adapted by using one of two strategies provided by the MR-Linac system: "adapt-to-position" (ATP) or "adapt-to-shape" (ATS) [13,14].

The ATP workflow involves rigid registration of the daily MRI to the reference CT to calculate positional shift and update the treatment isocenter of the plan. In ATP, no contour modifications are performed; instead, the daily adaptive plan is either recalculated or reoptimized directly from the reference plan to account for the isocenter shift and to maintain dose consistency. This workflow is most effective when anatomical changes between fractions are minimal, ensuring that the precision and conformity of dose delivery are maintained. ATP is similar to traditional image-guided radiotherapy (IGRT), utilizing daily MRI for alignment and treatment guidance, relying on reference CT anatomy for dose calculations. The ATS workflow uses deformable image registration (DIR) to propagate contours from the reference CT to the daily MRI, followed by manual adjustments if needed to reflect daily anatomical changes. A comprehensive re-optimization of the treatment plan is conducted based on the updated anatomy captured by the daily MRI, allowing for greater flexibility in dose distribution. ATS is particularly suitable for situations involving substantial anatomical changes, such as tumor shrinkage, weight loss, or shifts in the position of organs at risk. This approach is analogous to creating a new adaptive CT simulation and treatment plan, offering a higher degree of adaptation to meet the patient's current anatomical configuration.

The ATP workflow was chosen for every patient by default. The ATS workflow was chosen based on the following criteria: (1) substantial anatomic changes in nearby GI organs requiring recontouring to evaluate dose; (2) the OAR dosimetric goals (e.g., bowel dose) could not be met; and (3) changes in tumor size to an extent requiring CTV recontouring.

Before radiation delivery, each adaptive plan underwent an MU verification by using the RadCalc system. During beam delivery, internal anatomic motion was monitored in real time by using three orthogonal cine MR images centered at the tumor. At the completion of each fraction, an additional IMRT QA assessment was conducted on the adapted plan for the ATS workflow, serving as an extra measure of quality control.

3. Results

3.1. Adaptive Plan and Treatment Delivery

From August 2020 through April 2024, 34 patients were successfully treated with 1.5 T MR-Linac-based SBRT at MD Anderson Cancer Center. Only one patient (3%) did not complete the final fraction because of unresolvable logistic considerations, receiving 28 Gy of the prescribed 42 Gy; the other 33 patients successfully completed the intended treatment.

The [default] ATP workflow was used for most of the treatment fractions for all 34 patients. Nevertheless, a combination of online ATP and online ATS was required for 10 patients, with a minimum of one ATS during the treatment course to account for GI dose constraints. The adaptive plans were critical to meet the dosimetric goals set in the reference plans, ensuring precise dose delivery in these 10 patients. Figure 1 shows one example of an ATS plan dose overlaid on the daily MR image and compared with the reference plan dose. It was observed that the interfraction anatomical variability, particularly within the duodenum, required ATS in this specific case to maintain target dose and OAR sparing.

Across the treatment cohort, 102 fractions were planned, with 101 successfully delivered via MR-Linac. The single undelivered fraction resulted from a patient's decision to decline the final treatment session. Of the delivered fractions, 88 utilized ATP and 13 employed ATS, reflecting the specific needs for adaptation. The median duration of treatment was 56 min overall and was significantly shorter with ATP (median 54 min, range 38–97 min) than ATS (median 80, range 53–235 min).

3.2. Motion Management with the Compression Belt

The pneumatic compression belt was introduced into routine clinical practice for motion management of abdominal cancers to be treated with MR-Linac starting in July 2023. Before that, only 4D-CT was acquired for the tumor motion evaluation, without the compression belt. Tumor motion control with the compression belt in place was analyzed for 19 patients (9 with left and 10 with right kidney tumors); two examples are shown in Figure 2.

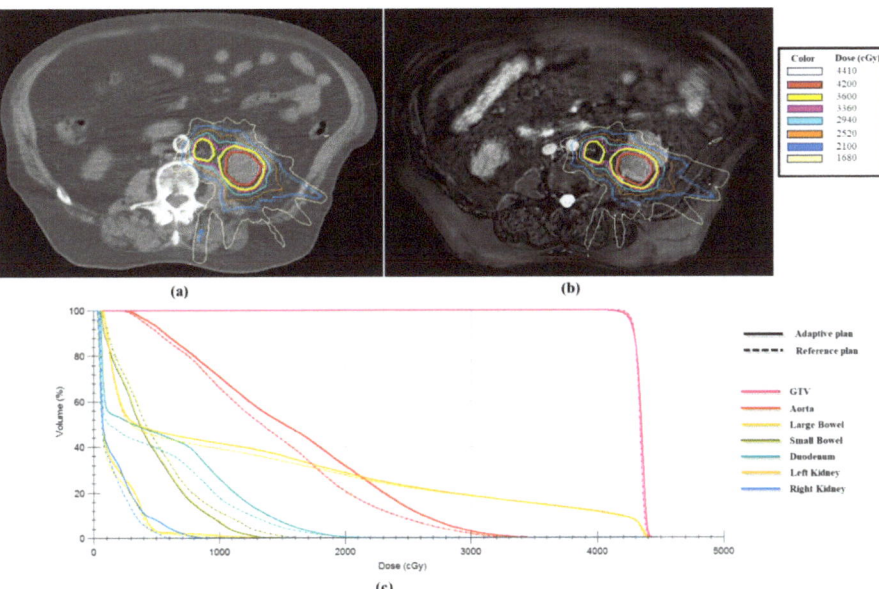

Figure 1. Illustration of an online adaptive plan for MR-guided SBRT. (**a**) Reference plan shown on the simulation CT image. (**b**) The adaptive plan for the 3rd fraction shown on the daily MR image. (**c**) The dose-volume histogram (DVH) comparing the reference plan (dashed lines) and the adaptive plan (solid lines).

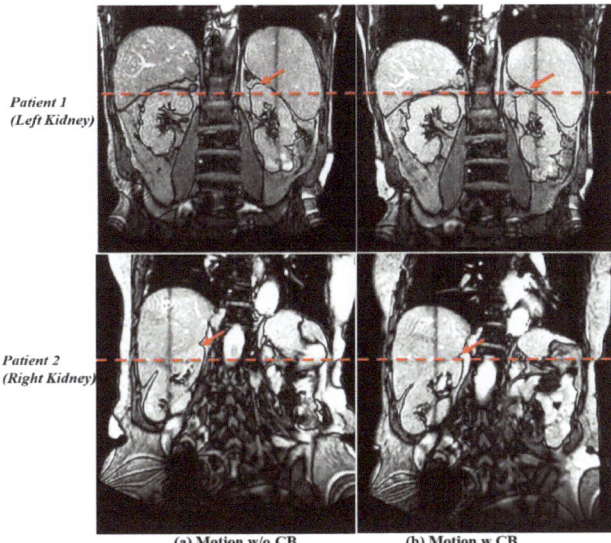

Figure 2. Examples of kidney target motion management with a compression belt (CB) in two patients undergoing magnetic resonance-guided stereotactic body radiation therapy. (**a**) Tumor motion without use of the belt was 18 mm for Patient 1 (top) and 13 mm for Patient 2 (bottom). (**b**) Tumor motion was significantly reduced with use of the belt to 7 mm for Patient 1 (with a left kidney tumor) and to 3 mm for Patient 2 (with a right kidney tumor), as shown by the dashed red lines and arrows.

Of these 19 patients, 16 (75%) displayed substantially reduced tumor motion with the compression belt. Mean cranial–caudal motion decreased from 12.1 mm (range 8–20 mm) without the belt to 5.0 mm (range 3–7 mm) with the belt (a mean 59% motion reduction). Indeed, the reduction in motion to <10 mm allowed these patients to undergo MR-Linac treatment. Daily motion assessment demonstrated a consistent mean motion of 6.3 mm (range 2.5–10.4 mm) when the belt was used. Of the 19 patients, one could not tolerate the belt, and tumor motion for two others could not be reduced to <10 mm, and those 3 patients were not treated with MR-Linac. Tumor motion for the 16 patients treated successfully with the compression belt and the MR-Linac is shown in Figure 3.

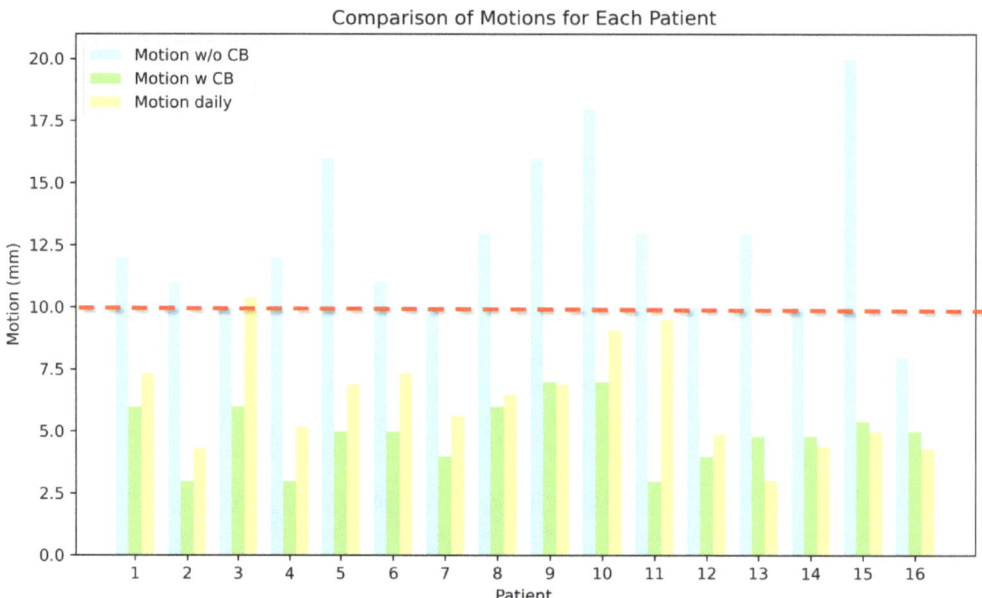

Figure 3. Comparison of respiratory-induced target motion in 16 patients, with and without use of a compression belt (CB) during MR-guided SBRT. Blue indicates cranio–caudal motion without the belt; green shows motion with the belt; and yellow indicates the average daily motion with the belt applied during treatment sessions. The red dashed line represents the clinical threshold of 10 mm, below which motion is considered sufficiently controlled to allow MR-Linac treatment. Although some patients experienced greater daily motion, it generally fell below the clinical thresholds for treatment, particularly if a belt was used during simulation.

3.3. Patient Outcomes

A total of 25 (73%) participants were treated for an upper urinary tract primary malignancy, 6 (18%) for an upper tract malignancy in a solitary kidney, and 3 (9%) for a non-genitourinary malignancy in the upper urinary tract. A total of 26 patients (77%) experienced an acute toxicity, and 4 (12%; one patient was lost to long-term follow-up) developed a late, likely radiation-attributable, toxicity per the Common Terminology Criteria for Adverse Events (CTCAE) v5.0. Acute toxicities included one or a combination of grade 1–2 fatigue (46%), nausea (31%), pain (abdominal, tumor, or chest wall; 15%), vomiting (4%), and/or diarrhea (4%), and these were typically self-resolving. Among long-term toxicities, patients described grade 1–2 nausea (18%), constipation (18%), fatigue (9%), diarrhea (9%), pain (abdominal; 9%), and irritative urinary symptoms (frequency; 9%); there was one instance (9%) of grade 2 hematuria with associated grade 2 urinary tract obstruction (9%); one patient (9%) developed possible treatment-related grade 3 pyelonephritis (reported as kidney infection as the most similar CTCAE v5.0 category). This was treated with brief hospitalization for observation and administration of intravenous antibiotics. No patient experienced treatment-related death or kidney failure, despite the aggressive application of SBRT.

4. Discussion

We report our single-institution clinical experience with using a 1.5 T MR-Linac to plan and deliver SBRT for either the primary management of RCC or UTUC or the consolidation of secondary kidney involvement by metastatic disease. To our knowledge, this is the largest series describing the technique, feasibility, and safety of this approach.

The seminal Multi-OutcoMe EvaluatioN of radiation Therapy Using the MR-Linac (MOMENTUM) study opened in 2019 as a multi-national collaborative database collecting clinical and technical data of patients treated on the Unity MR-Linac [15]. To date, only 24 participants have been included due to the challenges in patient recruitment, with most centers contributing <5 and just one having treated >10 individuals. Nonetheless, this initiative is imperative in providing an infrastructure for multicenter outcome reporting and highlights the importance of this study in contributing to the limited evidence base.

MR-guided radiotherapy provides superior soft-tissue contrast with enhanced visualization of the target and adjacent OARs, a capability particularly useful in the management of lesions within the upper urinary tract, which are moving and are in proximity to several radiosensitive gastrointestinal structures. Our 1.5 Tesla MR-Linac system enabled a high degree of confidence in achieving a conformal dose distribution while simultaneously meeting surrounding OAR dose constraints. It holds the potential to substantially contribute to the efficacy of SBRT and may enable further dose escalation, while mitigating the risk of toxicity. In our experience, the implementation of a pneumatic compression belt for patients receiving MRL-SBRT had a pivotal role in managing intrafraction motion due to respiration. It significantly reduced the cranial–caudal movement of the tumor (from 12.1 mm to 5.0 mm), thereby allowing for more stable, reproducible, and precise treatment delivery, critical components in SBRT. However, while most patients tolerated the compression belt well, a small subset required alternative motion management strategies, underscoring the need to develop additional approaches. All of the included patients were treated before comprehensive motion management (CMM) [16] was available in our Unity system. With CMM respiratory gating, the compression belt may still be useful to reduce motion and improve the duty cycle of gating treatment. The use of the compression belt is not limited to MR-Linac treatment. We have established the protocol of using the compression belt for general motion management of thoracic and abdominal cancer treatments subject to respiratory motion when breath-hold or other motion management approaches are not an option [17–19]. The compression belt is particularly useful for MR-Linac treatment before the CMM is available in the MR-Linac. The use of the compression belt helped enhance the precision of the dose delivery to moving targets, contributing to improved clinical outcomes by reducing radiation exposure to healthy surrounding tissues.

A notable concern with the use of the MR-Linac is the total treatment duration. Recorded median treatment time was 56 min. Fractions requiring ATS significantly extended the median treatment time to 80 min, compared with 54 min for those using solely ATP. This increased duration for ATS was due to the extensive processes required to propagate contours from the reference CT to the daily MR images, followed by thorough verification by the radiation oncologist. However, implementation of adaptive planning is critical in this application, as upper urinary targets are highly susceptible to daily anatomical changes and are located near critical structures like the bowel [20,21]. Although adaptive planning results in longer treatment times, the benefits of increased precision and safety are substantial. The anticipated integration of auto-contouring [22] and optimized workflows [9,23], as well as ongoing developments in automation and AI-driven processes, are expected to significantly reduce the time and resource demands of ATS strategies, thereby enhancing the usability of MRL-SBRT [24]. These advancements will reduce the need for specialized training and mitigate the challenges associated with longer treatment durations, making MR-Linac technology a feasible and efficient option for a broader range of clinical settings, including small centers with limited personnel, resources, and expertise [25].

Most patients (77%) experienced self-resolving grade 1–2 acute toxicities, with just four experiencing late toxicities of grades 1–2 (3 patients; 9%) and grade 3 (1 patient; 3%). These results are encouraging considering the 10% rate of grade 3 treatment-related adverse events (nausea and vomitting; abdominal, flank or tumour pain; colonic obstruction; and diarrhea) within TROG15.03 FASTRACK II and the aggregate grade 2 (5.3%) and grade 3 (2.7%) treatment-related effects reported in the systematic review and practice guidelines from the ISRS. We did not experience any grade 4+ toxicities as were reported in 1% of patients (gastritis, duodenal ulcer) in the 5-year update of the individual level meta-analysis from the IROCK group, nor did any patients require dialysis (reported previously as occuring in 1–4% of patients), despite the aggressive application of SBRT [26–28].

This analysis exhibits several strengths, as well as some limitations. It provides the largest single-institution experience with 1.5 T MRI-Linac-based SBRT for the treatment of upper urinary tract targets. Prior publications have reported outcomes from 0.35 T MRL SBRT for primary RCC [12] or have investigated the application of 1.5 T MRL in the management of upper abdominal [29] and prostate primary malignancies [30]. Moreover, nearly all patients were contoured and treated by two radiation oncologists at MD Anderson, using doses of 36–42 Gy in three fractions, and their final treatment plans underwent comprehensive intradepartmental peer review prior to delivery. Among the limitations of this study to be considered include first, the single-institution, retrospective nature of the analysis, which included patients from across the United States, and physician-recorded toxicities, carrying the potential for underreporting or not reporting toxicities experienced.

5. Conclusions

This study contributes to the workflow and evidence base supporting the safe use of 1.5 T MR Linac SBRT as a definitive treatment strategy for upper urinary tract malignancies occurring in patients who are precluded from surgical resection. The superior soft tissue discrimination, treatment monitoring potential, and precision of the MR-Linac-based approaches make them well suited to treating these complex lesions. Despite the promising outcomes, this single-institution, retrospective analysis is limited by the potential underreporting of toxicities. Future multicenter studies with extended follow-up are needed to further validate these results. Nevertheless, MR-Linac technology represents a significant advancement in precision radiotherapy, offering an effective, definitive treatment modality with the potential for dose escalation and enhanced tumor control, while minimizing toxicity.

Author Contributions: Conceptualization, A.C., C.T. and J.Y.; Methodology, Y.Z., A.C., Y.D., L.A.P., B.L., S.C. (Sian Cooper), R.W., A.T., C.H., S.C. (Seungtaek Choi), C.T. and J.Y.; Software, Y.Z.; Validation, Y.Z., A.C., O.M., C.H., C.T. and J.Y.; Formal analysis, Y.Z., A.C., C.T. and J.Y.; Investigation, Y.Z., C.T. and J.Y.; Data curation, Y.Z., A.C., Y.D., L.A.P., R.R., X.C., A.K., S.P., H.Y., E.D.S., K.B., J.W., S.B., B.L., M.M., O.M., H.M., S.C. (Seungtaek Choi), C.T. and J.Y.; Writing—original draft, Y.Z. and A.C.; Writing—review & editing, Y.Z., A.C., Y.D., L.A.P., X.C., S.P., H.Y., E.D.S., J.W., S.B., S.C. (Sian Cooper), R.W., A.T., O.M., C.H., S.C. (Seungtaek Choi), C.T. and J.Y.; Supervision, C.T. and J.Y.; Project administration, C.T. and J.Y. All authors have read and agreed to the published version of the manuscript.

Funding: This work was supported in part by a start-up fund from MD Anderson Cancer Center and through the National Cancer Institute, National Institutes of Health via Cancer Center Support (Core) Grant P30CA016672. Dr. Tree is supported by a Cancer Research UK Radiation Research Center of Excellence at The Institute of Cancer Research and The Royal Marsden NHS Foundation Trust (grant ref: A28724) and a Cancer Research UK Program Grant (ref: C33589/A28284).

Institutional Review Board Statement: This retrospective study was approved by the institutional review board (IRB 2022-0521).

Informed Consent Statement: Due to the retrospective nature of the research, informed consent was not required.

Data Availability Statement: The dataset is available through the MOMENTUM clinical trial.

Acknowledgments: Tree, Westley, and Cooper acknowledge NHS funding to the NIHR Biomedical Research Center at The Royal Marsden and The Institute of Cancer Research. The views expressed in this publication are those of the author(s) and not necessarily those of the NHS, the National Institute for Health Research, or the Department of Health and Social Care.

Conflicts of Interest: Dr. Tree reports institutional research funding from Elekta, Accuray, and Varian. Elekta supports The Royal Marsden research fellow program. Dr. Tree is the chair of the MR-Linac consortium steering committee and has received honoraria and/or travel assistance grants from Elekta, Janssen, Accuray, and Bayer. The other authors have no conflicts to disclose.

References

1. Ingrosso, G.; Becherini, C.; Francolini, G.; Lancia, A.; Alì, E.; Caini, S.; Teriaca, M.A.; Marchionni, A.; Filippi, A.R.; Livi, L.; et al. Stereotactic Body Radiotherapy (SBRT) in Combination with Drugs in Metastatic Kidney Cancer: A Systematic Review. *Crit. Rev. Oncol./Hematol.* **2021**, *159*, 103242. [CrossRef]
2. Rich, B.J.; Noy, M.A.; Dal Pra, A. Stereotactic Body Radiotherapy for Localized Kidney Cancer. *Curr. Urol. Rep.* **2022**, *23*, 371–381. [CrossRef] [PubMed]
3. Yamamoto, T.; Kawasaki, Y.; Umezawa, R.; Kadoya, N.; Matsushita, H.; Takeda, K.; Ishikawa, Y.; Takahashi, N.; Suzuki, Y.; Takeda, K.; et al. Stereotactic Body Radiotherapy for Kidney Cancer: A 10-Year Experience from a Single Institute. *J. Radiat. Res.* **2021**, *62*, 533–539. [CrossRef] [PubMed]
4. Evaluation of Kidney Motion and Target Localization in Abdominal SBRT Patients—Sonier—2016—Journal of Applied Clinical Medical Physics—Wiley Online Library. Available online: https://aapm.onlinelibrary.wiley.com/doi/full/10.1120/jacmp.v17i6.6406 (accessed on 21 November 2024).
5. Capitanio, U.; Montorsi, F. Renal Cancer. *Lancet* **2016**, *387*, 894–906. [CrossRef] [PubMed]
6. Lagendijk, J.J.W.; Raaymakers, B.W.; van Vulpen, M. The Magnetic Resonance Imaging-Linac System. *Semin. Radiat. Oncol.* **2014**, *24*, 207–209. [CrossRef] [PubMed]
7. Liney, G.P.; Whelan, B.; Oborn, B.; Barton, M.; Keall, P. MRI-Linear Accelerator Radiotherapy Systems. *Clin. Oncol.* **2018**, *30*, 686–691. [CrossRef]
8. Lagendijk, J.J.W.; Raaymakers, B.W.; Raaijmakers, A.J.E.; Overweg, J.; Brown, K.J.; Kerkhof, E.M.; van der Put, R.W.; Hårdemark, B.; van Vulpen, M.; van der Heide, U.A. MRI/Linac Integration. *Radiother. Oncol.* **2008**, *86*, 25–29. [CrossRef]
9. Zhao, Y.; Chen, X.; McDonald, B.; Yu, C.; Mohamed, A.S.R.; Fuller, C.D.; Court, L.E.; Pan, T.; Wang, H.; Wang, X.; et al. A Transformer-Based Hierarchical Registration Framework for Multimodality Deformable Image Registration. *Comput. Med. Imaging Graph.* **2023**, *108*, 102286. [CrossRef]
10. Kishan, A.U.; Ma, T.M.; Lamb, J.M.; Casado, M.; Wilhalme, H.; Low, D.A.; Sheng, K.; Sharma, S.; Nickols, N.G.; Pham, J.; et al. Magnetic Resonance Imaging–Guided vs Computed Tomography–Guided Stereotactic Body Radiotherapy for Prostate Cancer: The MIRAGE Randomized Clinical Trial. *JAMA Oncol.* **2023**, *9*, 365–373. [CrossRef]
11. Chuong, M.D.; Clark, M.A.; Henke, L.E.; Kishan, A.U.; Portelance, L.; Parikh, P.J.; Bassetti, M.F.; Nagar, H.; Rosenberg, S.A.; Mehta, M.P.; et al. Patterns of Utilization and Clinical Adoption of 0.35 Tesla MR-Guided Radiation Therapy in the United States—Understanding the Transition to Adaptive, Ultra-Hypofractionated Treatments. *Clin. Transl. Radiat. Oncol.* **2023**, *38*, 161–168. [CrossRef]
12. Tetar, S.U.; Bohoudi, O.; Senan, S.; Palacios, M.A.; Oei, S.S.; van der Wel, A.M.; Slotman, B.J.; van Moorselaar, R.J.A.; Lagerwaard, F.J.; Bruynzeel, A.M.E. The Role of Daily Adaptive Stereotactic MR-Guided Radiotherapy for Renal Cell Cancer. *Cancers* **2020**, *12*, 2763. [CrossRef] [PubMed]
13. Winkel, D.; Bol, G.H.; Kroon, P.S.; van Asselen, B.; Hackett, S.S.; Werensteijn-Honingh, A.M.; Intven, M.P.W.; Eppinga, W.S.C.; Tijssen, R.H.N.; Kerkmeijer, L.G.W.; et al. Adaptive Radiotherapy: The Elekta Unity MR-Linac Concept. *Clin. Transl. Radiat. Oncol.* **2019**, *18*, 54–59. [CrossRef]
14. Gupta, A.; Dunlop, A.; Mitchell, A.; McQuaid, D.; Nill, S.; Barnes, H.; Newbold, K.; Nutting, C.; Bhide, S.; Oelfke, U.; et al. Online Adaptive Radiotherapy for Head and Neck Cancers on the MR Linear Accelerator: Introducing a Novel Modified Adapt-to-Shape Approach. *Clin. Transl. Radiat. Oncol.* **2022**, *32*, 48–51. [CrossRef]
15. de Mol van Otterloo, S.R.; Christodouleas, J.P.; Blezer, E.L.A.; Akhiat, H.; Brown, K.; Choudhury, A.; Eggert, D.; Erickson, B.A.; Faivre-Finn, C.; Fuller, C.D.; et al. The MOMENTUM Study: An International Registry for the Evidence-Based Introduction of MR-Guided Adaptive Therapy. *Front. Oncol.* **2020**, *10*, 1328. [CrossRef]
16. Jassar, H.; Tai, A.; Chen, X.; Keiper, T.D.; Paulson, E.; Lathuilière, F.; Bériault, S.; Hébert, F.; Savard, L.; Cooper, D.T.; et al. Real-Time Motion Monitoring Using Orthogonal Cine MRI during MR-Guided Adaptive Radiation Therapy for Abdominal Tumors on 1.5 T MR-Linac. *Med. Phys.* **2023**, *50*, 3103–3116. [CrossRef]

17. Baker, R.; Han, G.; Sarangkasiri, S.; DeMarco, M.; Turke, C.; Stevens, C.W.; Dilling, T.J. Clinical and Dosimetric Predictors of Radiation Pneumonitis in a Large Series of Patients Treated With Stereotactic Body Radiation Therapy to the Lung. *Int. J. Radiat. Oncol. Biol. Phys.* **2013**, *85*, 190–195. [CrossRef]
18. Javadi, S.; Eckstein, J.; Ulizio, V.; Palm, R.; Reddy, K.; Pearson, D. Evaluation of the Use of Abdominal Compression of the Lung in Stereotactic Radiation Therapy. *Med. Dosim.* **2019**, *44*, 365–369. [CrossRef]
19. Moreira, A.; Li, W.; Berlin, A.; Carpino-Rocca, C.; Chung, P.; Conroy, L.; Dang, J.; Dawson, L.A.; Glicksman, R.M.; Hosni, A.; et al. Prospective Evaluation of Patient-Reported Anxiety and Experiences with Adaptive Radiation Therapy on an MR-Linac. *Tech. Innov. Patient Support Radiat. Oncol.* **2024**, *29*, 100240. [CrossRef]
20. Bohoudi, O.; Bruynzeel, A.M.E.; Senan, S.; Cuijpers, J.P.; Slotman, B.J.; Lagerwaard, F.J.; Palacios, M.A. Fast and Robust Online Adaptive Planning in Stereotactic MR-Guided Adaptive Radiation Therapy (SMART) for Pancreatic Cancer. *Radiother. Oncol.* **2017**, *125*, 439–444. [CrossRef]
21. Cusumano, D.; Boldrini, L.; Dhont, J.; Fiorino, C.; Green, O.; Güngör, G.; Jornet, N.; Klüter, S.; Landry, G.; Mattiucci, G.C. Artificial Intelligence in Magnetic Resonance Guided Radiotherapy: Medical and Physical Considerations on State of Art and Future Perspectives. *Phys. Medica* **2021**, *85*, 175–191. [CrossRef]
22. Li, Z.; Zhang, W.; Li, B.; Zhu, J.; Peng, Y.; Li, C.; Zhu, J.; Zhou, Q.; Yin, Y. Patient-Specific Daily Updated Deep Learning Auto-Segmentation for MRI-Guided Adaptive Radiotherapy. *Radiother. Oncol.* **2022**, *177*, 222–230. [CrossRef]
23. Zhao, Y.; Wang, H.; Yu, C.; Court, L.E.; Wang, X.; Wang, Q.; Pan, T.; Ding, Y.; Phan, J.; Yang, J. Compensation Cycle Consistent Generative Adversarial Networks (Comp-GAN) for Synthetic CT Generation from MR Scans with Truncated Anatomy. *Med. Phys.* **2023**, *50*, 4399–4414. [CrossRef]
24. Zarenia, M.; Zhang, Y.; Sarosiek, C.; Conlin, R.; Amjad, A.; Paulson, E. Deep Learning-Based Automatic Contour Quality Assurance for Auto-Segmented Abdominal MR-Linac Contours. *Phys. Med. Biol.* **2024**, *69*, 215029. [CrossRef]
25. Hall, W.A.; Paulson, E.S.; van der Heide, U.A.; Fuller, C.D.; Raaymakers, B.W.; Lagendijk, J.J.W.; Li, X.A.; Jaffray, D.A.; Dawson, L.A.; Erickson, B.; et al. The Transformation of Radiation Oncology Using Real-Time Magnetic Resonance Guidance: A Review. *Eur. J. Cancer* **2019**, *122*, 42–52. [CrossRef]
26. Siva, S.; Ali, M.; Correa, R.J.M.; Muacevic, A.; Ponsky, L.; Ellis, R.J.; Lo, S.S.; Onishi, H.; Swaminath, A.; McLaughlin, M.; et al. 5-Year Outcomes after Stereotactic Ablative Body Radiotherapy for Primary Renal Cell Carcinoma: An Individual Patient Data Meta-Analysis from IROCK (the International Radiosurgery Consortium of the Kidney). *Lancet Oncol.* **2022**, *23*, 1508–1516. [CrossRef]
27. Siva, S.; Bressel, M.; Sidhom, M.; Sridharan, S.; Vanneste, B.G.L.; Davey, R.; Montgomery, R.; Ruben, J.; Foroudi, F.; Higgs, B.; et al. Stereotactic Ablative Body Radiotherapy for Primary Kidney Cancer (TROG 15.03 FASTRACK II): A Non-Randomised Phase 2 Trial. *Lancet Oncol.* **2024**, *25*, 308–316. [CrossRef]
28. Siva, S.; Louie, A.V.; Kotecha, R.; Barber, M.N.; Ali, M.; Zhang, Z.; Guckenberger, M.; Kim, M.-S.; Scorsetti, M.; Tree, A.C.; et al. Stereotactic Body Radiotherapy for Primary Renal Cell Carcinoma: A Systematic Review and Practice Guideline from the International Society of Stereotactic Radiosurgery (ISRS). *Lancet Oncol.* **2024**, *25*, e18–e28. [CrossRef]
29. Hall, W.A.; Straza, M.W.; Chen, X.; Mickevicius, N.; Erickson, B.; Schultz, C.; Awan, M.; Ahunbay, E.; Li, X.A.; Paulson, E.S. Initial Clinical Experience of Stereotactic Body Radiation Therapy (SBRT) for Liver Metastases, Primary Liver Malignancy, and Pancreatic Cancer with 4D-MRI Based Online Adaptation and Real-Time MRI Monitoring Using a 1.5 Tesla MR-Linac. *PLoS ONE* **2020**, *15*, e0236570. [CrossRef]
30. Turkkan, G.; Bilici, N.; Sertel, H.; Keskus, Y.; Alkaya, S.; Tavli, B.; Ozkirim, M.; Fayda, M. Clinical Utility of a 1.5 T Magnetic Resonance Imaging-Guided Linear Accelerator during Conventionally Fractionated and Hypofractionated Prostate Cancer Radiotherapy. *Front. Oncol.* **2022**, *12*, 909402. [CrossRef]

Disclaimer/Publisher's Note: The statements, opinions and data contained in all publications are solely those of the individual author(s) and contributor(s) and not of MDPI and/or the editor(s). MDPI and/or the editor(s) disclaim responsibility for any injury to people or property resulting from any ideas, methods, instructions or products referred to in the content.

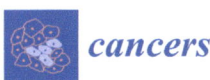

Article

Per-Irradiation Monitoring by kV-2D Acquisitions in Stereotactic Treatment of Spinal and Non-Spinal Bony Metastases Using an On-Board Imager of a Linear Accelerator

Ahmed Hadj Henni [1,*], Geoffrey Martinage [1,2], Lucie Lebret [1,2] and Ilias Arhoun [1]

1. Radiation Oncology Department, Centre Frederic Joliot, 76000 Rouen, France; geoffrey.martinage@centrefredericjoliot.fr (G.M.); lucie.lebret@centrefredericjoliot.fr (L.L.); ilias.arhoun@centrefredericjoliot.fr (I.A.)
2. Oncology Department, Clinique Saint Hilaire, 76000 Rouen, France
* Correspondence: ahadjhenni@gmail.com

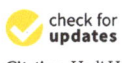

Citation: Hadj Henni, A.; Martinage, G.; Lebret, L.; Arhoun, I. Per-Irradiation Monitoring by kV-2D Acquisitions in Stereotactic Treatment of Spinal and Non-Spinal Bony Metastases Using an On-Board Imager of a Linear Accelerator. *Cancers* **2024**, *16*, 4267. https://doi.org/10.3390/cancers16244267

Academic Editors: Sam Beddar and Michael D. Chuong

Received: 15 November 2024
Revised: 10 December 2024
Accepted: 20 December 2024
Published: 22 December 2024

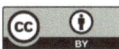

Copyright: © 2024 by the authors. Licensee MDPI, Basel, Switzerland. This article is an open access article distributed under the terms and conditions of the Creative Commons Attribution (CC BY) license (https:// creativecommons.org/licenses/by/ 4.0/).

Simple Summary: An on-board imager on a linear accelerator allows the acquisition of kV-2D images during irradiation. Overlaying specific structures on these images enables the visual verification of movement at regular frequencies. The aim of this study was to validate the method of the visual tracking of the target volume motion for the stereotactic treatment of bone metastases. To the best of our knowledge, this image-guided radiation therapy (IGRT) method has never been studied in non-spinal bony sites. The results were obtained using measurements from an anthropomorphic phantom and analysis of kV–cone beam computed tomography images from 29 patients treated at our institution. The results validated a visual tracking accuracy of 2.0 mm for spinal sites and 3.0 mm for non-vertebral bone locations. This method, based on an imaging device that is available on current linear accelerators, enables a robust IGRT strategy for performing bone stereotactic treatment at no additional cost to centers.

Abstract: Background/Objectives: An on-board imager on a linear accelerator allows the acquisition of kV-2D images during irradiation. Overlaying specific structures on these images enables the visual verification of movement at regular frequencies. Our aim was to validate this tracking method for the stereotactic treatment of bone metastases. Methods: Shifts in three translational directions were simulated using an anthropomorphic phantom. For these simulated shifts, planar images were acquired at different angles of incidence, with overlaid volumes of interest. A blinded test was then administered to the 18 participants to evaluate their decisions regarding whether to stop treatment. The results considered the experience of the operators. Quantitative analyses were performed on the intra-fractional images of 29 patients. Results: Participants analyzed each image with an average (standard deviation) decision time of 3.0 s (2.3). For offsets of 0.0, 1.0, 1.5, and 2.0 mm, the results were 78%, 93%, 90%, and 100% for the expert group and 78%, 70%, 79%, and 88% for the less-experienced group. Clinical feedback confirmed this guidance technique and extended it to non-spinal bony metastases. Sudden movements exceeding the 2.0 mm threshold occurred in 3.3% of the analyzed fractions, with a detection rate of 97.8% for vertebral locations. For non-vertebral bone locations, movements exceeding a threshold of 3.0 mm occurred in 3.5% of cases and were detected in 96.5%. Conclusions: The clinical use of planar OBI and superimposed structures for visual-image guidance in bone stereotactic treatment was validated using an anthropomorphic phantom and clinical feedback.

Keywords: bone SBRT; image-guided radiotherapy; intra-fraction motion; on-board imager; triggered kV imaging; kV-CBCT

1. Introduction

Stereotactic body radiotherapy (SBRT) is a technique based on delivering high doses of radiation with millimeter precision. However, these treatments are often associated with strong dose gradients and reduced margins to spare the normal tissues. The goal is to achieve a high biologically effective dose (BED) in a limited number of fractions to deliver ablative doses to the target in the treatment of patients with a localized tumor or oligometastasis. Spinal SBRT fits this definition, particularly because of the proximity of nerve structures (the spinal cord, cauda equina, and nerve roots) to the planning target volume (PTV). For this site, several prospective and retrospective studies have shown that a high BED results in local control rates of approximately 80–90% in one year [1–3]. The most commonly reported protocols in the literature are as follows: 16–24 Gy in 1 fraction, 24 Gy in 2 fractions, 24–27 Gy in 3 fractions, and 30–35 Gy in 5 fractions [4–6]. The complexity of dosimetric planning using intensity modulation to enable a high PTV conformation is correlated with irradiation using adapted immobilization systems and an image-guided radiation therapy (IGRT) strategy. The level of precision required could be of the order of 1 mm/2°, depending on the proximity of the organs at risk [7]. Wang et al. [7] performed a dosimetric study on 20 vertebral metastases and recommended this level of precision to maintain the risk of target volume coverage loss at <5% and the dose increase in organs at risk at <25%.

The appropriate choice of a non-invasive positioning system for the treatment of bone metastases currently guarantees, on average, very low positioning deviations [8]. However, several teams have questioned the relevance of intra-fraction imaging. Indeed, during the stereotactic treatment of bone metastases, the per-beam monitoring of the target movement shows that involuntary patient movements are possible and frequent [9,10].

For example, a study by Hadj Henni et al. [11], using kV-2D images acquired by a system not mounted on a linear accelerator, showed that these offsets could occur at any time during irradiation, with values sometimes exceeding 3 mm. These offsets were corrected at a frequency of ≤ 1 min and allowed to guarantee a positioning of <1 mm and <2° in all cases.

These results clearly demonstrate that an IGRT approach based solely on three-dimensional cone-beam computed tomography (3D-CBCT) pre- and post-treatment scans is not sufficient to ensure millimeter accuracy in bone SBRT. For the CyberKnife platform (Accuray Inc., Sunnyvale, CA, USA), an imaging system [12] consisting of two X-ray sources and two detectors installed on the floor and ceiling of the treatment room allows for the acquisition of two oblique kV-2D images, and, thus, the real-time monitoring of the target volume position. Linear accelerators, such as the Varian TrueBeam (Varian Medical System, Palo Alto, CA, USA), require the addition of an external kV-2D imaging system to benefit from the same technological capabilities as CyberKnife. The ExacTrac X-Ray 6D orthogonal imaging system fulfills this function perfectly [13], but its cost may not fit the center's budget. Systems based on tracking the patient's surface rather than the target volume are more accessible but have not been widely used for the SBRT of bone metastases [14,15]. All other technological options for real-time tumor position tracking require invasive fiducial implantation [16,17].

Varian TrueBeam machines are equipped with an on-board imager (OBI) system that enables the acquisition of 3D CBCT images that can be used to verify patient positioning between each beam of the treatment plan. This intra-fraction IGRT method, often described in the literature [18–21], increases treatment time, and, therefore, the possibility of patient movement [8]. OBI also offers the possibility of acquiring kV-2D images during irradiation using different triggers (Monitor Unit, degree, or time). In addition, when fiducial markers are implanted, this option (auto-beam hold) allows them to be detected, and the beam to be stopped automatically if they are outside a predefined tolerance zone [22,23]. In the absence of fiducial markers, which is the case in most bone SBRT treatments, only the visual monitoring of these planar images is possible.

Koo et al. [24] were among the first to propose a validated IGRT strategy based on this OBI option for thoracic and lumbar spinal stereotactic treatments. By overlaying the patient's anatomical structures (vertebral body and spinous process) previously delineated on the planning CT of these kV-2D images, this team was able to detect and correct the intra-fractional motion in 11 of 94 fractions.

The aim of our study was, first, to validate the feasibility of this approach on an anthropomorphic phantom, based on the visual tracking of the target vertebra as well as the inferior and superior vertebrae, using kV-2D imaging during motion irradiation. The choice of a vertebral phantom was motivated by the proximity of the spinal cord to the target volume in this case. Additionally, the effect of operator experience on the detection efficiency of millimeter-scale positional deviations was evaluated.

Clinical feedback from 29 patients validated this approach for guiding irradiation in spinal stereotactic treatment and allowed it to be extended to other extra-vertebral bone sites in a second phase. Structures that facilitate the visual detection of positioning discrepancies in extra-vertebral bone metastases have also been proposed for the clinical use of intra-fraction monitoring with an on-board imager. To the best of our knowledge, this image-guided radiation therapy method has never been studied in non-spinal bony sites.

2. Materials and Methods

2.1. Phantom Study

Prior to its use in routine clinical practice, a study was performed on a thoracic anthropomorphic phantom developed by RTSafe© (RTsafe P.C., Athens, Greece) (Figure 1) to evaluate the performance of visual tracking of the target volume position. Inspired by Koo et al. [24], offsets of 0.0, 1.0, 1.5, and 2.0 mm were simulated in three translational directions. On CT acquisition (Somatom Definition AS20 RT, Siemens©, Washington, DC, USA) of the phantom with a slice thickness of 1.0 mm, the target, overlying, and underlying vertebrae were delineated to serve as tracking structures of the positional offset in the vertical, longitudinal, and lateral directions. A full-arc treatment plan with X6 FFF (flattening filter-free) beam was simulated using TPS Eclipse (AcurosXB 15.6, 0.1 cm grid, Varian Medical Systems, Palo Alto, CA, USA) to enable experimental manipulation in the treatment room.

In this study, intra-fraction rotational deviations from the reference position were not considered. Numerous studies, such as those by Wang et al. [7] and GukenBerger et al. [25], have defined acceptable rotation thresholds (pitch, yaw, and roll) between $2°$ and $3.5°$ without significant dosimetric effects on the spinal cord. For vacuum bag positioning systems, these rotational corrections are well below thresholds [8,11].

For each translational deviation simulated at the accelerator, kV-2D images were acquired every $45°$ from $0°$ to $315°$ with the volumes of interest superimposed (Figure 1). A set of 35 randomly selected images was collected from the set of available images. Without knowing the occurrence and amplitude of the discrepancies, 18 operators (14 radiation therapist, 2 physicians, and 2 physicists) were asked to visually assess these discrepancies and to choose between the answers "Yes, error requiring treatment interruption and kV-CBCT acquisition" and "No, no treatment interruption".

They were also asked to record their decision-making times. Cases in which the errors were parallel to the acquisition angles of the OBI images could not be detected and were excluded from this test. However, images with an offset of 0.0 were retained. To familiarize users with this blind test, a preliminary self-training step was proposed. This consisted of 12 sample kV-2D images, including information on the acquisition angle, amplitude, and direction of the applied offsets.

The evaluation considered the experience of the operators, who were divided into two groups: referent and non-referent. The referent group comprised professionals directly involved in implementing the IGRT strategy for stereotactic bone treatment at our center. This group included two physicians, one radiation therapist, and one physicist.

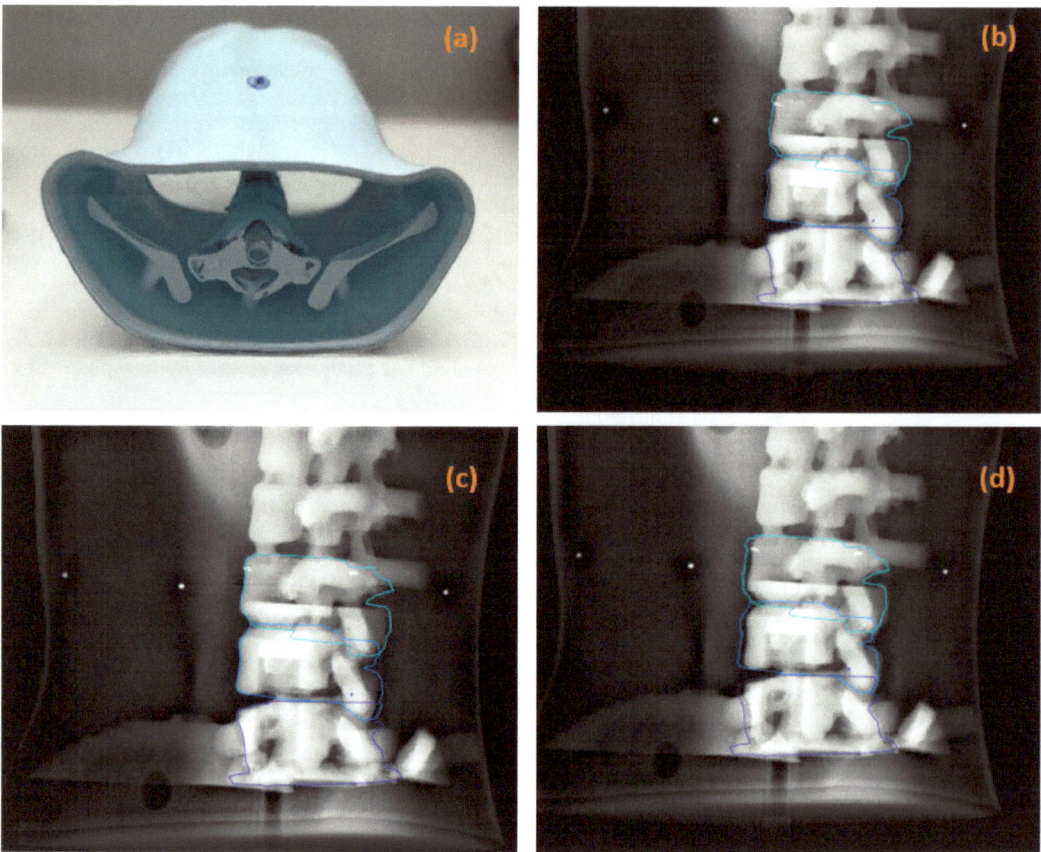

Figure 1. (**a**) RTSafe Spine© phantom. (**b**–**d**) Examples of kV-2D images analyzed by 18 participants during the anthropomorphic phantom test. The angle of incidence of the images was 135°, with deviations of (**b**) 0.0 mm, (**c**) 2.0 mm laterally, and (**d**) 2.0 mm vertically. Visual guidance structures were superimposed onto the images.

2.2. Patient Study

The data analyzed in this study were obtained from 29 patients treated at our center under stereotactic conditions for one or more bone metastases (35 tumor sites). The total dose was, in most cases (n = 33), 35 Gy in 5 fractions of 7 Gy (n = 33), delivered on one day out of two. The treatment period ranged from 03/2023 to 03/2024. Table 1 presents the treatment characteristics.

All patients were immobilized in the supine position using a vacuum bag system (Meicen©, Ektelesi Medical, Paris, France) below T3, with the arms raised on an indexed armrest. Above T3, a thermoplastic mask was used with the arms alongside the body. In addition to these devices, the knee and footrest were used. CT images (Somatom Definition AS20 RT, Siemens©) were acquired using a standardized protocol for bone stereotactic treatment, with a slice thickness of 1.0 mm.

Table 1. Patient and treatment characteristics. Abbreviations: ADK = adenocarcinoma; CCI = carcinoma; NET = neuroendocrine tumor; CCRCC = clear cell renal cell carcinoma; NA = not applicable; WHO = World Health Organization.

Patients	Site Treated	WHO Performance Status	Primary Cancer	Histological Types	Sex	21 Men
						8 Women
					Median Age (Years) (Range)	71 (47–85)
					Dose/Fractions	
1	Sacrum	0	Prostate	ADK	35 Gy/5 fr	
2	Right iliac wing	0	Prostate	ADK	35 Gy/5 fr	
3	Acromion	0	Breast	CCI	35 Gy/5 fr	
4	Right 10th rib	0	Prostate	ADK	35 Gy/5 fr	
5	Pubic symphysis	1	Breast	CCI	35 Gy/5 fr	
6	Right ischium	NA	Prostate	ADK	30 Gy/6 fr	
7	L5-S1	0	Prostate	ADK	36 Gy/6 fr	
8	T5	0	Prostate	ADK	35 Gy/5 fr	
9	Right iliac wing	0	Prostate	ADK	35 Gy/5 fr	
10	L5	NA	Breast	ADK	35 Gy/5 fr	
11	First right rib	0	Prostate	ADK	35 Gy/5 fr	
	Right 7th rib	0	Prostate	ADK	35 Gy/5 fr	
12	Left 10th rib	0	Kydney	CCRCC	35 Gy/5 fr	
13	Right ischium	0	Prostate	ADK	35 Gy/5 fr	
14	L4	0	Prostate	ADK	35 Gy/5 fr	
15	T12	1	Prostate	ADK	35 Gy/5 fr	
	Left 5th rib	1	Prostate	ADK	35 Gy/5 fr	
16	T12-L2 post-operative	NA	Breast	CCI	30 Gy/10 fr	
17	Right iliac wing	0	Prostate	ADK	35 Gy/5 fr	
	Right 6th rib	0	Prostate	ADK	35 Gy/5 fr	
	Left 6th rib	0	Prostate	ADK	35 Gy/5 fr	
18	T12	0	Breast	ADK	35 Gy/5 fr	
19	Right ischium	0	Prostate	ADK	35 Gy/5 fr	
20	T12	0	Prostate	ADK	35 Gy/5 fr	
21	Right posterior iliac wing	0	Prostate	ADK	35 Gy/5 fr	
	Right anterior iliac wing	0	Prostate	ADK	35 Gy/5 fr	
	T3	0	Prostate	ADK	35 Gy/5 fr	
22	L1	0	Breast	ADK	35 Gy/5 fr	
23	T12	0	Kidney	NET	35 Gy/5 fr	
24	C5	0	Prostate	ADK	35 Gy/5 fr	
25	Left ischium	0	Breast	ADK	35 Gy/5 fr	
26	T12	0	Breast	ADK	35 Gy/5 fr	
27	T11	1	Prostate	ADK	35 Gy/5 fr	
28	T2	0	Prostate	ADK	35 Gy/5 fr	
29	T1	0	Prostate	ADK	35 Gy/5 fr	

For spinal lesions, the gross target volume (GTV) was delineated by experienced physicians after the registration of various imaging modalities (CT, MRI with millimetric slices, and PET-CT when available). The clinical target volume (CTV) was delineated according to the international recommendations of Cox et al. [26]. In the case of epidural lesions, a distance of 3 mm was maintained between the spinal cord and the epidural lesion. For non-vertebral lesions, the CTV corresponded to a geometric extension of 5 mm from the GTV (which could be increased to 10 mm in certain cases) for bone disease and extra-osseous extensions (if extended at this level), respecting the anatomical barriers [27,28]. A 2 mm margin was applied from the CTV to obtain the PTV. This margin can be reduced to 0 mm in cases with proximity to the spinal cord. For non-vertebral bony lesions, the margin was 3 mm (potentially up to 5 mm). A margin of 2 mm was applied around the spinal cord volume and international dose constraints defined for the spinal cord volume were applied to the planning risk volumes of the spinal cord.

As the treatment did not involve the direct participation of the patient, no consent was required. All retrospective analyses were performed using fully anonymized data, in accordance with the ethical standards of our center and the 1964 Declaration of Helsinki.

All treatments were performed using volumetric modulated arc therapy according to our dosimetric protocol based on three coplanar arcs in 6 MV FFF photons at 1400 MU/min with collimator angles of 45°, 315°, and 95°. All treatment plans were calculated using the same planning system (Eclipse Acuros XB 15.6, 0.1 cm grid; Varian Medical Systems).

Irradiation was delivered in a bunker equipped with a TrueBeam 120 MLC (Varian Medical Systems, Palo Alto, CA, USA) and an OBI, which allowed kV-CBCT acquisitions as well as kV-2D images during irradiation. Patients were positioned on a 6D perfect pitch table.

The IGRT procedure involved acquiring a pretreatment kV-CBCT image with the application of the offsets obtained after the patient was placed on the table. The TrueBeam Varian v4.0 Intra-fraction Motion Review (IMR) application was used to acquire kV-2D images at a frequency of 7 s, for an average (standard deviation) of 2646 (740) MU per fraction, which allowed sufficient intra-fraction temporal tracking and decision time. Superimposed structures of the target vertebra and overlying and underlying vertebrae were used as visual guidance volumes for vertebral treatment. In the present study, the method of Koo et al. was extended to non-vertebral bony sites [24]. The initial tracking volumes covered the entire diseased bone and were then progressively adjusted. Borders and edges were then modified according to clinical feedback. Figure 2 summarizes the guidance volumes used at different sites contoured on CT images. Figure 3 shows some examples of kV-2D images acquired during irradiation and analyzed by operators at the treatment station.

The operators were instructed to stop the treatment if they considered correction of the patient's position necessary. kV-CBCT was then systematically performed to correct the patient's position, regardless of the actual offsets obtained. Intra-arc and post-treatment kV-CBCT were used to verify the decisions made by radiation therapists.

2.3. Analysis Method

Positioning errors were recorded using the Aria Offline Review module (ARIA 15.6; Varian Medical System, Palo Alto, CA, USA) for the lateral, vertical, and longitudinal translations. The kV-CBCT images acquired after the operators stopped the irradiation arc were used to measure real deviations. Without stops during each of the three arcs, the intra-arc and post-treatment kV-CBCT served the same purpose of quantifying the actual offsets.

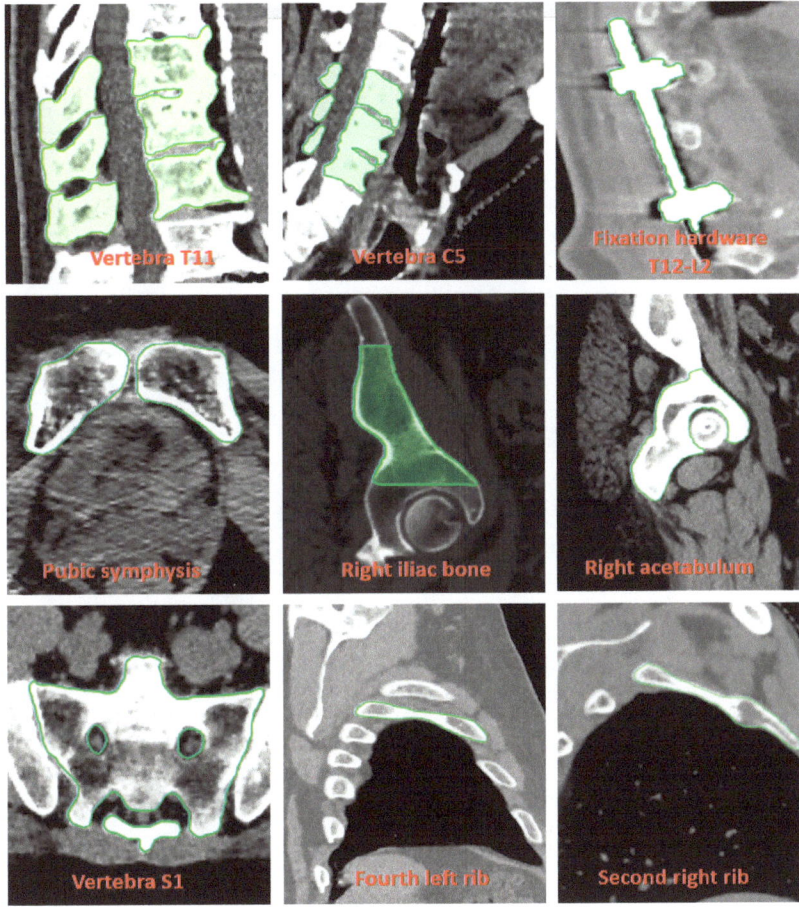

Figure 2. Examples of delineated structure types on millimeter-slice-thickness CT used for bone stereotactic IGRT based on kV acquisition during irradiation.

Five tolerance thresholds (1.0, 1.5, 2.0, 2.5, and 3.0 mm) were selected for data analysis. These thresholds were used to quantify the number of positioning deviations that exceeded the fixed tolerance (true positives (TP)) and were detected by the operators. True negatives (TN) corresponded to cases in which no deviation was visually observed by the radiation therapists and confirmed by subsequent kV-CBCT (intra-arc or post-treatment). False positives (FP) represented stops that were decided by the operator but whose deviations, as determined by kV-CBCT, were below the predefined threshold. Finally, false negatives (FN) corresponded to deviations above the threshold provided by the intra-arc or post-treatment kV-CBCT acquisition, but were not detected by the operators.

We have separated the analysis of vertebral localizations from that of extra-vertebral bone localizations to take account for the different margins used in these two cases.

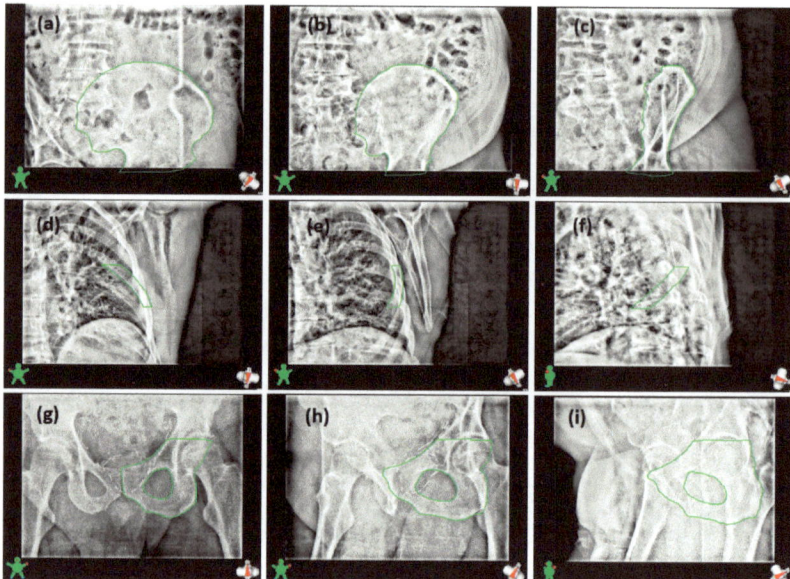

Figure 3. Examples of kV-2D images acquired during treatment fractions: (**a–c**) images of a right iliac wing acquired at 215.7°, 183.8°, and 147.9°; (**d–f**) images of a right fifth rib acquired at 188.3°, 147.7°, and 105.9°; and (**g–i**) images of a left ischium acquired at 359.3°, 29.4°, and 59.4°.

3. Results

3.1. Phantom Study

For all 18 participants, the average, minimum, and maximum scores were 81%, 65%, and 94%, respectively, of the 630 responses analyzed, with an average (standard deviation) decision time of 3.0 s (2.3). The referent group achieved 91% (89%, 94%) and 79% (65%, 89%) in the non-referent group. In this test, the detectability of phantom errors was proportional to their amplitudes. For offsets of 0.0, 1.0, 1.5, and 2.0 mm—independent of image incidence (Figure 4)—the results were 77.8%, 92.6%, 90.0%, and 100% for the expert group, and 77.8%, 69.6%, 79.3%, and 88.0% for the less experienced group.

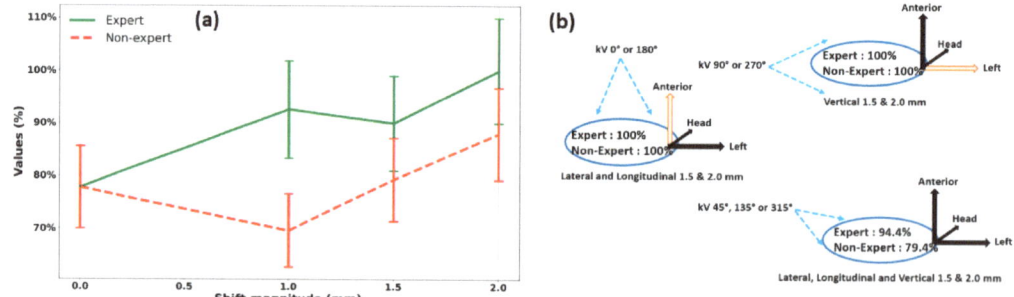

Figure 4. (**a**) Proportion (%) of correct responses to the anthropomorphic phantom test according to the amplitude of the shifts applied for the referent group (green solid line) and the less experienced group (red dashed line). (**b**) Evaluation of the acquisition incidence effect for offsets of 1.5 mm and 2.0 mm in the three translation directions.

The referent group showed a better ability to detect positioning errors as early as the 1.0 mm threshold, with 100% detectability at 2.0 mm versus 88.0% for the non-referent group. When no offset was applied, both groups did not hesitate to select the answer "Yes, error requiring treatment interruption, and kV-CBCT acquisition" in over 20% of cases. Both groups were aware that omitting positioning errors would be more detrimental to the patient than performing an additional kV-CBCT scan.

The effect of the acquisition incidence was also assessed (Figure 4) for offsets of 1.5 mm and 2.0 mm in the three translation directions. These errors were not detected when the directions were parallel to the OBI angle. In contrast, positioning errors of ≥1.5 mm were 100% detected when the image incidence was perpendicular to the displacement, regardless of the operator's skill level. When the angle of incidence was intermediate (45°, 135°, or 315°), errors were detected in 94% and 79% of the experts and non-experts, respectively.

3.2. Patient Study

In this section, 205 kV-CBCT images were retrospectively reviewed to determine the performance of the proposed IGRT method, which is based on the visual tracking of the target volume position by kV-2D imaging during irradiation with the help of a tumor-specific tracking volume (Figure 2). Of these 205 kV-CBCT, 92 related to vertebral locations and 113 to bony locations outside the vertebrae. Of the 165 available fractions, 135 were used in the present study.

For the vertebral locations and for the three vertical, longitudinal, and lateral directions, the median (maximum) absolute values of the positioning errors were 0.3 (3.6) mm, 0.4 (2.3) mm, and 0.5 (2.1) mm, respectively (Figure 5a). For non-spinal bony metastases and in the same order, the positioning errors were 0.5 (3.3) mm, 0.4 (2.1) mm, and 0.6 (4.8) mm (Figure 5c).

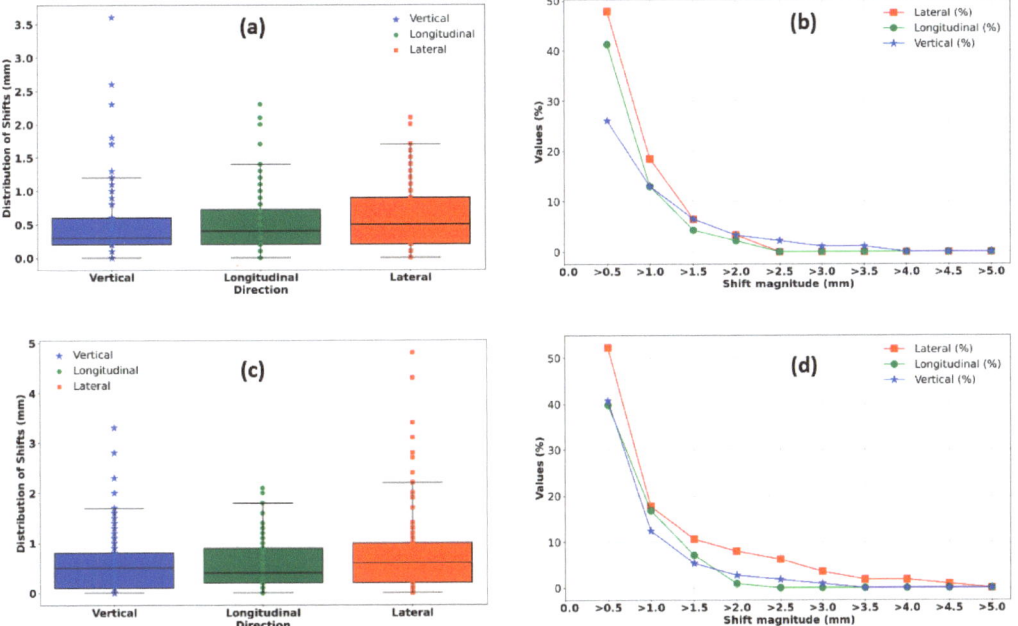

Figure 5. (**a**,**c**) Distribution of observed deviations for the three directions: vertical, longitudinal, and lateral for spinal locations and for non-spinal bony metastases, respectively. (**b**,**d**) Proportion (%) of observed deviations by direction and above a given threshold in millimeters for spinal locations and for non-spinal bony metastases, respectively.

The curves in Figure 5b,d show the proportion (%) of the positioning errors above a given threshold in the three directions. For the vertebral locations, the percentages of errors measured with kV-CBCT images above a particular threshold of 2.0 mm were 3.3%, 2.2%, and 3.3% in the vertical, longitudinal, and lateral directions, respectively. For the bony locations outside the vertebrae, the results for the same threshold and in the same order were 2.7%, 0.9%, and 8.0%. For the latter, taking into account the clinical margins used, the proportion of positioning errors greater than a 3 mm threshold was 0.9%, 0.0%, and 3.5% in the vertical, longitudinal, and lateral directions, respectively.

Table 2 shows the scores obtained by radiation therapists according to different tolerance thresholds using the previously defined IGRT method. The relevance of the decision to stop or not stop the beam during treatment, when the position of the target volume appeared suspicious, was verified using subsequent kV-CBCTs.

Table 2. Proportions of true positives (TP), true negatives (TN), false positives (FP), and false negatives (FN) according to the tolerance thresholds applied to the analysis of the operator's decisions in the treatment room. FN are shown in bold. Abbreviations: VB = vertebrae; NVB = non-vertebral bone.

92 and 113 kV-CBCT Scenarios for VB and NVB Sites, Respectively	Designation		Threshold				
			1.0 mm	1.5 mm	2.0 mm	2.5 mm	3.0 mm
Beam stop and subsequent kV-CBCT acquisition ≥ threshold	True Positives (TP)	VB	21 (22.8%)	14 (15.2%)	8 (8.7%)	2 (2.2%)	1 (1.1%)
		NVB	31 (27.4%)	14 (12.4%)	11 (9.7%)	11 (9.7%)	4 (3.5%)
No beam stop and kV-CBCT acquisition at end of arc < threshold	True Negatives (TN)	VB	42 (45.6%)	56 (60.9%)	57 (62.0%)	59 (64.1%)	59 (64.1%)
		NVB	45 (39.8%)	62 (54.9%)	67 (59.3%)	69 (61.1%)	70 (61.9%)
Beam stop and subsequent kV-CBCT acquisition < threshold	False Positives (FP)	VB	12 (13.0%)	19 (20.6%)	25 (27.2%)	31 (33.7%)	32 (34.8%)
		NVB	11 (9.7%)	28 (24.8%)	31 (27.4%)	35 (31.0%)	38 (33.6%)
No beam stop and kV-CBCT acquisition at end of arc ≥ threshold	**False Negatives (FN)**	**VB**	**17 (18.5%)**	**3 (3.3%)**	**2 (2.2%)**	**0 (0.0%)**	**0 (0.0%)**
		NVB	**26 (23.0%)**	**9 (8.0%)**	**4 (3.5%)**	**2 (1.8%)**	**1 (0.9%)**

FN were the only errors considered harmful to patients and are highlighted in Table 2. FP, which are considered less serious, involve the acquisition of a kV-CBCT of approximately 1.5 min in duration, with an average additional effective dose of 10–20 mSv [29]. For spinal locations and for thresholds of 1.0, 1.5, 2.0, 2.5, and 3.0 mm, the nondetection rates for deviations above these tolerances were 18.5%, 3.3%, 2.2%, 0.0%, and 0.0%, respectively. For non-spinal bony metastases and in the same order, the nondetection rates were 23.0%, 8.0%, 3.5%, 1.8%, and 0.9%.

4. Discussion

This study evaluated and validated the IGRT strategy used for the stereotactic treatment of bone metastases, based on the ability to generate periodic kV-2D images during irradiation with superimposed volumes, to facilitate the visual tracking of the target volume position.

The anthropomorphic phantom test confirmed the accuracy of this qualitative target volume tracking method and served as a training tool prior to its implementation in the clinical routine. An analysis of 18 participant responses—which were divided into two groups: referent and non-referent—showed the influence of operator experience on the performance of the proposed IGRT method. Without knowing the occurrence and amplitude of simulated errors of 0.0, 1.0, 1.5, and 2.0 mm in the three translation directions, and without considering the angle of incidence at which the kV-2D images were acquired, the referent group obtained an average correct response of 91% versus 79% for the non-referent group. The larger the offset, the higher the score. For an offset of 2.0 mm, regardless of the angle of image acquisition—except parallel to the direction of the error because it was undetectable—experienced operators achieved 100% success compared with 88% for less experienced operators. These results were significantly different from those reported by Koo et al. [24]. In their study, the detectability rates of the experienced and inexperienced groups were approximately 55% and 28%, respectively, for an offset of 2 mm. This difference can be explained by the experimental conditions and, more specifically, by the type of phantom used. The images of the anthropomorphic Alderson RANDO phantom (Alderson Research Laboratories, Inc., Long Island City, NY, USA) showed artifacts that prevented a good estimation of the simulated shifts. An equally plausible explanation is that the present study included pre-training before phantom testing, which was not the case in the study of Koo et al. [24]. This highlights the importance of training prior to implementing the new IGRT method. Additionally, it highlights the obvious limitations of the results obtained on the phantom compared with the real treatment.

For the experimental protocol used in this study, positioning errors of ≥ 1.5 mm were detected 100% of the time by all operators when the incidence of the planar image was perpendicular to the displacement. At intermediate angles (45°, 135°, and 315°), the success rate for expert participants was 94%, compared with 74% for the less experienced group. These results indicate that a deviation occurring at an acquisition angle parallel to its direction is likely to be detected at the maximum angle of 45°. With arm rotation speeds in the order of 6°/s, this type of misalignment is detected approximately 7–10 s later, corresponding to one or two new automatically triggered images.

Ong et al. [30] investigated the dosimetric impact of intra-fractional movements on the spinal cord for 6 MV and 6 MV FFF spinal stereotactic treatments. In their study, for 6 MV FFF beams, an offset of 2 mm for 10 s and 30 s induce an increase in Dmax at the spinal cord of 3% and 13%, respectively. The mean (SD) operator-decision time for the present study was 3 (2.3) s. Considering this result and that of Ong et al. [30], the triggering of kV-2D images by the IMR application was set every 7 s during the clinical routine.

During the clinical implementation, we decided to extend the IGRT method beyond the treatment of vertebral bones. The visual guide volume was defined for each site (Figure 2). Clinical cases of patients with orthopedic hardware in the spine are included in this list. Inspired by the study by Cetnar et al. [31], this device was used as a landmark (Figure 2).

The intra-fraction offset values are in the range reported in the literature. Although the majority of offsets were below our clinical threshold of 2 mm and 3 mm depending on the margins applied, our study confirmed the occurrence of sudden movements with amplitudes above these tolerance thresholds.

The rate of deviation of >2 mm and 3 mm, undetected by radiation therapists (FN), was approximately 2% and 1% for spinal locations and for non-spinal bony metastases respectively. These results helped to limit excessive undetected shifts and assumes no distinction between the expertise of the people and the incidence of the planar image in relation to the direction of movement. This result must also be weighed against the fact that movement may occur between the beam stop and kV-CBCT acquisition.

The results also showed that, for a tolerance threshold of 1.0 mm, the detectability (FN) decreased to 81.5% for spinal sites. This performance has not been validated in the clinical routine at our institution and does not allow for the margin reduction of the positioning uncertainty in this threshold. This finding and the limitations of this strategy should be compared with the performance of non-embedded accelerator systems with automatic registration during irradiation, which can guarantee an accuracy of the order of 1.0 mm [32] for the spinal treatment.

We have extended the methodology to non-vertebral bone locations, initially proposing guide volumes that cover the entire diseased bone and then progressively adjusting the boundaries and edges according to clinical feedback. Each team implementing our methodology must use its own clinical feedback to find the most relevant guide volumes. Several image parameters, such as kV, mAs, or filters selected by the operators at the treatment console, can impact the performance of this IGRT strategy. This impact has not been studied in this manuscript. Nevertheless, the results in Table 2 showed that, for spinal sites, eight offsets greater than 2 mm were corrected (true positives) by kV-CBCT acquired immediately after stopping treatment. No CBCT at the end of the arc (false negatives) was greater than 2.5 mm. For non-vertebral bone locations, four offsets greater than 3.0 mm were corrected and only one kV-CBCT at the end of the arc was greater than 3.0 mm.

The tracking volumes shown in Figure 2 were manually delineated, adding a time-consuming step to the treatment plan. This was compounded by the fact that the present study was performed using a CT scanner with a slice thickness of 1.0 mm. The effect of CT slice thickness on the performance of this IGRT method has been investigated by several authors [33]. For example, Koo et al. [24] reported a decrease in detectability of >10% for a 2 mm threshold when comparing the 1.0 mm and 3.0 mm CT scans. Therefore, to maintain the accuracy of the IGRT method, the thickness of the dosimetric scans was not increased. Automatic segmentation strategies reduce the time required for this task while harmonizing the delineation of the positioning structures.

Notably, this method is expertise-dependent and requires maximum operator concentration in the workplace. Therefore, training is a key factor in the effectiveness of monitoring qualitative target volume positions. At least two radiation therapists supervised the irradiation fraction and 2D kV images. To limit interruptions, we established a procedure to clearly signal the progress of stereotactic bone treatment. During these treatments, only those directly involved were present, a "stereotactic treatment in progress" flag was installed, and telephone calls were turned off.

Automated beam stopping is possible with this type of machine [23], but it requires the implantation of fiducials, as in the case of prostate cancer treatment. A major step forward in the management of motion in bone SBRT is the development of an automated beam stop by the manufacturer, which should be available with the IMR application and based on bone registration. Currently, the only alternative is external imaging devices based on bone registration [13].

To date, many centers use kV-CBCT imaging only before the start of each arc, and, at best, between each arc. However, this adds time to the treatment fraction and delays the detection of patient motion. TPS Eclipse can provide the exact timing of the stops that occur during the irradiation arcs. This information will allow the investigation to continue by estimating the dosimetric impact on the target volume and OAR according to the IGRT strategy used, with or without kV-2D imaging during irradiation.

5. Conclusions

The use of OBI kV-2D imaging for the visual guidance of spinal and non-spinal bony stereotactic radiation was validated using anthropomorphic phantom and clinical data. The results confirmed a visual accuracy of 2 mm for spinal stereotactic treatment and 3 mm for non-spinal stereotactic treatment. These results were consistent with the positioning uncertainty margins used. The study also proposed structures to guide the visual monitoring of the target volume position for different treated sites. The proposed method, based on an imaging device that is always available on current linear accelerators, enables a robust IGRT strategy for performing bone stereotactic treatment at no additional cost to centers.

Author Contributions: A.H.H.: conceptualization, formal analysis, investigation, methodology, software, supervision, validation, writing—original draft, and writing—review and editing. G.M.: investigation, validation, and writing—review and editing. L.L.: investigation, validation, and writing—review, and editing. I.A.: conceptualization, formal analysis, investigation, methodology, software, validation, and writing—review, and editing. All authors have read and agreed to the published version of the manuscript.

Funding: This research received no external funding.

Institutional Review Board Statement: Not applicable.

Informed Consent Statement: Informed consent was waived due to retrospective nature of the study. Informed consent was waived due to retrospective nature of the study.

Data Availability Statement: The original contributions of this study are included in the article. Further inquiries can be directed to the corresponding authors.

Conflicts of Interest: The authors declare that this research was conducted in the absence of commercial or financial relationships that could be construed as potential conflicts of interest.

References

1. Gong, Y.; Xu, L.; Zhuang, H.; Jiang, L.; Wei, F.; Liu, Z.; Li, Y.; Yu, M.; Ni, K.; Liu, X. Efficacy and safety of different fractions in stereotactic body radiotherapy for spinal metastases: A systematic review. *Cancer Med.* **2019**, *8*, 6176–6184. [CrossRef]
2. De la Pinta, C. SBRT in non-spine bone metastases: A literature review. *Med. Oncol.* **2020**, *37*, 119. [CrossRef]
3. Palma, D.A.; Olson, R.; Harrow, S.; Gaede, S.; Louie, A.V.; Haasbeek, C.; Mulroy, L.; Lock, M.; Rodrigues, G.B.; Yaremko, B.P.; et al. Stereotactic Ablative Radiotherapy for the Comprehensive Treatment of Oligometastatic Cancers: Long-Term Results of the SABR-COMET Phase II Randomized Trial. *J. Clin. Oncol. Off. J. Am. Soc. Clin. Oncol.* **2020**, *38*, 2830–2838. [CrossRef] [PubMed]
4. Pougnet, I.; Jaegle, E.; Garcia, R.; Tessier, F.; Faivre, J.C.; Louvel, G.; Gross, E.; Gonzague, L.; Benchalal, M.; Ducteil, A.; et al. État des lieux de la radiothérapie en conditions stéréotaxiques vertébrale en France en 2016 [Spinal stereotactic body radiotherapy: French assessment in 2016]. *Cancer Radiother. J. Soc. Fr. Radiother. Oncol.* **2017**, *21*, 276–285. [CrossRef]
5. Bhattacharya, I.S.; Hoskin, P.J. Stereotactic body radiotherapy for spinal and bone metastases. *Clin. Oncol.* **2015**, *27*, 298–306. [CrossRef] [PubMed]
6. Guckenberger, M.; Mantel, F.; Gersten, P.C.; Flickinger, J.C.; Sahgal, A.; Létourneau, D.; Grills, I.S.; Jawad, M.; Fahim, D.K.; Shin, J.H.; et al. Safety and efficacy of stereotactic body radiotherapy as primary treatment for vertebral metastases: A multi-institutional analysis. *Radiat. Oncol.* **2014**, *9*, 226. [CrossRef] [PubMed]
7. Wang, H.; Shiu, A.; Wang, C.; O'Daniel, J.; Mahajan, A.; Woo, S.; Liengsawangwong, P.; Mohan, R.; Chang, E.L. Dosimetric effect of translational and rotational errors for patients undergoing image-guided stereotactic body radiotherapy for spinal metastases. *Int. J. Radiat. Oncol. Biol. Phys.* **2008**, *71*, 1261–1271. [CrossRef] [PubMed]
8. Hadj Henni, A.; Gensanne, D.; Roge, M.; Hanzen, C.; Bulot, G.; Colard, E.; Thureau, S. Evaluation of inter- and intra-fraction 6D motion for stereotactic body radiation therapy of spinal metastases: Influence of treatment time. *Radiat. Oncol.* **2021**, *16*, 168. [CrossRef] [PubMed]
9. Li, W.; Sahgal, A.; Foote, M.; Millar, B.-A.; Jaffray, D.A.; Letourneau, D. Impact of immobilization on intrafraction motion for spine stereotactic body radiotherapy using cone beam computed tomography. *Int. J. Radiat. Oncol. Biol. Phys.* **2012**, *84*, 520–526. [CrossRef]
10. Agazaryan, N.; Tenn, S.E.; Desalles, A.A.F.; Selch, M.T. Image-guided radiosurgery for spinal tumors: Methods, accuracy and patient intrafraction motion. *Phys. Med. Biol.* **2008**, *53*, 1715–1727. [CrossRef] [PubMed]
11. Hadj Henni, A.; Gensanne, D.; Bulot, G.; Roge, M.; Mallet, R.; Colard, E.; Daras, M.; Hanzen, C.; Thureau, S. ExacTrac X-ray 6D imaging during stereotactic body radiation therapy of spinal and nonspinal metastases. *Technol. Cancer Res. Treat.* **2023**, *22*, 15330338231210786. [CrossRef] [PubMed]
12. Kurup, G. CyberKnife: A new paradigm in radiotherapy. *J. Med. Phys.* **2010**, *35*, 63–64. [CrossRef]
13. Montgomery, C.; Collins, M. An evaluation of the BrainLAB 6D ExacTrac/Novalis Tx system for image-guided intracranial radiotherapy. *J. Radiother. Pract.* **2017**, *16*, 326–333. [CrossRef]
14. Covington, E.L.; Fiveash, J.B.; Wu, X.; Brezovich, I.; Willey, C.D.; Riley, K.; Popple, R.A. Optical surface guidance for submillimeter monitoring of patient position during frameless stereotactic radiotherapy. *J. Appl. Clin. Med. Phys.* **2019**, *20*, 91–98. [CrossRef] [PubMed]
15. Covington, E.L.; Stanley, D.N.; Fiveash, J.B.; Thomas, E.M.; Marcrom, S.R.; Bredel, M.; Willey, C.D.; Riley, K.O.; Popple, R.A. Surface guided imaging during stereotactic radiosurgery with automated delivery. *J. Appl. Clin. Med. Phys.* **2020**, *21*, 90–95. [CrossRef] [PubMed]
16. Bell, L.J.; Eade, T.; Kneebone, A.; Hruby, G.; Alfieri, F.; Bromley, R.; Grimberg, K.; Barnes, M.; Booth, J.T. Initial experience with intra-fraction motion monitoring using Calypso guided volumetric modulated arc therapy for definitive prostate cancer treatment. *J. Med. Radiat. Sci.* **2017**, *64*, 25–34. [CrossRef]
17. Kupelian, P.; Willoughby, T.; Mahadevan, A.; Djemil, T.; Weinstein, G.; Jani, S.; Enke, C.; Solberg, T.; Flores, N.; Liu, D.; et al. Multi-institutional clinical experience with the Calypso System in localization and continuous, real-time monitoring of the prostate gland during external radiotherapy. *Int. J. Radiat. Oncol. Biol. Phys.* **2007**, *67*, 1088–1098. [CrossRef]
18. Hyde, D.; Lochray, F.; Korol, R.; Davidson, M.; Wong, C.S.; Ma, L.; Sahgal, A. Spine stereotactic body radiotherapy utilizing cone-beam CT image-guidance with a robotic couch: Intrafraction motion analysis accounting for all six degrees of freedom. *Int. J. Radiat. Oncol. Biol. Phys.* **2012**, *82*, e555–e562. [CrossRef] [PubMed]
19. Finnigan, R.; Lamprecht, B.; Barry, T.; Jones, K.; Boyd, J.; Pullar, A.; Burmeister, B.; Foote, M. Inter- and intra-fraction motion in stereotactic body radiotherapy for spinal and paraspinal tumours using cone-beam CT and positional correction in six degrees of freedom. *J. Med. Imaging Radiat. Oncol.* **2016**, *60*, 112–118. [CrossRef]
20. Dahele, M.; Slotman, B.; Verbakel, W. Stereotactic body radiotherapy for spine and bony pelvis using flattening filter free volumetric modulated arc therapy, 6D cone-beam CT and simple positioning techniques: Treatment time and patient stability. *Acta Oncol.* **2016**, *55*, 795–798. [CrossRef]

21. Graadal Svestad, J.; Ramberg, C.; Skar, B.; Paulsen Hellebust, T. Intrafractional motion in stereotactic body radiotherapy of spinal metastases utilizing cone beam computed tomography image guidance. *Phys. Imaging Radiat. Oncol.* **2019**, *12*, 1–6. [CrossRef]
22. Chasseray, M.; Dissaux, G.; Lucia, F.; Boussion, N.; Goasduff, G.; Pradier, O.; Bourbonne, V.; Schick, U. Kilovoltage intrafraction monitoring during normofractionated prostate cancer radiotherapy. *Cancer Radiother.* **2020**, *24*, 99–105. [CrossRef] [PubMed]
23. Korpics, M.C.; Rokni, M.; Degnan, M.; Aydogan, B.; Liauw, S.L.; Redler, G. Utilizing the TrueBeam Advanced Imaging Package to monitor intrafraction motion with periodic kV imaging and automatic marker detection during VMAT prostate treatments. *J. Appl. Clin. Med. Phys.* **2020**, *21*, 184–191. [CrossRef]
24. Koo, J.; Nardella, L.; Degnan, M.; Andreozzi, J.; Yu, H.M.; Penagaricano, J.; Johnstone, P.A.S.; Oliver, D.; Ahmed, K.; Rosenberg, S.A.; et al. Triggered kV Imaging During Spine SBRT for Intrafraction Motion Management. *Technol. Cancer Res. Treat.* **2021**, *20*, 15330338211063033. [CrossRef] [PubMed]
25. GuckenBerger, M.; Meyer, J.; Wilbert, J.; Baier, K.; Bratengeier, K.; Vordermark, D.; Flentje, M. Precision required for dose-escalated treatment of spinal metastases and implications for image-guided radiation therapy (IGRT). *Radiother. Oncol.* **2007**, *84*, 56–63. [CrossRef] [PubMed]
26. Cox, B.W.; Spratt, D.E.; Lovelock, M.; Bilsky, M.H.; Lis, E.; Ryu, S.; Sheehan, J.; Gerszten, P.C.; Chang, E.; Gibbs, I.; et al. International Spine Radiosurgery Consortium consensus guidelines for target volume definition in spinal stereotactic radiosurgery. *Int. J. Radiat. Oncol. Biol. Phys.* **2012**, *83*, e597–e605. [CrossRef]
27. Dunne, E.M.; Sahgal, A.; Lo, S.S.; Bergman, A.; Kosztyla, R.; Dea, N.; Chang, E.L.; Chang, U.K.; Chao, S.T.; Faruqi, S.; et al. International consensus recommendations for target volume delineation specific to sacral metastases and spinal stereotactic body radiation therapy (SBRT). *Radiother. Oncol. J. Eur. Soc. Ther. Radiol. Oncol.* **2020**, *145*, 21–29. [CrossRef] [PubMed]
28. Nguyen, T.K.; Chin, L.; Sahgal, A.; Dagan, R.; Eppinga, W.; Guckenberger, M.; Kim, J.H.; Lo, S.S.; Redmond, K.J.; Siva, S.; et al. International Multi-institutional Patterns of Contouring Practice and Clinical Target Volume Recommendations for Stereotactic Body Radiation Therapy for Non-Spine Bone Metastases. *Int. J. Radiat. Oncol. Biol. Phys.* **2022**, *112*, 351–360. [CrossRef] [PubMed]
29. Kan, M.W.K.; Leung, L.H.T.; Wong, W.; Lam, N. Radiation dose from cone beam computed tomography for image-guided radiation therapy. *Int. J. Radiat. Oncol. Biol. Phys.* **2008**, *70*, 272–279. [CrossRef] [PubMed]
30. Ong, C.L.; Dahele, M.; Cuijpers, J.P.; Senan, S.; Slotman, B.J.; Verbakel, W.F.A.R. Dosimetric impact of intrafraction motion during RapidArc stereotactic vertebral radiation therapy using flattened and flattening filter-free beams. *Int. J. Radiat. Oncol. Biol. Phys.* **2013**, *86*, 420–425. [CrossRef] [PubMed]
31. Cetnar, A.J.; Degnan, M.; Pichler, J.; Jain, S.; Morelli, S.; Thomas, E.; Elder, J.B.; Scharschmidt, T.J.; Palmer, J.D.; Blakaj, D.M. Implementation of triggered kilovoltage imaging for stereotactic radiotherapy of the spine for patients with spinal fixation hardware. *Phys. Imaging Radiat. Oncol.* **2023**, *25*, 100422. [CrossRef]
32. Wu, J.; Wu, J.; Ballangrud, Å.; Mechalakos, J.; Yamada, J.; Lovelock, D.M. Frequency of large intrafractional target motions during spine stereotactic body radiation therapy. *Pract. Radiat. Oncol.* **2020**, *10*, e45–e49. [CrossRef]
33. Bellon, M.R.; Siddiqui, M.S.; Ryu, S.; Chetty, I.J. The effect of longitudinal CT resolution and pixel size (FOV) on target delineation and treatment planning in stereotactic radiosurgery. *J. Radiosurg. SBRT* **2014**, *3*, 149–163. [PubMed] [PubMed Central]

Disclaimer/Publisher's Note: The statements, opinions and data contained in all publications are solely those of the individual author(s) and contributor(s) and not of MDPI and/or the editor(s). MDPI and/or the editor(s) disclaim responsibility for any injury to people or property resulting from any ideas, methods, instructions or products referred to in the content.

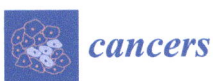 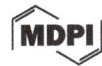

Article

Evolving Trends and Patterns of Utilization of Magnetic Resonance-Guided Radiotherapy at a Single Institution, 2018–2024

Robert A. Herrera [1,*], Eyub Y. Akdemir [1], Rupesh Kotecha [1,2], Kathryn E. Mittauer [1,2], Matthew D. Hall [1,2], Adeel Kaiser [1,2], Nema Bassiri-Gharb [1,2], Noah S. Kalman [1,2], Yonatan Weiss [1], Tino Romaguera [1,2], Diane Alvarez [1,2], Sreenija Yarlagadda [1], Ranjini Tolakanahalli [1,2], Alonso N. Gutierrez [1,2], Minesh P. Mehta [1,2] and Michael D. Chuong [1,2,*]

[1] Department of Radiation Oncology, Miami Cancer Institute, Miami, FL 33176, USA; eyub.akdemir@baptisthealth.net (E.Y.A.); rupeshk@baptisthealth.net (R.K.); kathrynm@baptisthealth.net (K.E.M.); matthewha@baptisthealth.net (M.D.H.); nema.bassirigharb@baptisthealth.net (N.B.-G.); noahk@baptisthealth.net (N.S.K.); yonatan.weiss@baptisthealth.net (Y.W.); antinogenesr@baptisthealth.net (T.R.); dianeal@baptisthealth.net (D.A.); sreenija.yarlagadda@baptisthealth.net (S.Y.); ranjinit@baptisthealth.net (R.T.); alonsog@baptisthealth.net (A.N.G.); mineshm@baptisthealth.net (M.P.M.)
[2] Herbert Wertheim College of Medicine, Florida International University, Miami, FL 33199, USA
* Correspondence: robertoherr@baptisthealth.net (R.A.H.); michaelchu@baptisthealth.net (M.D.C.)

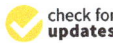

Academic Editor: Hideya Yamazaki

Received: 30 November 2024
Revised: 2 January 2025
Accepted: 7 January 2025
Published: 10 January 2025

Citation: Herrera, R.A.; Akdemir, E.Y.; Kotecha, R.; Mittauer, K.E.; Hall, M.D.; Kaiser, A.; Bassiri-Gharb, N.; Kalman, N.S.; Weiss, Y.; Romaguera, T.; et al. Evolving Trends and Patterns of Utilization of Magnetic Resonance-Guided Radiotherapy at a Single Institution, 2018–2024. *Cancers* **2025**, *17*, 208. https://doi.org/10.3390/cancers17020208

Copyright: © 2025 by the authors. Licensee MDPI, Basel, Switzerland. This article is an open access article distributed under the terms and conditions of the Creative Commons Attribution (CC BY) license (https://creativecommons.org/licenses/by/4.0/).

Simple Summary: Magnetic resonance-guided radiotherapy (MRgRT) is expanding worldwide thanks to advances in soft tissue imaging, continuous visualization of the target and normal organs-at-risk during treatment, automated intelligently gated beam delivery within predefined targeting boundaries, and on-table adaptive replanning, all of which permit improved treatment efficacy, toxicity reduction, and shortened fractionation regimens. This, however, is still a nascent technology which can be more time- and resource-intensive than standard radiotherapy, and hence its optimal utilization and deployment remain in constant flux and evolution. We retrospectively analyzed our institutional MRgRT utilization across 823 treatment courses over a 6-year period, which predominantly included abdominal and pelvic tumors treated with dose-escalated ultra-hypofractionation.

Abstract: Background/Objectives: Over the past decade, significant advances have been made in image-guided radiotherapy (RT) particularly with the introduction of magnetic resonance (MR)-guided radiotherapy (MRgRT). However, the optimal clinical applications of MRgRT are still evolving. The intent of this analysis was to describe our institutional MRgRT utilization patterns and evolution therein, specifically as an early adopter within a center endowed with multiple other technology platforms. **Materials/Methods:** We retrospectively evaluated patterns of MRgRT utilization for patients treated with a 0.35-Tesla MR-Linac at our institution from April 2018 to April 2024. We analyzed changes in utilization across six annualized periods: Period 1 (April 2018–April 2019) through Period 6 (April 2023–April 2024). We defined ultra-hypofractionation (UHfx) as 5 or fewer fractions with a minimum fractional dose of 5 Gy. Electronic health records were reviewed, and data were extracted related to patient, tumor, and treatment characteristics. **Results**: A total of 823 treatment courses were delivered to 712 patients treated for 854 lesions. The most commonly treated sites were the pancreas (242 [29.4%]), thorax (172; 20.9%), abdominopelvic lymph nodes (107; 13.0%), liver (72; 8.7%), and adrenal glands (68; 8.3%). The median total prescribed dose of 50 Gy in five fractions (fxs) was typically delivered in consecutive days with automatic beam gating in inspiration breath hold. The median biologically effective dose ($\alpha/\beta = 10$, BED10) was 94.4 Gy with nearly half (404, 49.1%)

of all courses at a prescribed BED10 ≥ 100 Gy, which is widely regarded as a highly effective ablative dose. Courses in Period 6 vs. Period 1 more often had a prescribed BED10 ≥ 100 Gy (60.2% vs. 41.6%; $p = 0.004$). Of the 6036 total delivered fxs, nearly half (2643, 43.8%) required at least one fx of on-table adaptive radiotherapy (oART), most commonly for pancreatic tumors (1081, 17.9%). UHfx was used in over three quarters of all courses (630, 76.5%) with 472 (57.4%) of these requiring oART for at least one fraction. The relative utilization of oART increased significantly from Period 1 to Period 6 (37.6% to 85.0%; $p < 0.001$); a similar increase in the use of UHfx (66.3% to 89.5%; $p < 0.001$) was also observed. The median total in-room time for oART decreased from 81 min in Period 1 to 45 min in Period 6, while for non-oART, it remained stable around 40 min across all periods. **Conclusions**: Our institution implemented MRgRT with a priority for targeting mobile extracranial tumors in challenging anatomic locations that are frequently treated with dose escalation, require enhanced soft-tissue visualization, and could benefit from an ablative radiotherapy approach. Over the period under evaluation, the use of high-dose ablative doses (BED10 ≥ 100 Gy), oART and UHfx (including single-fraction ablation) increased significantly, underscoring both a swift learning curve and ability to optimize processes to maximize throughput and efficiency.

Keywords: MR-guided radiotherapy; MRgRT; stereotactic ablative radiotherapy; on-table adaptive radiation therapy; stereotactic body radiotherapy; SBRT; SMART; ART; ultra-hypofractionated; treatment patterns

1. Introduction

Contemporary image-guided radiotherapy (IGRT) relies on kilovoltage/megavoltage (kV/MV) portal imaging and/or cone-beam computed tomography (MV or kvCT)-based techniques to ensure appropriate patient positioning and target localization. However, these imaging modalities may provide a suboptimal visualization of gross disease and organs-at-risk (OARs) due to limitations in visualizing low-density structures, especially when adjacent or abutting [1]. Magnetic resonance (MR)-guided radiotherapy (MRgRT) is a novel technology featuring advanced imaging and rapid replanning capabilities using on-table images [2] that may improve clinical outcomes by facilitating safe dose escalation and reducing toxicity, especially for tumors in challenging anatomic locations [3,4] that have suboptimal outcomes when treated with CT-guided linear accelerators (Linacs) [3,5–9].

In 2018, our institution became one of the first worldwide adopters of a 0.35-Tesla (T) MR-Linac (ViewRay Inc., Cleveland, OH, USA) [10]. The 0.35-T MR-Linac has several advanced capabilities including continuous intrafraction multi-planar MR imaging [2], automatic beam gating [11], and the ability to deliver on-table adaptive radiotherapy (oART) [6,7]. There has been increasing worldwide MRgRT adoption, and different centers have deployed this technology with differing clinical goal: some focusing on prostate and breast tumors and others focusing on mobile intrathoracic and intraabdominal tumors [12–15]. Our center has multiple technology platforms, and the goal of incorporating this technology was to implement ablative dosing approaches for mobile tumors, especially susceptible to respiratory incursions, and not suitable for CT-guided approaches because of soft-tissue resolution limitations. Inherently, this focused the indications toward UHfx and oART. These approaches evolved with technology and software improvements as well as with process-based efficiencies and improved learning and QA. We therefore evaluated changes in MRgRT utilization at our institution over a 6-year period with a focus on identifying specific clinical scenarios that might especially benefit from MRgRT, and we also sought to understand whether throughput efficiencies could be achieved with experience.

2. Materials and Methods

This single-institution retrospective analysis evaluated patients treated with MRgRT on a 0.35-T MRIdian-Linac between April 2018 and April 2024. Patient demographics, tumor, and treatment data as well as treatment time distributions (e.g., total in-room time [TIRT] and total delivery time [TDT]) were collected (Table 1). We defined TIRT as the time spent inside the treatment room, while TDT was the time from first beam-on to treatment completion. To evaluate trends over time, treatment courses were divided into six consecutive 12-month periods. Patients receiving multiple MRgRT treatment courses for local recurrences or distant tumor sites were treated as distinct cases.

Table 1. Baseline characteristics of patients treated with magnetic resonance-guided radiotherapy. Abbreviations: GTV, gross tumor volume; CTV, clinical tumor volume; PTV, planning tumor volume; BED, biological effective dose.

		Tumor Sites						
Characteristics	Treatment Courses (n = 823)	Pancreas (n = 242)	Thorax (n = 172)	Abdominopelvic Lymph Node (n = 107)	Liver (n = 72)	Adrenal Glands (n = 68)	Prostate (n = 17)	Other (n = 146)
Age—yr								
Median (range)	69.0 (7.0–94.0)	71.0 (21.0–94.0)	71.0 (15.0–94.0)	67.0 (31.0–90.0)	68.0 (7.0–88.0)	64.0 (28.0–85.0)	63.5 (59.0–76.0)	69.0 (8.0–93.0)
≥65 yr—no. (%)	528 (64.2)	165 (20.0)	123 (14.9)	58 (7.0)	43 (5.2)	32 (3.9)	8 (1.0)	99 (12.0)
Sex—no. (%)								
Female	379 (46.1)	116 (14.1)	76 (9.2)	70 (8.5)	31 (3.8)	27 (3.3)	0 (0.0)	59 (7.2)
Male	444 (53.9)	126 (15.3)	96 (11.7)	37 (4.5)	41 (5.0)	41 (5.0)	16 (1.9)	87 (10.6)
Race or ethnic group—no. (%)								
Asian	13 (1.6)	7 (0.9)	3 (0.4)	2 (0.2)	0 (0.0)	0 (0.0)	0 (0.0)	1 (0.1)
Black	58 (7.0)	19 (2.3)	10 (1.2)	7 (0.9)	8 (1.0)	5 (0.6)	0 (0.0)	9 (1.1)
White	724 (88.0)	204 (24.8)	154 (18.7)	96 (11.7)	62 (7.5)	61 (7.4)	16 (1.9)	131 (15.9)
Other	10 (1.2)	3 (0.4)	3 (0.4)	2 (0.2)	0 (0.0)	0 (0.0)	0 (0.0)	2 (0.2)
Unknown/Declined	18 (2.2)	9 (1.1)	2 (0.2)	0 (0.0)	2 (0.2)	2 (0.2)	0 (0.0)	3 (0.4)
Hispanic or Latino ethnic group—no (%)								
Yes	452 (54.9)	111 (13.5)	98 (11.9)	70 (8.5)	45 (5.5)	44 (5.3)	7 (0.9)	77 (9.4)
No	371 (45.1)	131 (15.9)	74 (9.0)	37 (4.5)	27 (3.3)	24 (2.9)	9 (1.1)	69 (8.4)
Treatment Summary								
Prescribed dose—Gy								
Median (range)	50.0 (16.0–76.0)	50.0 (20.0–76.0)	50.0 (30.0–60.0)	42.0 (25.0–62.0)	50.0 (30.0–60.0)	50.0 (25.0–60.0)	40.0 (37.0–74.0)	40.0 (16.0–68.0)
Prescribed fractions								
Median (range)	5 (1–41)	5 (1–33)	5 (1–30)	5 (1–34)	5 (1–28)	5 (1–6)	5 (5–41)	6 (1–36)
Radiotherapy duration—days								
Median (range)	8 (1–67)	7 (1–64)	10 (1–65)	8 (1–54)	7 (1–39)	8 (1–27)	10 (7–59)	10 (1–67)
Prescribed BED10—Gy								
Median (range)	94.4 (28.0–200.0)	100.0 (37.5–104.6)	100.0 (36.0–149.6)	72.0 (37.5–100.0)	100.0 (48.0–200.0)	100.0 (48.0–132.0)	72.0 (64.4–87.4)	63.7 (28.0–100.8)

Table 1. Cont.

Characteristics	Treatment Courses (n = 823)	Tumor Sites						
		Pancreas (n = 242)	Thorax (n = 172)	Abdominopelvic Lymph Node (n = 107)	Liver (n = 72)	Adrenal Glands (n = 68)	Prostate (n= 17)	Other (n = 146)
Fractions—no. (%)								
Total delivered	6036 (100.0)	1353 (22.4)	1460 (24.2)	631 (10.5)	396 (6.6)	307 (5.1)	91 (1.5)	1798 (29.8)
Total adapted	2643 (43.8)	1081 (17.9)	484 (8.0)	423 (7.0)	110 (1.8)	235 (3.9)	0 (0.0)	310 (5.1)
On-table adaptive courses—no. (%)	515 (62.6)	219 (26.6)	54 (6.6)	91 (11.1)	28 (3.4)	58 (7.0)	0 (0.0)	65 (7.9)
Treatment fractionation—no. (%)								
Daily	653 (79.3)	236 (28.7)	109 (13.2)	92 (11.2)	58 (7.0)	35 (4.3)	5 (0.6)	118 (14.3)
Every other day	165 (20.0)	6 (0.7)	63 (7.7)	14 (1.7)	14 (1.7)	33 (4.0)	11 (1.3)	24 (2.9)
Twice daily	3 (0.4)	0 (0.0)	0 (0.0)	1 (0.1)	0 (0.0)	0 (0.0)	0 (0.0)	2 (0.02)
Weekly	2 (0.2)	0 (0.0)	0 (0.0)	0 (0.0)	0 (0.0)	0 (0.0)	0 (0.0)	2 (0.02)
Respiratory motion management—no. (%)								
Breath-hold	687 (83.5)	235 (28.6)	160 (19.4)	69 (8.4)	69 (8.4)	67 (8.1)	1 (0.1)	86 (10.4)
Free breathing	118 (14.3)	4 (0.5)	7 (0.9)	35 (4.3)	2 (0.2)	1 (0.1)	13 (1.6)	56 (6.8)
Unknown	18 (2.2)	3 (0.4)	5 (0.6)	3 (0.4)	1 (0.1)	0 (0.0)	2 (0.2)	4 (0.5)
Abdominal compression—no. (%)								
Yes	54 (6.6)	9 (1.1)	16 (1.9)	6 (0.7)	11 (1.3)	8 (1.0)	0 (0.0)	4 (0.5)
No	769 (93.4)	233 (28.3)	156 (19.0)	101 (12.3)	61 (7.4)	60 (7.3)	16 (1.9)	142 (17.3)
Target volume—cc.								
GTV—Median	18.7	33.3	8.8	10.3 (0.8–1062.0)	14.5	15.4	8.7 (8.7–8.7)	284
(range)	(0.4–1062.0)	(1.1–854.4)	(1.0–232.4)		(0.6–808.0)	(1.1–296.9)		(0.4–714.8)
CTV—Median	64.9	110.2	17.9	31.1 (1.6–439.0)	22.2	20.3	49.6	1605
(range)	(1.5–1450.6)	(4.7–535.4)	(2.6–410.9)		(1.5–129.3)	(6.5–142.3)	(27.7–68.6)	(2.5–1450.6)
PTV—Median	45.7	63.4	29.9	25.7 (2.4–1225.2)	40.5	37.2	90.9	79.5
(range)	(2.4–2296.5)	(3.0–979.4)	(4.9–506.0)		(4.7–618.3)	(7.7–377.4)	(34.5–124.9)	(5.1–2296.5)
Target mean dose coverage BED10—Gy								
GTV—Median	108.2	113.3	121.2	93.7 (81.3–110.7)	118.6	113.2	26.5	69.0
(IQR)	(84.3–120.9)	(92.9–118.3)	(87.0–150.3)		(104.7–125.7)	(90.4–122.4)	(26.5–26.5)	(56.4–88.0)
CTV—Median	91.4	93.7	121.1	87.1 (68.9–97.9)	119.9	98.0	79.0	62.1
(IQR)	(71.7–116.6)	(85.7–103.4)	(110.2–157.6)		(106.2–123.8)	(85.8–111.2)	(76.6–83.1)	(45.1–71.6)
PTV—Median	100.1	106.8	113	85.7 (76.0–102.3)	112.6	106.3	76.5	63.4
(IQR)	(77.4–113.3)	(90.3–112.4)	(81.1–144.9)		(92.7–116.5)	(83.6–114.3)	(74.8–80.8)	(51.2–82.9)
Total in-room time—mins.								
Median (IQR)	51.0 (39.0–64.0)	58.0 (46.0–71.0)	45.0 (37.0–56.0)	55.0 (43.5–68.5)	49.0 (42.8–61.3)	55.5 (49.0–68.5)	45.0 (35.8–49.3)	37.5 (31.0–52.0)
Total delivery time—mins.								
Median (IQR)	15.0 (12.0–20.0)	16.0 (13.0–19.8)	17.0 (13.0–22.0)	13 (11.0–16.0)	17.5 (14.0–23.3)	17.0 (13.0–21.0)	15.0 (12.8–18.3)	12.0 (10.0–16.0)

Because we expected a steep learning curve for efficiently and safely treating on the MR-Linac, we began our MRgRT program in April 2018 with a plan to not treat with oART for several months. As such, we delayed implementing oART until September 2018 [6]. A treatment course was classified as oART if at least one fraction (fx) required on-table replanning.

In July 2022, our MR-Linac was upgraded with the A3i system (A3i, 510K approval December 2021) that featured enhanced automation, real-time 3D multi-planar tracking, the BrainTx™ package [16], and a parallel adaptive workflow [17]. Our daily oART workflow is detailed in Figure 1, and Figure 2 provides an example showing the importance of oART for a patient receiving an ablative dose to a mesenteric lymph node. Daily changes in the patient's position of the small and large bowel relative to the GTV caused dose constraint violations, reducing the target dose coverage and requiring each fraction to be replanned.

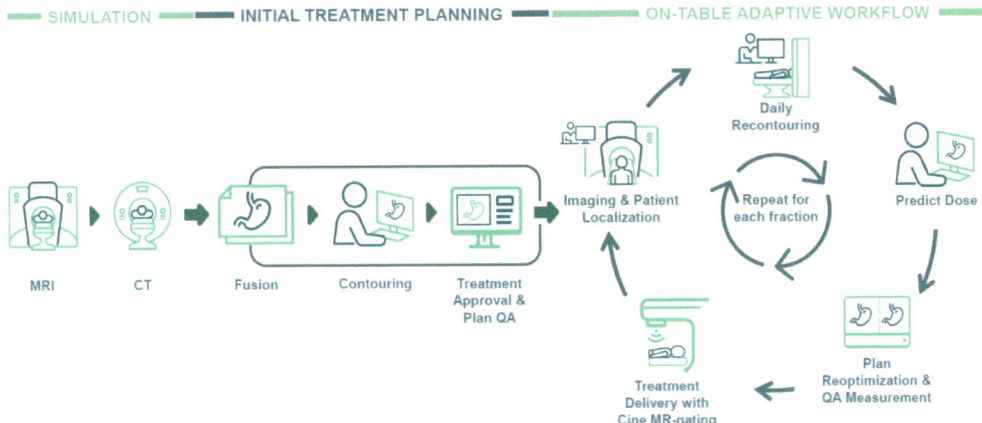

Figure 1. Clinical workflow of magnetic resonance-guided radiotherapy employing on-table adaptive processes. Abbreviations: MRI, magnetic resonance imaging; CT, computer tomography; QA, quality assurance.

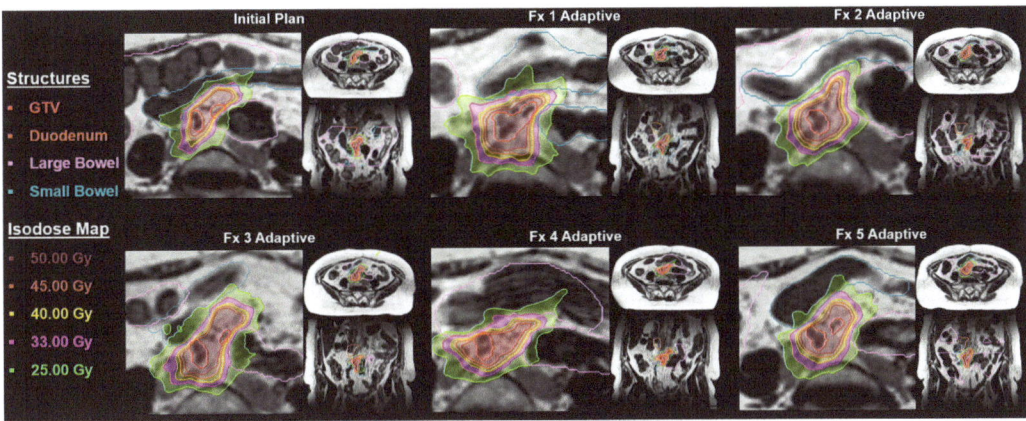

Figure 2. Representation of an on-table adaptive radiotherapy plan for a mesenteric lymph node treated to 50 Gy in 5 fractions. Note the GTV had significant inter-fractional anatomical shifts, necessitating plan adaptation to ensure the preservation of adjacent critical structures and avoidance of any potential violation of organs-at-risk. Abbreviations: GTV, gross tumor volume, Fx, fraction.

Treatment prescription schedules were recalculated and expressed as biological effective dose for tumors, using an α/β of 10 (BED10) [18]. We defined ultra-hypofractionation (UHfx) as courses with five (5) or fewer fxs with a minimum fx size of 5 Gy. Target volumes included a gross tumor volume (GTV), a planning target volume (PTV) with a typical 3 mm expansion (up to 5 mm), and based on specific clinical considerations, a clinical target volume (CTV). To evaluate the anatomic relationship between treated lesions and nearby dose-limiting OARs (e.g., stomach, bowel), we expanded the GTV isotropically by 3 mm and 5 mm. The overlap volumes between the expanded GTV and adjacent OARs was analyzed to estimate areas at risk of underdosing, serving as a surrogate for planning difficulty. Treatment courses were categorized into six 12-month periods, starting from Period 1 (April 2018–April 2019) to Period 6 (April 2023–April 2024).

Patient, disease, and treatment characteristics were summarized using descriptive statistics. Statistical analyses were performed using Microsoft Excel 2022 (Microsoft Corporation, Redmond, WA, USA) and SPSS version 27.0 (IBM, SPSS Statistics, Chicago, IL, USA) with comparisons performed using the Mann–Whitney U test. $p < 0.05$ was considered as statistically significant.

3. Results

3.1. Patient Cohort

A total of 854 lesions were treated across 823 treatment courses in 712 patients with 6038 delivered fractions. The median age was 69 years (range, 7–94) with the majority being male (444 [53.9%]), White (724 [88.0%]), and Hispanic (452 [54.9%]). Overall, 473 patients (57.5%) underwent treatment to the primary tumor, while 325 (39.5%) received treatment for oligometastatic and 25 (3.0%) for polymetastatic lesions. A total of 40 (4.9%) courses were delivered for re-irradiation, and 18 (2.2%) were delivered as a dose-escalated boost following treatment on a different treatment platform, either proton or photon.

The most frequent sites treated were the pancreas (242 [29.4%]), thorax (172 [20.9%]), abdominopelvic lymph nodes (107 [13.0%]), liver (72 [8.7%]), and adrenal glands (68 [8.3%]). Other (146 [17.7%]) tumor sites included the esophagus (18 [2.2%]), stomach (14 [1.7%]), colorectal (12 [1.5%]), ampulla of vater/bile duct (11 [1.3%]), bone—non-spine (11 [1.3%]), abdominal wall (8 [1.0%]), bone—spine (8 [1.0%]), brain (7 [0.9%]), head and neck (7 [0.9%]), kidneys (7 [0.9%]), mesentery/omentum (5 [0.6%]), vagina (5 [0.6%]), bladder (4 [0.5%]), gallbladder (4 [0.5%]), retroperitoneum (4 [0.5%]), breast (2 [0.2%]), celiac plexus (2 [0.2%]), cervix (2 [0.2%]), paraspinal (2 [0.2%]), pelvic mass (2 [0.2%]), supraclavicular (2 [0.2%]), uterus (2 [0.2%]), axilla (1 [0.1%]), cardiophrenic lymph node (1 [0.1%]), endometrium (1 [0.1%]), inferior vena cave tumor thrombus (1 [0.1%]), ovaries (1 [0.1%]), porta hepatis (1 [0.1%]), and pulmonary artery (1 [0.1%]). The baseline characteristics of patients and tumors are summarized in Table 1.

The number of treatment courses delivered modestly increased over time: 101 in Period 1, 126 in Period 2, 144 in Period 3, 157 in Period 4, 162 in Period 5, and 133 in Period 6. Throughout all periods, the distribution of treated sites remained consistent (Figure 3).

3.2. Trends in MR-Guided Radiotherapy

The median prescription dose was 50 Gy (range, 16–76) in a median of 5 fxs (range, 1–41) delivered over a median of 8 days (range, 1–67). The median prescribed BED10 was 94.4 Gy (range, 28.0–200.0). Almost half of all patients (404, 49.1%) were prescribed a highly ablative BED10 $\geq$ 100 Gy, while almost one third (249, 30.3%) received a BED10 $\geq$ 70 Gy. Most patients were treated daily (653 [79.3%]) and in breath-hold (687 [83.5%]). An abdominal compression belt (54 [6.6%]) was used for patients who did not tolerate treatment in breath-hold. The median target volumes were 18.7 cc (range, 0.4–1062.0) for GTV, 64.9 cc (range, 1.5–1450.6) for CTV, and 45.7 cc (range, 2.4–2296.5) for PTV.

A total of 6036 fxs were delivered, with 2643 (43.8%) fxs requiring on-table adaptive replanning. The distribution of fxs by treated site was 1353 (22.4%) for pancreas, 1460 (24.2%) for thorax, 631 (10.5%) for abdominopelvic lymph nodes, 307 (5.1%) for adrenal glands, 396 (6.6%) for liver, 91 (1.5%) for prostate, and 1798 (29.8%) for other. Among the 2643 fxs that underwent oART, the distribution was 1081 (17.9%) for pancreas, 484 (8.0%) for thorax, 423 (7.0%) in abdominopelvic lymph nodes, 235 (3.9%) for adrenal glands, 110 (1.8%) for liver, and 310 (5.1%) for other.

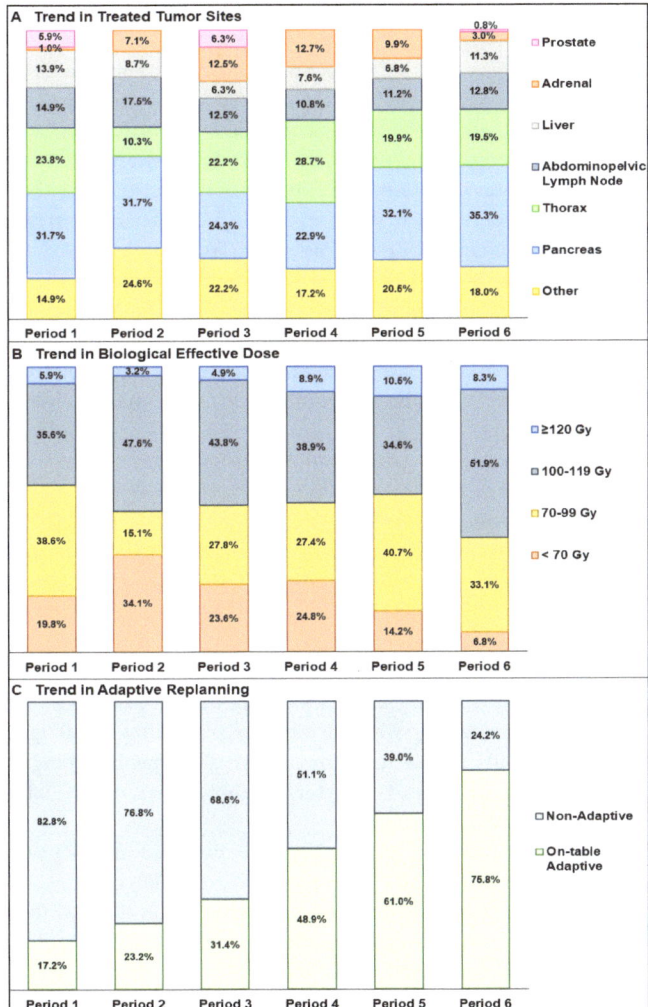

Figure 3. Trends in the use of magnetic resonance-guided radiotherapy by disease site (**A**), biological effective dose (**B**), and on-table adaptive vs. non-adaptive fractions (**C**) (Periods 1–6).

Although the vast majority of all courses (778, 94.6%) were multi-fractionated regimens prescribed to a median dose of 50 Gy (range, 16–76; median [range] BED10: 91.7 [18.8–132.0] Gy), a small proportion, (45, 5.5%) of courses were treated with a median single-fx ablative dose of 30 Gy (range, 16–40; median [range] BED10: 120.0 [41.6–200.0] Gy). Among the 45 single-fx courses, the treated sites included thorax (16, 35.6%), liver (9, 20.0%), adrenal glands (7, 15.6%), pancreas (6, 13.3%), abdominopelvic lymph nodes (5, 11.1%), bone—spine (1, 2.2%), and celiac plexus (1, 2.2%).

The median oART prescription was 50 Gy (18–68) in 5 fx (1–36) over 7 days (1–56) in 515 (62.6%) courses. Most treatment courses were delivered daily (427 [51.9%]) in breath-hold (464 [56.4%]). Among the 515 courses, the median BED10 was 100.0 Gy (range, 36.0–157.5) with 277 patients (53.8%) treated with a BED10 ≥ 100 Gy, and an additional 171 (33.2%) were ≥70 Gy. The most commonly treated courses with oART were pancreas

(219 [26.6%]), abdominopelvic lymph nodes (91 [11.1%]), adrenal glands (58 [7.0%]), thorax (62 [7.3%]), liver (28 [3.4%]), and other (65 [7.9%]).

One significant pattern of interperiodic temporal evolution was a significant increase in oART, increasing from 168 fxs (19.0%) in Period 1 to 615 fxs (78.9%) in Period 6 (Figure 3). Notably, the percentage of fxs treated with oART for thorax increased from 0.7% to 21.2%, while for pancreas, it rose from 12.7% to 29.0% between Periods 1 and 6. A second significant interperiodic evolutionary change between Periods 1 and 6 was the increase in the use of UHfx courses from 66.3% to 89.5%. Treatment courses that utilized both UHfx and oART increased from 29.7% in Period 1 to 76.7% in Period 6.

The number of courses using oART also substantially increased from 37.6% in Period 1 to 85.0% in Period 6. oART courses nearly doubled from 44.7% to 77.2% from Periods 1–3 to Periods 4–6. When comparing the use of oART across the overall treated sites by period, the use of oART for pancreatic courses had increased from 25.0% in Period 1 to 33.6% in Period 6, while the rate for thoracic tumors had risen from 1.0% in Period 1 to 16.1% in Period 6.

Overlapping dose-limiting OARs within a 3 mm GTV expansion were seen in 58.8% (484) of courses, increasing to 65.9% (542) when a 5 mm GTV expansion was applied. In oART courses, 42.9% (353) of courses had overlap with dose-limiting OARs within the 3 mm GTV expansion, while 48.1% (396) showed overlap within the 5 mm GTV expansion. Pancreatic courses showed the highest overlap with 24.2% (199) of courses showing overlap within the 3 mm GTV expansion and 26.2% (216) within the 5 mm GTV expansion.

The median TDT and TIRT were 15.0 min (IQR, 12.0–20.0) and 51.0 min (IQR, 39.0–64.0), respectively. TIRT was ≤60 min for 573 courses (69.6%) with 408 (49.6%) completed in ≤50 min, 228 (27.7%%) in ≤40 min, and 63 (7.7%) in ≤30 min. The median TDT for free-breathing was 12.0 min (IQR, 9.0–15.0) vs. 16.0 min (IQR, 13.0–21.0) for breath-hold ($p < 0.001$). Similarly, the median TIRT for free-breathing was 43.0 min (IQR, 33.0–55.0) vs. 52.0 min (IQR, 41.0–65.0) for breath-hold ($p < 0.001$). Table 1 presents the TDT and TIRT based on tumor site.

The median TDT for non-adaptive RT and oART was 14.0 min (IQR, 10.0–19.0) and 16.0 min (IQR, 13.0–20.0), respectively ($p < 0.001$), while the median TIRT was 40.0 min (IQR, 32.0–50.0) for non-adaptive RT and 57.0 min (IQR, 47.0–69.0) for oART ($p < 0.001$). Over time, significant improvements were seen in oART with a median TIRT, decreasing from 81.0 min in Period 1 to 45.0 min in Period 6, while TDT decreased slightly from 18.5 min to 16.0 min. Figure 4 presents the TIRT of oART across the six-year period.

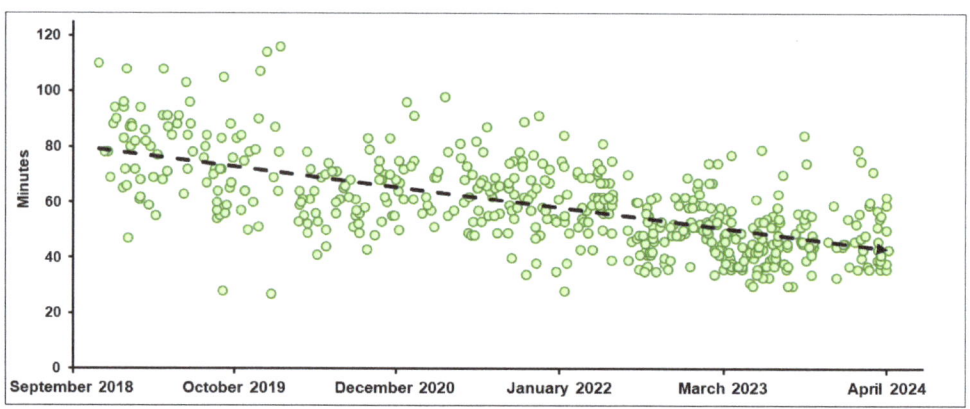

Figure 4. Trend in median overall total in-room time (min) for on-table adaptive radiotherapy treatment courses (Periods 1–6).

4. Discussion

We treat a high volume of patients with definitive dose-escalated RT across multiple stereotactic body radiation therapy (SBRT) platforms (TrueBeam [Varian Medical Systems Inc., Palo Alto, CA, USA], CyberKnife [Accuray Inc., Sunnyvale, CA, USA], Tomotherapy [Accuray Inc., Sunnyvale, CA, USA], MRIdian Linac) as well as pencil beam scanning proton therapy. These technologies are all located in the same building, and they are not restricted for use by only a subset of physicians, which facilitates our ability to use a robust peer review process to actively triage patients from the entire practice to the treatment platform that we expect will provide the best therapeutic ratio.

We became an early adopter of the MRIdian Linac in early 2018, and our initial treatment strategy was to attempt significant dose escalation using UHfx to tumors in challenging anatomic locations that we could not safely dose escalate in the same manner using our other treatment devices either because of suboptimal X-ray or CT image guidance and/or the inability to either effectively manage motion or offer oART. Our initial intent was to primarily treat tumors in the abdomen and pelvis based on emerging dose-escalated outcomes from MRIdian cobalt centers demonstrating both safety and encouraging efficacy and also because tumors in these locations are most significantly limited by motion and soft-tissue resolution issues not easily addressed by other technologies [7,19].

While most institutions do not yet offer the MR-Linac platform, there is growing interest in MRgRT that likely has been spurred by increasing clinical evidence demonstrating improved outcomes over conventional forms of RT, specifically in terms of improved local control using high ablative dosing.

In 2022, patterns of utilization analysis from 16 U.S. MRIdian centers indicated that MRgRT was predominantly delivered with UHfx (70.3%) and while oART (38.5%) was relatively uncommon with an average of 1.7 adapted fractions/course, this had grown by a compounded annual rate of 88.5% by the end of 2020 [12]. The most frequently treated sites in the U.S. were the pancreas (20.7%), liver (16.5%), prostate (12.5%), breast (11.5%), lung (9.4%), and "other" organs (10.4%). Similarly, drawing on reports from 21 centers in Europe and Asia, delivering over 46,000 fxs, UHfx schedules constituted 63.5% of courses, with 57.8% requiring oART. The most commonly treated sites were the prostate (23.5%), liver (14.5%), lung (12.3%), pancreas (11.2%), and breast (8.0%) [20].

Since we have been treating with MRgRT for more than half a decade, and because we had specifically focused on minimizing utilization for prostate cancer, the most common use-case as demonstrated in the global survey, our experiential evolution would provide valuable use-case lessons to the radiation oncology community in understanding the value and changing patterns of MRgRT utilization, even in the setting of having access to almost every other major advanced radiotherapeutic platform, thereby specifically identifying patients deriving the greatest benefit from MRgRT. As shown in Figure 2, MRgRT is especially beneficial for patients with highly mobile tumors, particularly in the abdominal and pelvic regions. It allows real-time adjustments for both inter- and intra-fractional motion, improving target volume coverage and positioning to enhance dosimetric parameters. These tumors are highly sensitive to respiratory motion and are often unsuitable for MV or kV CT-guided methods, which are limited by poor soft-tissue resolution and primarily address only inter-fractional motion.

Our MRgRT experience predominantly includes unresectable abdominal tumors that were routinely treated with dose escalation, UHfx, and oART. Abdominal tumors comprised nearly two thirds of all treatment courses in our 6-year experience, predominantly those in the pancreas, and also frequently involving abdominal lymph nodes, liver, and adrenal glands. We published favorable clinical outcomes from our early experience using this approach for various challenging clinical scenarios (e.g., 50 Gy/5 fx for metastatic mesenteric nodules refractory to systemic therapy) [21], and this may have contributed to our steadily increasing volumes across each treatment period that increasingly included patients seeking out MRgRT from outside of south Florida. Our increasing volume, specifically of locally advanced pancreatic cancer, was also likely influenced by favorable outcomes from a recently published phase 2 trial that evaluated the feasibility of ablative 5-fraction stereotactic magnetic resonance-guided on-table adaptive radiation therapy (SMART) for borderline resectable and locally advanced pancreatic cancer; no acute grade ≥ 3 gastrointestinal toxicities definitely related to MRgRT were reported with a very favorable 2-year OS of >50% from diagnosis [22,23]. This aligns with the growing evidence supporting RT as a key component in pancreatic cancer treatment [19,22,24]. Because of the encouraging outcomes that we observed in treating challenging abdominal and pelvic tumors, we increasingly triaged thoracic patients who may specifically benefit with the use of MRgRT, such as central and ultra-central tumors that are at risk for toxicity with non-dose-reduced CT-guided SBRT [25,26]. Additionally, we also frequently utilized the MRIdian Linac for treating peripheral lung tumors with SBRT, especially for those patients either with very poor pulmonary function (such as idiopathic pulmonary fibrosis) or those with peridiaphragmatic lesions subject to 4D-CT verified significant motion. The ability to treat these patients with automatic beam gating, in breath-hold, eliminated the need for an internal target volume (ITV), resulting in significant reduction in normal lung volume irradiated and thus reducing the risk of toxicity.

While UHfx was common in our initial MRgRT experience, the COVID-19 pandemic sharply increased UHfx within our MRgRT program [27,28]. Prior to the pandemic (Period 2), 65.9% of courses were UHfx, rising to 76.4% during the pandemic and reaching almost 90% of all courses in Period 6. The COVID-19 pandemic also led us to consider single-fraction SBRT for the first time [29], which has been increasingly utilized in our practice most commonly for lung and liver metastases. We recently completed the multi-center phase 2 SMART ONE trial of single-fraction SBRT using the MRIdian Linac for tumors in the chest, abdomen, and pelvis, and our initial publication reports feasibility, safety, and efficacy [30]. Since the pandemic, the use of single-fraction SBRT has progressively increased from 5 courses in Period 3 to 12 in Period 4, 20 in Period 5, and 8 in Period 6.

Treatment times on an MR-Linac are typically longer than on a standard linac, which is in large part because delivery uses a step-and-shoot approach but also because all treatments typically incorporate automatic beam gating on the MRIdian Linac and also because the dose-per-fraction is typically very high and the need for precision delivery is significantly greater [31,32]. Reducing treatment times and increasing machine throughput has been a priority for MRgRT centers to improve tolerability for patients—especially those treated with oART (Figure 1). In 2017, Henke et al. reported a median oART TIRT of 79 min for abdominal malignancies treated with a MRIdian cobalt device [7], while Tetar et al. demonstrated an average oART TIRT of 44.7 min for 140 prostate cancer treatments [33]. In 2020, Gungor et al. analyzed 166 oART treatment courses using MRIdian, reporting a median TIRT of 45 min [34]. Prior to our A3i upgrade that introduced several advanced capabilities including a parallel oART workflow allowing physician, physicist/dosimetrist, and radiation therapy to work in parallel on different monitors, we observed a median TIRT of 65 min (IQR, 57–75) across 286 oART courses compared to 47 min (IQR, 40–54) afterwards: a relative time savings of 27.7%. As expected, non-oART treatment times remained stable. When considering all patients treated since 2018, we observed decreasing TIRT that likely was related to technological improvements and also attributable to the development of standardized treatment workflows related to oART as well as increasing experience among all MRgRT team members [35].

There are several limitations of this study including its retrospective design and that our MRgRT utilization is very specific and may not be generalizable to others. For example, we do not treat a high volume of prostate cancer with MRgRT due to having robust referral patterns for abdominal tumors that cannot be safely treated with dose escalation and UHfx on our other treatment machines, and because we have several other very effective prostate cancer treatment platforms. For context, MRgRT has recently been demonstrated to reduce toxicity over CT-guided RT for prostate cancer patients in the randomized MIRAGE trial [3]. Another limitation is our use of a uniform BED α/β ratio of 10, which may not fully account for histology-dependent variations. Lastly, ViewRay, Inc. filed for Chapter 11 bankruptcy in 2023 that resulted in a more limited use of our MR-Linac because of concerns regarding machine downtime and lack of device servicing for a period of time; with recent corporate restructuring, some of these concerns have eased to a certain extent.

5. Conclusions

In conclusion, since the inception of our MRgRT program in 2018, we have intentionally prioritized treatment on the MRIdian Linac for patients who would benefit from significant dose escalation above what can be safely delivered on our other advanced radiation treatment systems. The unique capabilities of the MRIdian Linac enable not only safe dose escalation that frequently requires oART, especially for abdominal and pelvic tumors, but also the routine use of UHfx and increasingly single-fraction SBRT. Important reasons for our program's success include our early decision to develop a standardization of patient selection and oART workflows as well as robust training and credentialing of all staff who are involved in MRgRT within our department.

Author Contributions: Conceptualization, R.A.H. and M.D.C.; methodology, R.A.H.; formal analysis, R.A.H., investigation, R.A.H. and M.D.C., data curation, R.A.H., writing—original draft preparation, R.A.H.; writing—review and editing, R.A.H., E.Y.A., R.K., A.K., M.D.H., Y.W., N.S.K., S.Y., K.E.M., N.B.-G., T.R., D.A., R.T., A.N.G., M.P.M. and M.D.C.; visualization, R.A.H.; supervision, M.D.C.; project administration, R.A.H. and M.D.C. All authors have read and agreed to the published version of the manuscript.

Funding: This research received no external funding.

Institutional Review Board Statement: The study was conducted in accordance and approved by the Institutional Review Board of Miami Cancer Institute at Baptist Health (IRB #1880120).

Informed Consent Statement: There was no consent due to the retrospective nature of the study.

Data Availability Statement: Research data are stored in an institutional repository and will be made available upon request to the corresponding authors.

Conflicts of Interest: R.K. reports consulting fees from Viewray Inc. outside the submitted work; grants or contracts from Viewray Inc. outside the submitted work; honoraria from Viewray Inc. outside the submitted work; participation on data safety/advisory boards for Viewray Inc. outside the submitted work; and support for meetings/travel from Viewray Inc. outside the submitted work. The following authors have declared no relevant conflicts of interest, R.A.H., E.Y.A, K.E.M., A.K., M.D.H., N.B.-G., N.S.K., Y.W., T.R., D.A., S.Y., R.T., A.N.G., M.P.M., M.D.C.

References

1. Srinivasan, K.; Mohammadi, M.; Shepherd, J. Applications of linac-mounted kilovoltage Cone-beam Computed Tomography in modern radiation therapy: A review. *Pol. J. Radiol.* **2014**, *79*, 181–193. [PubMed]
2. Hall, W.A.; Paulson, E.S.; van der Heide, U.A.; Fuller, C.D.; Raaymakers, B.W.; Lagendijk, J.J.W.; Li, X.A.; Jaffray, D.A.; Dawson, L.A.; Erickson, B.; et al. The transformation of radiation oncology using real-time magnetic resonance guidance: A review. *Eur. J. Cancer* **2019**, *122*, 42–52. [CrossRef]

3. Kishan, A.U.; Ma, T.M.; Lamb, J.M.; Casado, M.; Wilhalme, H.; Low, D.A.; Sheng, K.; Sharma, S.; Nickols, N.G.; Pham, J.; et al. Magnetic Resonance Imaging–Guided vs Computed Tomography–Guided Stereotactic Body Radiotherapy for Prostate Cancer: The MIRAGE Randomized Clinical Trial. *JAMA Oncol.* **2023**, *9*, 365–373. [CrossRef] [PubMed]
4. Werensteijn-Honingh, A.M.; Kroon, P.S.; Winkel, D.; van Gaal, J.C.; Hes, J.; Snoeren, L.M.W.; Timmer, J.K.; Mout, C.C.P.; Bol, G.H.; Kotte, A.N.; et al. Impact of magnetic resonance-guided versus conventional radiotherapy workflows on organ at risk doses in stereotactic body radiotherapy for lymph node oligometastases. *Phys. Imaging Radiat. Oncol.* **2022**, *23*, 66–73. [CrossRef]
5. Hoegen, P.; Katsigiannopulos, E.; Buchele, C.; Regnery, S.; Weykamp, F.; Sandrini, E.; Ristau, J.; Liermann, J.; Meixner, E.; Forster, T.; et al. Stereotactic magnetic resonance-guided online adaptive radiotherapy of adrenal metastases combines high ablative doses with optimized sparing of organs at risk. *Clin. Transl. Radiat. Oncol.* **2023**, *39*, 100567. [CrossRef] [PubMed]
6. Chuong, M.D.; Bryant, J.; Mittauer, K.E.; Hall, M.; Kotecha, R.; Alvarez, D.; Romaguera, T.; Rubens, M.; Adamson, S.; Godley, A.; et al. Ablative 5-Fraction Stereotactic Magnetic Resonance–Guided Radiation Therapy with On-Table Adaptive Replanning and Elective Nodal Irradiation for Inoperable Pancreas Cancer. *Pract. Radiat. Oncol.* **2021**, *11*, 134–147. [CrossRef]
7. Henke, L.; Kashani, R.; Robinson, C.; Curcuru, A.; DeWees, T.; Bradley, J.; Green, O.; Michalski, J.; Mutic, S.; Parikh, P.; et al. Phase I trial of stereotactic MR-guided online adaptive radiation therapy (SMART) for the treatment of oligometastatic or unresectable primary malignancies of the abdomen. *Radiother. Oncol.* **2018**, *126*, 519–526. [CrossRef]
8. Bruynzeel, A.M.E.; Tetar, S.U.; Oei, S.S.; Senan, S.; Haasbeek, C.J.A.; Spoelstra, F.O.B.; Piet, A.H.; Meijnen, P.; van der Jagt, M.A.B.; Fraikin, T.; et al. A Prospective Single-Arm Phase 2 Study of Stereotactic Magnetic Resonance Guided Adaptive Radiation Therapy for Prostate Cancer: Early Toxicity Results. *Int. J. Radiat. Oncol. Biol. Phys.* **2019**, *105*, 1086–1094. [CrossRef] [PubMed]
9. Chin, R.-I.; Schiff, J.P.; Bommireddy, A.; Kang, K.H.; Andruska, N.; Price, A.T.; Green, O.L.; Huang, Y.; Korenblat, K.; Parikh, P.J.; et al. Clinical outcomes of patients with unresectable primary liver cancer treated with MR-guided stereotactic body radiation Therapy: A Six-Year experience. *Clin. Transl. Radiat. Oncol.* **2023**, *41*, 100627. [CrossRef]
10. Klüter, S. Technical design and concept of a 0.35 T MR-Linac. *Clin. Transl. Radiat. Oncol.* **2019**, *18*, 98–101. [CrossRef] [PubMed]
11. Mutic, S.; Dempsey, J.F. The ViewRay System: Magnetic Resonance–Guided and Controlled Radiotherapy. *Semin. Radiat. Oncol.* **2014**, *24*, 196–199. [CrossRef]
12. Chuong, M.D.; Clark, M.A.; Henke, L.E.; Kishan, A.U.; Portelance, L.; Parikh, P.J.; Bassetti, M.F.; Nagar, H.; Rosenberg, S.A.; Mehta, M.P.; et al. Patterns of utilization and clinical adoption of 0.35 Tesla MR-guided radiation therapy in the United States—Understanding the transition to adaptive, ultra-hypofractionated treatments. *Clin. Transl. Radiat. Oncol.* **2023**, *38*, 161–168. [CrossRef] [PubMed]
13. Parikh, P.J.; Lee, P.; Low, D.; Kim, J.; Mittauer, K.E.; Bassetti, M.F.; Glide-Hurst, C.; Raldow, A.; Yang, Y.; Portelance, L.; et al. Stereotactic MR-Guided On-Table Adaptive Radiation Therapy (SMART) for Patients with Borderline or Locally Advanced Pancreatic Cancer: Primary Endpoint Outcomes of a Prospective Phase II Multi-Center International Trial. *Int. J. Radiat. Oncol. Biol. Phys.* **2022**, *114*, 1062–1063. [CrossRef]
14. Ristau, J.; Hörner-Rieber, J.; Buchele, C.; Klüter, S.; Jäkel, C.; Baumann, L.; Andratschke, N.; Schüler, H.G.; Guckenberger, M.; Li, M.; et al. Stereotactic MRI-guided radiation therapy for localized prostate cancer (SMILE): A prospective, multicentric phase-II-trial. *Radiat. Oncol.* **2022**, *17*, 75. [CrossRef] [PubMed]
15. Henke, L.E.; Contreras, J.A.; Green, O.L.; Cai, B.; Kim, H.; Roach, M.C.; Olsen, J.R.; Fischer-Valuck, B.; Mullen, D.F.; Kashani, R.; et al. Magnetic Resonance Image-Guided Radiotherapy (MRIgRT): A 4.5-Year Clinical Experience. *Clin. Oncol.* **2018**, *30*, 720–727. [CrossRef] [PubMed]
16. Snyder, K.C.; Mao, W.; Kim, J.P.; Cunningham, J.; Chetty, I.J.; Siddiqui, S.M.; Parikh, P.; Dolan, J. Commissioning, clinical implementation, and initial experience with a new brain tumor treatment package on a low-field MR-linac. *J. Appl. Clin. Med. Phys.* **2023**, *24*, e13919. [CrossRef]
17. Votta, C.; Iacovone, S.; Turco, G.; Carrozzo, V.; Vagni, M.; Scalia, A.; Chiloiro, G.; Meffe, G.; Nardini, M.; Panza, G.; et al. Evaluation of clinical parallel workflow in online adaptive MR-guided Radiotherapy: A detailed assessment of treatment session times. *Tech. Innov. Patient Support Radiat. Oncol.* **2024**, *29*, 100239. [CrossRef] [PubMed]
18. Jones, B.; Dale, R.G.; Deehan, C.; Hopkins, K.I.; Morgan, D.A.L. The Role of Biologically Effective Dose (BED) in Clinical Oncology. *Clin. Oncol.* **2001**, *13*, 71–81.
19. Rudra, S.; Jiang, N.; Rosenberg, S.A.; Olsen, J.R.; Roach, M.C.; Wan, L.; Portelance, L.; Mellon, E.A.; Bruynzeel, A.; Lagerwaard, F.; et al. Using adaptive magnetic resonance image-guided radiation therapy for treatment of inoperable pancreatic cancer. *Cancer Med.* **2019**, *8*, 2123–2132. [CrossRef] [PubMed]
20. Slotman, B.J.; Clark, M.A.; Özyar, E.; Kim, M.; Itami, J.; Tallet, A.; Debus, J.; Pfeffer, R.; Gentile, P.; Hama, Y.; et al. Clinical adoption patterns of 0.35 Tesla MR-guided radiation therapy in Europe and Asia. *Radiat. Oncol.* **2022**, *17*, 146. [CrossRef] [PubMed]
21. Chuong, M.D.; Alvarez, D.; Romaguera, T.; Mittauer, K.E.; Adamson, S.; Gutierrez, A.N.; Luciani, G.; Guerrero, H.; Ucar, A. Case report of ablative magnetic resonance-guided stereotactic body radiation therapy for oligometastatic mesenteric lymph nodes from bladder cancer. *Ther. Radiol. Oncol.* **2020**, *4*, 20. [CrossRef]

22. Parikh, P.J.; Lee, P.; Low, D.A.; Kim, J.; Mittauer, K.E.; Bassetti, M.F.; Glide-Hurst, C.K.; Raldow, A.C.; Yang, Y.; Portelance, L.; et al. A Multi-Institutional Phase 2 Trial of Ablative 5-Fraction Stereotactic Magnetic Resonance-Guided On-Table Adaptive Radiation Therapy for Borderline Resectable and Locally Advanced Pancreatic Cancer. *Int. J. Radiat. Oncol. Biol. Phys.* **2023**, *117*, 799–808. [CrossRef]
23. Chuong, M.D.; Lee, P.; Low, D.A.; Kim, J.; Mittauer, K.E.; Bassetti, M.F.; Glide-Hurst, C.K.; Raldow, A.C.; Yang, Y.; Portelance, L.; et al. Stereotactic MR-guided on-table adaptive radiation therapy (SMART) for borderline resectable and locally advanced pancreatic cancer: A multi-center, open-label phase 2 study. *Radiother. Oncol.* **2023**, *191*, 110064. [CrossRef]
24. Krishnan, S.; Chadha, A.S.; Suh, Y.; Chen, H.-C.; Rao, A.; Das, P.; Minsky, B.D.; Mahmood, U.; Delclos, M.E.; Sawakuchi, G.O.; et al. Focal Radiation Therapy Dose Escalation Improves Overall Survival in Locally Advanced Pancreatic Cancer Patients Receiving Induction Chemotherapy and Consolidative Chemoradiation. *Int. J. Radiat. Oncol. Biol. Phys.* **2016**, *94*, 755–765. [CrossRef]
25. Finazzi, T.; Haasbeek, C.J.A.; Spoelstra, F.O.B.; Palacios, M.A.; Admiraal, M.A.; Bruynzeel, A.M.E.; Slotman, B.J.; Lagerwaard, F.J.; Senan, S. Clinical Outcomes of Stereotactic MR-Guided Adaptive Radiation Therapy for High-Risk Lung Tumors. *Int. J. Radiat. Oncol. Biol. Phys.* **2020**, *107*, 270–278. [CrossRef] [PubMed]
26. Palma, D.A.; Olson, R.; Harrow, S.; Gaede, S.; Louie, A.V.; Haasbeek, C.; Mulroy, L.; Lock, M.; Rodrigues, P.G.B.; Yaremko, B.P.; et al. Stereotactic ablative radiotherapy versus standard of care palliative treatment in patients with oligometastatic cancers (SABR-COMET): A randomised, phase 2, open-label trial. *Lancet* **2019**, *393*, 2051–2058. [CrossRef]
27. Spencer, K.; Jones, C.M.; Girdler, R.; Roe, C.; Sharpe, M.; Lawton, S.; Miller, L.; Lewis, P.; Evans, M.; Sebag-Montefiore, D.; et al. The impact of the COVID-19 pandemic on radiotherapy services in England, UK: A population-based study. *Lancet Oncol.* **2021**, *22*, 309–320. [CrossRef]
28. Thomson, D.J.; Yom, S.S.; Saeed, H.; El Naqa, I.; Ballas, L.; Bentzen, S.M.; Chao, S.T.; Choudhury, A.; Coles, C.E.; Dover, L.; et al. Radiation Fractionation Schedules Published During the COVID-19 Pandemic: A Systematic Review of the Quality of Evidence and Recommendations for Future Development. *Int. J. Radiat. Oncol. Biol. Phys.* **2020**, *108*, 379–389. [CrossRef]
29. Ng, S.S.W.; Ning, M.S.; Lee, P.; McMahon, R.A.; Siva, S.; Chuong, M.D. Single-Fraction Stereotactic Body Radiation Therapy: A Paradigm During the Coronavirus Disease 2019 (COVID-19) Pandemic and Beyond? *Adv. Radiat. Oncol.* **2020**, *5*, 761–773. [CrossRef]
30. Chuong, M.D.; Mittauer, K.E.; Bassetti, M.F.; Glide-Hurst, C.; Rojas, C.; Kalman, N.S.; Tom, M.; Rubens, M.; Crosby, J.; Burr, A.; et al. Phase 2 Trial of Stereotactic MR-Guided Adaptive Radiation Therapy in One Fraction (SMART ONE). *Int. J. Radiat. Oncol. Biol. Phys.* **2024**, *120*, S163–S164. [CrossRef]
31. Bohoudi, O.; Bruynzeel, A.M.E.; Senan, S.; Cuijpers, J.P.; Slotman, B.J.; Lagerwaard, F.J.; Palacios, M.A. Fast and robust online adaptive planning in stereotactic MR-guided adaptive radiation therapy (SMART) for pancreatic cancer. *Radiother. Oncol.* **2017**, *125*, 439–444. [CrossRef] [PubMed]
32. Sahin, B.; Zoto Mustafayev, T.; Gungor, G.; Aydin, G.; Yapici, B.; Atalar, B.; Ozyar, E. First 500 Fractions Delivered with a Magnetic Resonance-guided Radiotherapy System: Initial Experience. *Cureus* **2019**, *11*, e6457. [CrossRef]
33. Tetar, S.U.; Bruynzeel, A.M.E.; Lagerwaard, F.J.; Slotman, B.J.; Bohoudi, O.; Palacios, M.A. Clinical implementation of magnetic resonance imaging guided adaptive radiotherapy for localized prostate cancer. *Phys. Imaging Radiat. Oncol.* **2019**, *9*, 69–76. [CrossRef]
34. Güngör, G.; Serbez, İ.; Temur, B.; Gür, G.; Kayalılar, N.; Mustafayev, T.Z.; Korkmaz, L.; Aydın, G.; Yapıcı, B.; Atalar, B.; et al. Time Analysis of Online Adaptive Magnetic Resonance-Guided Radiation Therapy Workflow According to Anatomical Sites. *Pract. Radiat. Oncol.* **2021**, *11*, e11–e21. [CrossRef] [PubMed]
35. Chetty, I.J.; Cai, B.; Chuong, M.D.; Dawes, S.L.; Hall, W.A.; Helms, A.R.; Kirby, S.; Laugeman, E.; Mierzwa, M.; Pursley, J.; et al. Quality and Safety Considerations for Adaptive Radiation Therapy: An ASTRO White Paper. *Int. J. Radiat. Oncol. Biol. Phys.* **2024**, in press. [CrossRef]

Disclaimer/Publisher's Note: The statements, opinions and data contained in all publications are solely those of the individual author(s) and contributor(s) and not of MDPI and/or the editor(s). MDPI and/or the editor(s) disclaim responsibility for any injury to people or property resulting from any ideas, methods, instructions or products referred to in the content.

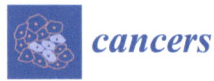

Article

Advanced External Beam Stereotactic Radiotherapy for Skull Base Reirradiation

He Wang [1,*], Fahed M. Alsanea [1], Dong Joo Rhee [1], Xiaodong Zhang [1], Wei Liu [2], Jinzhong Yang [1], Zhifei Wen [3], Yao Zhao [1], Tyler D. Williamson [4], Rachel A. Hunter [4], Peter A. Balter [1], Tina M. Briere [1], Ronald X. Zhu [1], Anna Lee [5], Amy C. Moreno [5], Jay P. Reddy [5], Adam S. Garden [5], David I. Rosenthal [5], Gary B. Gunn [5] and Jack Phan [5]

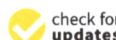

Academic Editor: Brigitta G. Baumert

Received: 24 December 2024
Revised: 29 January 2025
Accepted: 31 January 2025
Published: 5 February 2025

Citation: Wang, H.; Alsanea, F.M.; Rhee, D.J.; Zhang, X.; Liu, W.; Yang, J.; Wen, Z.; Zhao, Y.; Williamson, T.D.; Hunter, R.A.; et al. Advanced External Beam Stereotactic Radiotherapy for Skull Base Reirradiation. *Cancers* 2025, 17, 540. https://doi.org/10.3390/cancers17030540

Copyright: © 2025 by the authors. Licensee MDPI, Basel, Switzerland. This article is an open access article distributed under the terms and conditions of the Creative Commons Attribution (CC BY) license (https://creativecommons.org/licenses/by/4.0/).

[1] Radiation Physics, University of Texas M.D. Anderson Cancer Center, Houston, TX 77030, USA; fmalsanea@mdanderson.org (F.M.A.); drhee1@mdanderson.org (D.J.R.); xizhang@mdanderson.org (X.Z.); jyang4@mdanderson.org (J.Y.); yzhao15@mdanderson.org (Y.Z.)
[2] Medical Physics, Mayo Clinic College of Medicine and Science, Phoenix, AZ 85054, USA
[3] Radiation Oncology, Hoag Memorial Hospital, Hoag Cancer Center, Newport Beach, CA 92663, USA
[4] Radiation Therapeutic Physics, University of Texas M.D. Anderson Cancer Center, Houston, TX 77030, USA
[5] Radiation Oncology, University of Texas M.D. Anderson Cancer Center, Houston, TX 77030, USA; jphan@mdanderson.org (J.P.)
* Correspondence: hewang@mdanderson.org

Simple Summary: Skull base stereotactic radiotherapy (RT) is particularly challenging due to prior radiation and the proximity of several critical organs. This study reviewed four advanced external beam RT modalities and their corresponding or available modern treatment planning systems (TPSs). The plan quality and potentials were evaluated in terms of target coverage and dose gradient. The steepest border gradient was used to assess the fall-off speed achievable near the target to spare adjacent critical structures, while the volume gradient was used to evaluate dose spread at a distance. Gamma Knife demonstrated the highest border gradient, followed by small-spot-size proton beams and CyberKnife. The proton beam exhibited the least dose spread in the low-dose region.

Abstract: Background/Objectives: Stereotactic body radiation therapy (SBRT) for skull base reirradiation is particularly challenging, as patients have already received substantial radiation doses to the region, and nearby normal organs may have approached their tolerance limit from prior treatments. In this study, we reviewed the characteristics and capabilities of four advanced external beam radiation delivery systems and four modern treatment planning systems and evaluated the treatment plan quality of each technique using skull base reirradiation patient cases. Methods: SBRT plans were generated for sixteen skull base reirradiation patients using four modalities: the GK plan for the Elekta Leksell Gamma Knife Perfexion/ICON, the CyberKnife (CK) plan for the Accuray CyberKnife, the intensity-modulated proton therapy (IMPT) plan for the Hitachi ProBeat-FR proton therapy machine, and the volumetric-modulated arc therapy (VMAT) plan for the Varian TrueBeam STx. These plans were evaluated and compared using two novel gradient indices in addition to traditional dosimetry metrics for targets and organs at risk (OARs). The steepest border gradient quantified the percent prescription dose fall-off per millimeter at the boundary between the target and adjacent critical structures. This gradient index highlighted the system's ability to spare nearby critical OARs. The volume gradient assessed the extent of dose spread outside the target toward the patient's body. Results: All plans achieved comparable target coverage and conformity, while IMPT and VMAT demonstrated significantly better uniformity. The GK plans exhibited the highest border gradient, up to 20.9%/mm, followed by small-spot-size IMPT plans and CK plans. Additionally, IMPT plans showed the benefit of reduced dose spread in low-dose regions and the lowest maximum and mean doses to the brainstem and carotid artery. Conclusions: The advanced external beam radiotherapy modalities evaluated in this study are well-suited for SBRT in skull base reirradiation, which demands precise targeting of tumors with highly conformal doses and steep dose gradients to protect nearby normal structures.

Keywords: stereotactic body radiation therapy; reirradiation; skull base cancer; external beam radiation therapy; Gamma Knife; CyberKnife; proton therapy; dose gradient; intensity-modulated proton therapy; volumetric modulated radiation therapy

1. Introduction

The treatment of skull base cancer is complex and usually presents unique challenges due to the intricate anatomy and the proximity of various critical structures, such as the brainstem, optic apparatus, major vessels, and numerous cranial nerves. Typically, a multidisciplinary approach is required, involving a combination of surgery, radiation therapy, and sometimes chemotherapy or targeted therapies, to improve local control and survival rates [1–7].

Radiation therapy (RT) is commonly employed in the treatment of skull base cancers for patients who are surgically unresectable, have residual tumors following surgical resection, or possess physical or medical conditions that pose a high risk for surgery. Notably, stereotactic radiation therapy (SBRT) has emerged as an attractive option for localized residual or recurrent tumors [8–10]. SBRT delivers highly conformal ablative radiation in a small number of fractions over a short time period, typically within two weeks, in contrast to the 6–7 weeks required for conventional head and neck cancer treatment.

Reirradiation of skull base recurrences is among the most challenging cases as the patients have already received a significant radiation dose to the same region, and surrounding normal organs may have reached their tolerance dose from prior RT [11,12]. Several modern external beam radiation delivery systems are used for SBRT treatment to provide precise targeting of tumors with highly conformal doses and steep dose gradients, thereby minimizing damage to surrounding healthy tissues. These advanced systems include Gamma Knife (Elekta Instruments AB, Stockholm, Sweden) [13,14], CyberKnife (Accuray, Inc., Sunnyvale, CA, USA) [15–17], linear accelerators (LINACs) [18], Tomotherapy (TomoTherapy Inc., Madison, WI, USA) [19,20], and proton therapy machines [21,22]. Despite their differences in design, radiation sources, and delivery strategies, these systems all provide effective SBRT treatment.

In addition to the precise targeting requirements, treatment planning systems (TPSs) face similar challenges, particularly in ensuring dose calculation accuracy for small fields and providing the optimization tools necessary to achieve dosimetric goals [23–25]. The combination of a high-precision radiation delivery system and an optimal planning solution is crucial to achieving optimal treatment outcomes while minimizing toxicities.

Recent studies have demonstrated comparable overall survivals and relatively lower incidences of severe toxicities with SBRT in the reirradiation setting compared to conventional fractionated radiation therapy [26,27]. To achieve optimal sparing of organs at risk (OARs) without compromising target coverage, much stricter dose constraints are typically employed during the treatment planning process. In this context, the dose gradient at the boundary between the target and adjacent critical structures plays a pivotal role in the SRS/SRT/SBRT field. However, the traditionally used gradient index—commonly defined as the ratio of the 50% isodose line volume to the 100% isodose line volume [28]—does not adequately capture the sharpness of dose fall-off and its spatial relationship to critical structures. This limitation underscores the need for more refined metrics to evaluate dose gradients, particularly in complex treatment scenarios involving close proximity of targets to critical structures.

While numerous vendors and modalities of radiation treatment machines and various treatment planning systems are available, this study focused on reviewing the SBRT capabilities of a select group of advanced external beam RT delivery modalities and RT treatment planning systems, and investigated their dosimetric potentials, including novel gradient metrics, using skull base SBRT cases.

2. Materials and Methods

The outcomes of external beam radiation treatment are closely correlated with the delivery systems and treatment planning systems. For skull base SBRT, the requirements of these systems play a pivotal role in achieving precise targeting while maximizing normal tissue sparing. Before conducting the comparison of achievable treatment plans, we summarized the characteristics side-by-side in tables for the systems that were used in this study. The information is primarily sourced from vendor specifications.

2.1. External Beam Radiation Delivery Systems

The requirements for an external beam delivery system used for SBRT include mechanical and radiation accuracy, small-field collimation, volumetric imaging capability, and treatment efficiency. Table 1 compares the features and capabilities of four advanced systems used in this study: Elekta Leksell Gamma Knife Perfexion/ICON, Accuray CyberKnife M6/S7, Hitachi ProBeat-FR (representative of the proton therapy machines), and Varian TrueBeam STx (representative of LINAC machine).

LINACs are the most used external beam radiation therapy modality due to their versatility in radiation techniques, beam energies, and dose rates, enabling the treatment of various types and locations of cancer [42,43]. The TrueBeam STx is one of the premier LINAC machines, and it is highly regarded for its capabilities in SBRT. The Gamma Knife is specifically designed with a head frame to treat small intracranial lesions with high precision in single-fraction stereotactic radiosurgery (SRS). The advanced ICON version integrates cone-beam computed tomography (CBCT) and motion management, allowing for frameless and fractionated treatment. The CyberKnife is a robotic system capable of delivering radiation beams from nearly any angle, with real-time imaging for motion tracking. Both Gamma Knife and CyberKnife are dedicated SRS/SBRT machines. Proton beam therapy is renowned for its "Bragg peak", which allows energy deposition within the tumor while protecting surrounding healthy tissue and organs with no exit dose. The Hitachi ProBeat-FR, with its small spot sizes, is well-suited for SBRT.

Table 1 also lists the references for commissioning and quality assurance of these machines. The test and tolerances must adhere to the recommendations for the SRS/SBRT procedures.

Image guidance is the key element in stereotactic RT to enhance the precision and accuracy of radiation delivered to target while minimizing exposure to the surrounding healthy tissues. Fast kV volumetric imaging, such as cone-beam CT (CBCT), is the typical onboard imaging system on radiation modalities, as seen in Gamma Knife ICON, TrueBeam, and ProBeat. However, these systems lack the capability for real-time tracking. CyberKnife does not use CBCT technology; instead, it employs advanced live X-ray imaging that can continuously track the target during treatment and can perform real-time adaptations to compensate for patient motion. In addition to onboard imaging systems, several advanced technologies can be integrated with radiation delivery systems to facilitate efficient and accurate patient setup verification as well as motion tracking. These include BrainLab

Exactrac systems (X-ray and surface tracking) [44,45], CT-on-rail imaging [46], and surface guidance systems [47–49] such as VisionRT, C-Rad, etc. Modern techniques have recently emerged that integrate MRI and PET with LINACs, providing superior visualization of tumors at functional level [50,51], allowing biology-guided radiotherapy [52,53], and helping to improve radiation treatment outcomes.

Table 1. Representative external beam radiation therapy modalities for SBRT settings.

Modalities and Models	Leksell Gamma Knife Perfexion/ICON™	CyberKnife M6/S7	TrueBeam STx	Proton ProBeat-FR
Manufacturers	Elekta	Accuray	Varian	Hitachi
Radiation source/energy	192 sealed Co-60 sources (1.17 MeV and 1.33 MeV)	6 MeV photons on robotic arm	6 MeV, 10 MeV, 6 MeV FFF, 10 MeV FFF Photon on C arm	72.5 MeV–221.8 MeV proton
Mechanical and radiation accuracy	Sub-millimeter	Sub-millimeter	Sub-millimeter	Sub-millimeter
Collimation	Eight-sector crown-shaped collimator	Fixed cone, Iris collimator, InCise MLC	Jaw, high-definition MLC	Aperture, focused collimator
Maximum field size	1.6 cm (shot size)	Fixed cone, Iris collimator: 6 cm MLC: 12 cm × 10 cm	Jaw: 40 cm × 40 cm MLC: 22 cm × 40 cm	30 cm × 40 cm
Beam delivery	Combination of 4, 8, and 16 mm beams (shots)	Beamlets from hundreds of unique angles	Fixed-angle IMRT beams, VMAT	Passive scattering, Spot scanning (IMPT, spot size ~0.5 cm)
Dose rate	2.0 Gy/min (before source change)—3.6 Gy/min (new source)	400–1000 MU/min	400–600 MU/min (6 MeV, 10 MeV photon), 1400 MU/min (6 MeV FFF), 2400 MU/min (10 MeV FFF photon)	480 MU/min **
Onboard imaging *	CBCT (ICON) [29,30]	kV imagers	2D kV/MV and CBCT, 4D CBCT	2D KV and CBCT
Motion management	ICON: high-definition motion management [31,32]	Synchrony respiratory tracking system [33]	External gating system	External gating system
6 DoF setup/motion correction	6 DoF treatment plan adaptation	6 DoF delivery arm	6 DoF couch	6 DoF couch
Commissioning and quality assurance	Petti 2021 (TG 178) [34], Hu 2022 [35]	Sharma 2007 (TG 135) [36], Dieterich 2011 [37]	Klein 2009 (TG 142) [38], Hanley 2021 (TG 198) [39]	Arjomandy 2019 (TG 185) [40], Farr 2021 [41]

DoF: Degree of Freedom; VMAT: volumetric modulated arc therapy; IMRT: intensity-modulated radiation therapy; IMPT: intensity-modulated proton therapy; SBRT: stereotactic body radiation therapy; TG: AAPM Task Group; FF: flattening filter; FFF: flattening filter free; CBCT: cone-beam computed tomography; MLC: multi-leaf collimator. * External imaging systems, such as X-ray imaging (BrainLab's Exactrac), CT-on-rail, and surface imaging (BrainLab's Exactrac Dynamic, Vision RT's Align RT, C-Rad, etc.), can be integrated into radiation delivery systems, as is currently seen with the TrueBeam STx and ProBeat. ** $\geq$1.25 Gy/min with discrete scanning for the following settings: range: 20 g/cm^2; target volume: 1 L; and dose: 2 Gy).

2.2. Radiation Treatment Planning Systems

The treatment planning system is also crucial for generating high-precision SBRT plans to ensure effective and safe skull base cancer treatment. Corresponding to the RT delivery systems listed in Table 1, we compare the features and capabilities of four TPS systems in Table 2: the Leksell GammaPlan® for Gamm Knife Perfexion/ICON (GK), the Accuray Precision® for CyberKnife (CK), and RayStation® (RaySearch Laboratories) for both proton ProBeat and TrueBeam STx modalities. Plans from these four systems will be evaluated for our skull base reirradiation cases.

In summary, GammaPlan and Accuray Precision are the dedicated TPSs designed for Leksell Gamm Knife and CyberKnife, respectively, both specializing in non-isocentric treatment planning for SRS/SBRT patients. RayStation TPS supports multiple treatment modalities and offers several powerful tools that make it a superior choice for external beam radiation therapy. These include a multi-criteria optimization tool that helps users understand the tradeoffs between conflicting objectives using Pareto planes, an adaptive planning tool that can enhance the efficiency of adaptive treatment workflow, robust optimization that is particularly beneficial for particle beam therapy, and an advanced scripting tool that facilitate the automation of processing.

Table 2. Representative treatment planning systems for RT modalities in Table 1.

Treatment Planning Systems	Leksell GammaPlan	Accuray Precision	RayStation—IMRT/VMAT	RayStation—Proton
Manufacturers	Elekta	Accuray	RaySearch	RaySearch
Planning image	CT (pre-RT), MRI	CT	CT	CT
Isocenter(s) per prescription	Non-isocentric	Non-isocentric	Isocentric	Isocentric
Dose calculation engine	TMR10, convolution	Ray Tracing, FSPB (MLC), Monte Carlo (MLC)	CC Convolution, Monte Carlo	Monte Carlo
inhomogeneity correction	Yes, in convolution when using CT and tumor < 2 cm distance from skin	Yes	Yes	Yes
Optimization	Traditional inverse planning, LDO optimizer [54,55]	VOLO optimizer [56]	DMPO, MCO, robust optimization	DMPO, MCO, robust optimization
Adaptative planning	No	Yes, through PreciseART	Yes	Yes

CC: collapsed cone; LDO: lightning dose optimizer; DMPO: direct machine parameter optimization; MCO: multi-criteria optimization; FSPB: finite-size pencil beam.

Many additional capabilities common to all these TPS include multi-modality imaging fusion, inverse planning, non-coplanar beam geometry, and dose-volume histogram (DVH) analysis.

2.3. Patients and Treatment Plan Generation

Sixteen patients who underwent SBRT for skull base reirradiation on IRB-approved trials (SOAR 2016-1065; PA14-0198) were randomly selected. Nine patients received treatment on Varian TrueBeam STx with a prescription dose (Rx) of 45 Gy delivered in 5 fractions. Seven patients were treated on Elekta Leksell Gamma Knife Perfexion, receiving prescription doses ranging from 21 Gy to 27 Gy in 3 fractions. The mean initial treatment prescription was 66 Gy (range: 60 to 70 Gy) in 30–33 fractions. The mean reirradiation interval was 23 months (range: 3 to 57 months). Table 3 presents detailed patient and SBRT treatment information, with the primary target volume ranging from 2.1 cm^3 to 36.4 cm^3.

Treatment plans were generated using the four TPSs in Table 2 for treatment machines specified in Table 1. Identical target volumes were used for planning consistency. The proton plans were generated in RayStation R12A for Hitachi ProBeat-FR utilizing 3 to 5 non-coplanar beams with intensity modulation proton therapy (IMPT) technique and the Monte Carlo dose calculation engine. Robust optimization was applied with a 2 mm setup uncertainty and 2.5% range uncertainty. The volumetric modulated arc therapy (VMAT) plans were generated in RayStation R11A with 2 to 3 arcs for Varian TrueBeam STx using the collapsed cone convolution dose calculation engine. GK plans were manually created in Leksell Gamma Plan 10.1 for Leksell Gamma Knife Perfexion, while CyberKnife plans were created in Accuray Precision for the CyberKnife M6 employing multi-leaf collimators (MLC) and Monte Carlo dose calculation engine. All plans were generated by experienced medical physicists or dosimetrists.

The planning goals aimed to achieve comparable or improved target coverage while adhering to clinical dose constraints for critical organs or structures. The general clinical goals for 3- and 5-fraction reirradiation treatment plans are listed in Table 4. The constraints for OARs were much stricter than those for conventional treatment due to reirradiation. Evaluation includes comparing the target coverage, Paddick conformity index (PCI) [57], and homogeneity index (HI). HI is calculated as (D2-D98)/D50, where Dx represents the dose to x% of the volume in cumulative DVH. PCI values are ≤1.0, with 1.0 indicating perfect conformity; HI values are ≥0.0, with 0.0 indicating perfect uniformity.

Table 3. Detailed treatment site, target volume, and prescription for patients treated with SBRT.

Patient	Site	Anatomical/Clinical Region	Target Volume (cm^3)	Prescription (Gy)	Number of Fractions
1	Petroclival Occiput	Posterior Cranial Fossa	36.4	45	5
2	Petroclival Occiput	Posterior Cranial Fossa	36.4	24	3
3	Petroclival Occiput	Posterior Cranial Fossa	29.8	21	3
4	V3/Ovale	Central Skull Base	29.6	45	5
5	Clivus	Central Skull Base	26.1	45	5
6	Ethmoid/Cribiform	Anterior Cranial Fossa	25.7	45	5
7	Nasopharynx	Retropharynx	21.6	45	5
8	Cavernous Sinus	Central Skull Base	20.7	45	5
9	Retropharyngeal Node	Retropharynx	16.3	45	5
10	Cavernous Sinus	Central Skull Base	15	27	3
11	Cavernous Sinus	Central Skull Base	10.5	21	3
12	Petroclival	Posterior Cranial Fossa	9.2	24	3
13	Retropharyngeal	Retropharynx	9	45	5
14	Retropharyngeal	Retropharynx	7.4	45	5
15	Dura	Intracranial	2.6	24	3
16	Petroclival	Posterior Cranial Fossa	2.1	21	3

Table 4. Clinical goals and dose constraints used in SBRT plans for skull base reirradiation.

Structures	Clinical Goals/Dose Constraints	
PTVs	V100% > 95% Dmax < 120%	
OARs	No hot spot if in target, as low as reasonably achievable if outside of or away from target	
	21–27 Gy/3 fractions	40–45 Gy/5 fractions
Brainstem	Dmax < 10 Gy	Dmax < 13 Gy
Spinal cord	Dmax < 9 Gy	Dmax < 12 Gy
Optic apparatus	Dmax < 9 Gy	Dmax < 12 Gy
Carotids	Dmax < 20 Gy	Dmax < 30 Gy
Cochlea	Dmax < 21 Gy	Dmax < 21 Gy
Temporal lobe	Dmax < 18 Gy V12 Gy < 3 cm^3	Dmax < 27 Gy V18 Gy < 3 cm^3

SBRT: stereotactic body radiation therapy; PTV: planning target volume; OAR: organ at risk; V100: volume receiving 100% of prescription dose; VxGy: volume receiving x Gy; Dmax: maximum dose.

Traditional dose gradient analysis typically employs a single gradient index, calculated as the ratio of volume enclosed by the 50% Rx isodose line (IDL) to the volume enclosed by 100% IDL [28]. In skull base SBRT, multiple critical OARs may be in close proximity to or overlapping with the radiation target, necessitating a balance between the target coverage and OAR sparing. Of particular interest is the speed of dose fall-off at the boundary, which is crucial for estimating or predicting the target coverage versus normal tissue sparing. Given the use of different radiation sources and collimations across RT modalities, the rate of dose fall-off may vary. Therefore, our study is designed to evaluate two new gradient indices, both as functions of percent prescription dose (%Rx), enabling their application across different prescribed doses.

Steepest border gradient (SBG). SBG is defined as the highest percent of Rx dose fall-off per mm (%/mm) at the %Rx isodose line. It serves to evaluate the rapidity of dose fall-off at the boundary between the target and adjacent critical structures. An in-house developed script was employed to detect the shortest distance from the x% prescription isodose line IDL (%Rx) to the prescription isodose line IDL (Rx). Distances to IDL (Rx) were recorded for isodose lines ranging from 50% to 90% of the prescription dose; then, they were converted to %/mm.

Volume gradient (VG). VG is defined as VOL (%Rx)/TV, where VOL (%Rx) represents the volume enclosed by the IDL (%Rx), and TV is the volume of the primary target. VG assesses the speed of dose-volume spread-out, which is pertinent to the integral dose considerations. VG values were recorded from the 100% Rx IDL down to the 20% Rx IDL. The value of VG at 100% Rx IDL correlates with the RTOG conformity index [58], while the traditional gradient index [28] can be derived from VG values at 50% Rx IDL and 100% Rx IDL.

Both the SBG and VG are influenced by factors such as beam penumbra, beam angle arrangement, and the optimization constraints controlling the gradient-related parameters. These metrics will be compared across plans generated for the four RT modalities.

The maximum dose (defined as the dose to hottest 0.01 cm^3) and mean dose to the brainstem and the ipsilateral carotid arteries were recorded and normalized to the prescription dose. These metrics were compared among the RT plans. The brainstem and carotid arteries are among the most critical OARs in the majority of skull base reirradiation cases.

The above plan quality metrics were evaluated and compared among the four treatment plans. All plans were normalized to meet similar dose constraints on critical OARs while achieving best possible target coverage. Statistical analysis was performed using the Wilcoxon signed-rank test for comparison in IBM SPSS Statistics 24. A p-value < 0.05 was considered statistically significant.

3. Results

The delivery systems listed in Table 1 are well-suited for SBRT in skull base reirradiation, enabling precise targeting. The treatment planning systems outlined in Table 2 can achieve adequate dose gradients to spare adjacent critical structures through effective optimization. Figure 1 illustrates the dose distributions of representative SBRT plans generated using CK, GK, VMAT, and IMPT techniques.

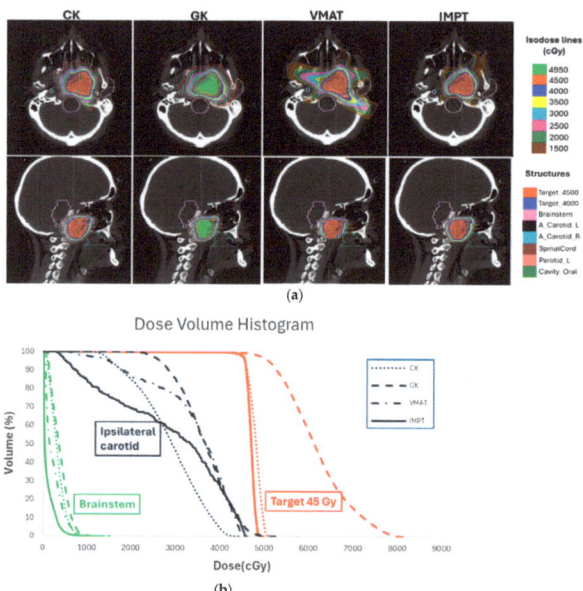

Figure 1. A representative case showing SBRT plans from CyberKnife (CK), Gamma Knife (GK), intensity-modulated proton therapy (IMPT), and volumetric modulated arc therapy (VMAT) techniques. The patient initially received 70 Gy in 33 fractions in 2013 and underwent a VMAT SBRT for left nasopharynx recurrence in 2015 (20-month intervals). (**a**) The transverse view (top row) and sagittal view (bottom row) of the plan dose distributions. Several organs at risk surround the target, and the plans were generated to meet clinical goals outlined in Table 4. (**b**) Dose-volume histograms of the primary target, brainstem, and ipsilateral carotid for the same patient.

Figure 2 displays the target coverage, PCI, and HI for the primary target of all 16 patients. The target coverage and PCI show comparable results across all four plans ($p > 0.05$). However, the HI is notably lower for IMPT and VMAT plans compared to CK and GK plans ($p < 0.01$), indicating superior uniformity in dose distribution for IMPT and VMAT.

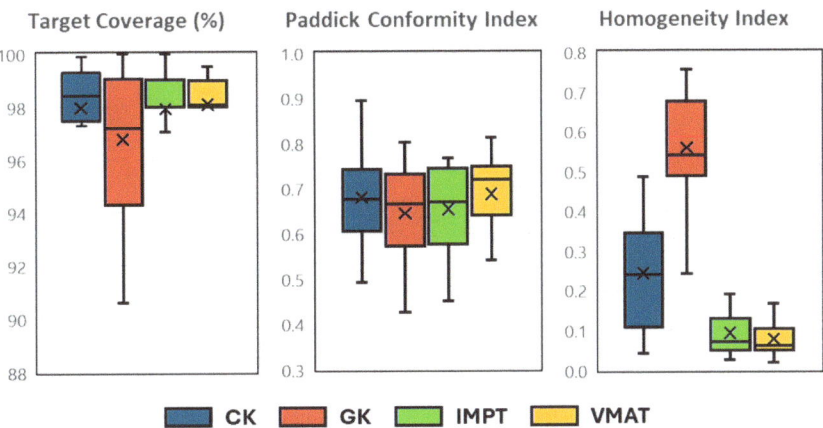

Figure 2. Comparison of primary target coverage, Paddick conformity index, and homogeneity index for CyberKnife (CK), Gamma Knife (GK), intensity-modulated proton therapy (IMPT), and volumetric modulated arc therapy (VMAT).

Figure 3 compares the SBG and VG among the four plans. Given the stringent brainstem dose constraints in skull base reirradiation, the highest dose gradient typically occurred at the boundary between the brainstem and the target. Analysis of the SBG reveals that for GK plans, the first 10% dose fall-off occurred within approximately 0.5 mm, resulting in an SBG as high as 20.9%/mm (Figure 3(left)). In contrast, CK, IMPT, and VMAT plans showed a 10% dose fall-off within about 1 mm, corresponding to 10.2%/mm to 12.8%/mm. At the 50% Rx isodose line, the mean fall-off speed decreased to 16.6% for GK plans, while the other three plans showed an increase. This variation is linked to plan normalization: GK plans typically prescribe 50% of the maximum dose, positioning the Rx isodose line at the steepest gradient of the dose profile. In contrast, VMAT and IMPT plans often prescribe to the shoulder (90% or above) of the dose profile, placing the steepest gradient at a lower isodose line location. Overall, GK plans showed the highest SBG compared to the other three techniques ($p < 0.05$) between 100% and 50% Rx IDLs. A 50% dose drop occurred in approximately 3 mm for the GK plan, compared to around 4 mm for IMPT, CK, and VMAT plans.

Figure 3 (right) illustrates the volume gradient comparison among the four techniques. At the 100% Rx isodose line, GK and IMPT plans covered a larger volume. As distances increased from the target, CK and VMAT plans showed an increase in volume for the 50% Rx isodose line, whereas IMPT maintained a larger volume than GK. By the 20% Rx isodose line, IMPT plans exhibited significantly lower volumes compared to the other techniques ($p < 0.05$).

Figure 4 compares the OAR doses among the four treatment plans. The brainstem was within 5 mm distance of the target for 9 out of 16 patients and within 2 mm for 4 out of 16 patients. The ipsilateral carotid artery partially overlapped with the target in 12 out of 16 patients and was within 2 mm of the target in 3 out of 16 patients. Due to the stringent dose constraints for the brainstem, plans typically exhibited sharp dose gradients toward it. Comparing the four techniques, IMPT plans demonstrated superior maximum and mean doses to the brainstem ($p < 0.05$). The mean dose to the ipsilateral carotid artery was comparable across all techniques, but the CK, IMPT, and VMAT plans achieved better adherence to the clinical goal of avoiding hot spots within the carotid artery compared to the GK plans ($p < 0.05$).

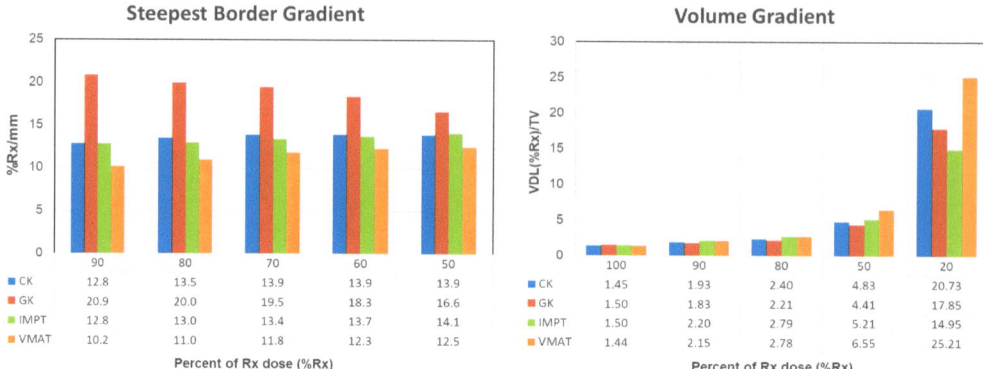

Figure 3. Comparison of the steepest border gradient (**left**) and volume gradient (**right**) for CyberKnife (CK) Gamma Knife (GK), intensity-modulated proton therapy (IMPT), and volumetric modulated arc therapy (VMAT).

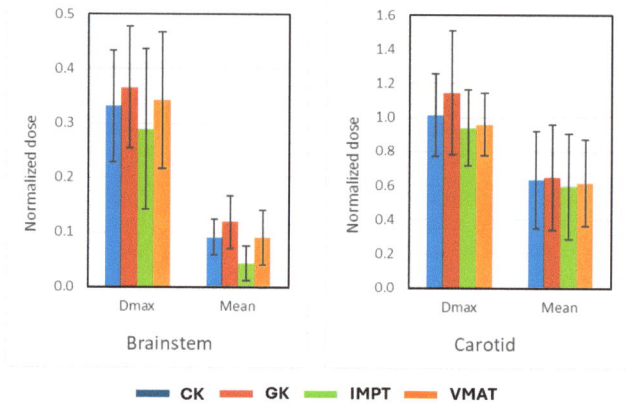

Figure 4. Comparison of the brainstem (**left**) and carotid (**right**) dose with one standard deviation for CyberKnife (CK), Gamma Knife (GK), intensity-modulated proton therapy (IMPT), and volumetric modulated arc therapy (VMAT). Doses are normalized to prescription doses.

The comparison of the above plan quality metrics is also summarized in Table 5. Table 5 also compared the beam-on-time and delivery time across the four treatment techniques. Notably, for CK and GK, the beam-on-time and delivery time were identical, as they continuously delivered all shots or beamlets. For IMPT and VMAT plans, the delivery time encompasses the duration from initiating the first beam to completing all beams, including time for field changes and verification, image acquisition before each beam, and couch rotation for non-coplanar beams. The beam-on-time calculations were based on specific delivery dose rates: 3 Gy/min for GK and 600 MU/min for VMAT plans.

Table 5. Dosimetric comparison of treatment plans for four external beam RT systems based on 16 skull base SBRT patients.

Technique	Primary Target Coverage (%)	PCI	HI	Beam-on-Time (min)	Delivery Time (min)	SBG @90%Rx (%/mm)	SBG @50%Rx (%/mm)
CK	98	0.68	0.24	24.3 *	24.3	12.8	13.9
GK	96.8	0.64	0.56	71.3 *	71.3	20.9	16.6
IMPT	97.9	0.65	0.09	2.2	12.1	12.8	14.1
VMAT	98.1	0.69	0.08	4.4	6.1	10.2	12.5

CK: CyberKnife; GK: Gamma Knife; IMPT: intensity-modulated proton therapy; VMAT: volumetric modulated arc therapy; PCI: Paddick conformity index; HI: homogeneity index; SBG: steepest border gradient. * Based on treatment time reported in the treatment planning system.

4. Discussion

Skull base recurrences are associated with high mortality rates and severe morbidity due to the local destruction of surrounding critical organs [11]. Typically, reirradiation is the only viable option for unresectable recurrences. However, reirradiation of the skull base tumors presents significant challenges. The proximity of critical structures, including the brainstem, spinal cord, optic apparatus, cochlea, major vessels, and numerous cranial nerves, increases the risk of severe radiation-induced toxicities. These structures may have already received a dose close to tolerance in the initial radiation therapy, which is typically 60–70 Gy in 30–35 fractions. Moreover, the separations between the tumors and vital structures may be only submillimeter, which necessitates an intricate balance between delivering a sufficient tumoricidal dose and sparing multiple critical structures, each with distinct dose tolerances. These complexities underscore the importance of advanced techniques and precise radiation delivery systems to minimize the risk of devastating outcomes while maximizing treatment efficacy.

In this study, we compared four external beam radiation techniques for SBRT with those used for skull base reirradiation. As shown in Table 4, the dose constraints were significantly stricter for reirradiation to minimize post-radiation complications. Specifically, we introduced a novel gradient concept to evaluate and compare the performance of these techniques in skull base SBRT and identified the potential gradient each technique could achieve in terms of OAR sparing. The steepest border gradient, expressed as the sharpest dose fall-off speed (%Rx/mm), evaluates each system's ability to achieve the steepest dose gradient when critical structures are near or adjacent to the target. This metric is particularly valuable in balancing target coverage with OAR sparing. It provides essential guidance during the treatment planning process by defining achievable planning goals for each system. Additionally, it offers a deeper understanding of the dosimetric consequences of daily patient setup errors.

Complementing the steepest border gradient, the volume gradient, which is similar to the traditional gradient index, was utilized to assess the dose spread throughout the patient's body outside the target volume. This measure further aids in understanding the overall dose distribution and minimizing unnecessary radiation exposure to healthy tissues.

For the other commonly used metrics for plan evaluation, all techniques achieved comparable target coverage and conformity, while VMAT and IMPT demonstrated superior homogeneity. LINAC-based SBRT emerged as the most utilized technique due to its versatility in treating various cancer types and its specific features that are well-suited for SBRT. However, the dose spread was highest in VMAT plans, which necessitates careful design before planning to minimize unintended dose exposure to healthy tissues, especially when non-coplanar arcs are used.

GK demonstrated the most effective capability in creating the steepest immediate dose fall-off at the boundary of the target, thereby sparing critical structures that are proximal or abutting. Following GK, IMPT also showed significant benefits in limiting dose spread beyond the 50% Rx isodose line. However, the efficacy of proton treatment depends on the target location and the number of beams utilized. In our study, proton beams utilized extended-range shifters located closer to the patient for more superficial targets, without the use of apertures, which are known to further reduce dose spread both locally and at a distance, according to references [59–62]. The larger volume observed for the isodose lines from 100% to 50% in IMPT plans was influenced by robust optimization techniques employed during planning, which also impacted the CI for IMPT. Typically, a 2 mm margin was used to account for patient position uncertainty in robust optimization. Online daily adaptation strategies may help reduce this uncertainty through daily imaging and provide additional benefits by minimizing radiation exposure to surrounding tissues.

The size of the proton spot is crucial for stereotactic radiation therapy. In our previous study, we utilized IMPT for head and neck SBRT using an early version of ProBeat, which had a spot size greater than 1 cm [63]. Plans with larger spot sizes did not demonstrate clear benefits in target coverage and gradient enhancement typical of proton treatment. However, the current Probeat-FR system features a spot size of approximately 5 mm, making it suitable for stereotactic treatment. The smaller spot size improves the proton system's ability to achieve a steep border gradient, with optimal volume gradient observed outside the 50% Rx isodose line as well.

While the primary focus of this study is not on dose calculation algorithms, the dosimetry accuracy of the TPSs must be meticulously assessed for small-field radiation [64], especially in the region of a high dose gradient. Monte Carlo-based dose calculation is renowned for its widely accepted accuracy, and it has overcome the computational time through the use of GPUs in RayStation for proton plans [65,66]. The VMAT plans generated in RayStation for this study employ the collapsed cone-based algorithm, which has demonstrated accuracy within 3% [67–69] for small-field irradiation. The TPSs for GK and CK are specially designed for SRS/SBRT. CK utilizes Monte Carlo dose calculation for MLC-based plans, while GK requires a CT scan to use a convolution algorithm to account for heterogeneity in dose calculation [34,70]. It is crucial to note that the accuracy of dose calculation in these TPSs is contingent upon the precision of beam modeling during the TPS commissioning. This accuracy should be thoroughly validated through comprehensive end-to-end testing, with particular attention to small field scenarios [71].

We used the same target volumes across all techniques in this study, applying a 2 mm margin to skull base lesions based on our patient setup protocol [72]. Similar immobilization techniques were assumed for the four techniques evaluated, facilitating hypofractionated treatment for skull base reirradiation. Additionally, some patients had subclinical risk target volumes contoured around the primary target to receive lower doses aimed at covering sites of potential high risks. These contouring decisions were made by the attending physicians based on their clinical judgment, balancing outcomes, and potential toxicities [12,27]. Advanced online adaptation techniques, such as MR-LINAC and Ethos, hold promise for further enhancing treatment procedures and reducing radiation to normal tissues, potentially allowing for reduced target margins.

The beam-on-time for IMPT was highly promising compared to the other techniques. This is due to the current synchrotron proton beam plans being delivered using discrete spot scanning and multi-energy extraction [73]. Discrete spot scanning involves delivering the specified dose for each spot location in a step-by-step manner. Once the spot dose is delivered, the irradiation stops, and the scanning magnets setting is changed to the next location. The purpose of multi-energy extraction is to reduce the possible energy layer switching time and, thus, significantly reduce the proton dose delivery time. This is achieved by delivering several energy layers in one single spill. In contrast, with the single energy layer extraction scheme, the synchrotron would need to decelerate and accelerate between each energy layer, taking approximately 2 s. The energy layer switch time is only 0.5 s with multi-energy extraction techniques. Furthermore, with continuous scanning (i.e., raster scanning), the estimated delivery dose rate could increase by up to 30%.

The beam-on-time represents the continuous radiation time without human interaction. For all four modalities in this study, this was based on estimates from the treatment planning systems. GK and CK deliver all radiation shots or beamlets in a single setup session, meaning the beam-on-time was equivalent to the overall delivery time. Although the beam-on-time has been significantly improved for IMPT on the proton ProBeat-FR system, the additional time for couch and gantry rotation, as well as imaging verification, added up to 2 min for each beam switch, extending the overall delivery time. The beam switch for VMAT typically takes around 1 min. Among the modalities, VMAT plans had the most efficient delivery time, followed by IMPT plans. GK treatments are particularly advantageous for small lesions but may require significantly longer delivery times for larger lesions.

Several studies have compared treatment plans across different delivery modalities in the context of stereotactic radiotherapy [74–79]. However, most of these studies typically involve comparisons of only 2–3 delivery systems or comparisons of techniques or treatment modes from the same modality. Almost all of them rely on the traditional gradient index to evaluate plans, which provides limited insight into the steepness of dose fall-off near critical structures. To date, there is only one publication similar to our study that compared GK, CK, VMAT, and proton therapy. That study used different planning systems for VMAT and proton plans and employed different delivery systems for proton therapy [78]. In addition, their comparison primarily focused on intracranial cases, where the target border gradient was less crucial than in skull base scenarios, making the steepness of dose gradients less of a priority. This distinction underscores the unique value of our study in addressing the challenges of skull base reirradiation.

Although we introduced the steepest dose gradient for the most challenging skull base reirradiation scenarios, it is evident that this information can also be applied to other SBRT sites with a similar CT intensity range, such as spinal stereotactic radiotherapy, where strict dose constraints are essential. Moreover, this gradient information provides a deeper understanding of the potential dose distribution of radiotherapy and its impact on critical structures nearby. It can further serve as a valuable tool in decision-making, helping to determine whether radiotherapy or surgery alone or in combination with other treatment modalities is the best approach to achieve optimal cancer control while maintaining a better quality of life post-treatment [4,5,7,80].

While all four of these advanced external beam radiotherapy modalities are suitable for skull base SBRT, the choice depends on several factors beyond the proximity of tumors to critical structures. These factors include patient conditions, availability of techniques, treatment costs, insurance coverage, and more. Proton therapy is often more expensive and less widely available compared to photon-based techniques. GK and CK are dedicated SRS/SBRT modalities, while LINAC machines are versatile, efficient, and widely used for treating various tumors. GK is more suitable for small intracranial lesions, whereas CK and VMAT plans are superior for irregularly shaped tumors. The integration of other modern techniques, such as MRI [51], with these modalities can further enhance treatment outcomes. Additionally, the choice is typically guided by a multidisciplinary team, including radiation oncologists, medical physicists, neurosurgeons, and other specialists.

The limitations of this study include the lack of clinical outcome data to demonstrate the benefit of sharp dose fall-off, the absence of proton aperture to further improve dose gradient and limit dose spread, and a potentially small sample size, which did not capture the effects of tumor shape or multiple lesions on the border gradient metric. Severe toxicities following skull base reirradiation, such as bone or soft tissue necrosis, carotid artery bleeding, cranial nerve damage, and others, could potentially be reduced or even avoided if these critical structures are carefully contoured and spared in the treatment plans using the knowledge of border gradients from this study. At the time of this manuscript, an aperture for head and neck stereotactic radiotherapy on the ProBeat-FR system has not been developed at our institution. However, other institutions have implemented this technique [61,81], demonstrating its advantages. The outcome following skull base reirradiation SBRT and the development of SBRT-specific apertures will be the focus of our future research.

5. Conclusions

External beam stereotactic radiotherapy plays an essential role in skull base reirradiation, as it requires steep dose gradients to protect nearby normal structures. The four advanced modalities evaluated in this study demonstrated their suitability for this challenging task. The treatment plans achieved comparable target coverage and dose conformity across the four techniques while meeting similar clinical objectives for protecting adjacent critical structures. The IMPT and VMAT plans demonstrated superior target dose uniformity, whereas the GK plans showed significant inhomogeneity.

Based on the steepest border gradient, GK plans achieved the fastest dose fall-off at the target-OAR border, with a 50% dose drop occurring in approximately 3 mm, compared to around 4 mm for IMPT, CK, and VMAT plans. This border gradient can provide essential guidance during the treatment planning process by defining achievable planning goals to balance effective tumor control with reduced toxicities. This is particularly crucial in situations where nearby OAR tolerance is critical, such as in skull base reirradiation SBRT. The volume gradient showed comparable dose spread-out within 50% prescription isodose lines among the four techniques, whereas IMPT plans demonstrated significantly reduced dose spread into low-dose regions, which is beneficial for minimizing unnecessary radiation exposure to healthy tissues.

Author Contributions: Conceptualization, H.W., F.M.A., X.Z., W.L. and J.P.; Data Curation, H.W., D.J.R., Z.W. and Y.Z.; Formal Analysis, H.W., F.M.A. and D.J.R.; Investigation, H.W., F.M.A., X.Z., J.Y., T.D.W. and R.A.H.; Methodology, H.W., F.M.A., W.L., P.A.B., T.M.B., R.X.Z., A.L., A.C.M., J.P.R., A.S.G., D.I.R., G.B.G. and J.P.; Project Administration, H.W. and J.P.; Resources, H.W., F.M.A., D.J.R., J.Y., Y.Z., T.D.W. and R.A.H.; Software, H.W., F.M.A., D.J.R., Z.W., Y.Z., T.D.W. and R.A.H.; Supervision, J.P.; Validation, H.W., F.M.A., T.M.B. and P.A.B.; Writing—Original Draft, H.W. and F.M.A.; Writing—Review and Editing, D.J.R., X.Z., W.L., J.Y., Z.W., Y.Z., T.D.W., R.A.H., P.A.B., T.M.B., R.X.Z., A.L., A.C.M., J.P.R., A.S.G., D.I.R., G.B.G. and J.P. All authors have read and agreed to the published version of the manuscript.

Funding: This research received no external funding.

Institutional Review Board Statement: This study was approved by the Institutional Review Board (SOAR 2016-1065, approved 3/1/2017; PA14-0198, approved 6/20/2014) of M.D. Anderson Cancer Center (Houston, TX, USA).

Informed Consent Statement: Patient consent was waived since this was a retrospective study.

Data Availability Statement: The data presented in this study are available on request from the corresponding author.

Conflicts of Interest: The authors declare no conflicts of interest.

References

1. Iannalfi, A.; Riva, G.; Ciccone, L.; Orlandi, E. The role of particle radiotherapy in the treatment of skull base tumors. *Front. Oncol.* **2023**, *13*, 1161752. [CrossRef] [PubMed]
2. Moraes, F.Y.; Chung, C. Radiation for skull base meningiomas: Review of the literature on the approach to radiotherapy. *Chin. Clin. Oncol.* **2017**, *6* (Suppl. S1), S3. [CrossRef] [PubMed]
3. Palmer, J.D.; Gamez, M.E.; Ranta, K.; Ruiz-Garcia, H.; Peterson, J.L.; Blakaj, D.M.; Prevedello, D.; Carrau, R.; Mahajan, A.; Chaichana, K.L.; et al. Radiation therapy strategies for skull-base malignancies. *J. Neuro-Oncol.* **2020**, *150*, 445–462. [CrossRef] [PubMed]
4. De Simone, M.; Choucha, A.; Dannhoff, G.; Kong, D.S.; Zoia, C.; Iaconetta, G. Treating Trigeminal Schwannoma through a Transorbital Approach: A Systematic Review. *J. Clin. Med.* **2024**, *13*, 3701. [CrossRef] [PubMed]
5. De Simone, M.; Conti, V.; Palermo, G.; De Maria, L.; Iaconetta, G. Advancements in Glioma Care: Focus on Emerging Neurosurgical Techniques. *Biomedicines* **2023**, *12*, 8. [CrossRef] [PubMed]
6. Bin-Alamer, O.; Mallela, A.N.; Palmisciano, P.; Gersey, Z.C.; Elarjani, T.; Labib, M.A.; Zenonos, G.A.; Dehdashti, A.R.; Sheehan, J.P.; Couldwell, W.T.; et al. Adjuvant stereotactic radiosurgery with or without postoperative fractionated radiation therapy in adults with skull base chordomas: A systematic review. *Neurosurg. Focus* **2022**, *53*, E5. [CrossRef]
7. Choucha, A.; Troude, L.; Morin, L.; Fernandes, S.; Baucher, G.; De Simone, M.; Lihi, A.; Mazen, K.; Alseirihi, M.; Passeri, T.; et al. Management of large Trigeminal Schwannoma: Long-term oncologic and functional outcome from a multicentric retrospective cohort. *Acta Neurochir.* **2024**, *166*, 440. [CrossRef]
8. Krengli, M.; Apicella, G.; Deantonio, L.; Paolini, M.; Masini, L. Stereotactic radiation therapy for skull base recurrences: Is a salvage approach still possible? *Rep. Pract. Oncol. Radiother.* **2015**, *20*, 430–439. [CrossRef]
9. Mohamad, I.; Karam, I.; El-Sehemy, A.; Abu-Gheida, I.; Al-Ibraheem, A.; Al-Assaf, H.; Aldeheim, M.; Alghamdi, M.; Alotain, I.; Ashour, M.; et al. The Evolving Role of Stereotactic Body Radiation Therapy for Head and Neck Cancer: Where Do We Stand? *Cancers* **2023**, *15*, 5010. [CrossRef]
10. Mori, Y.; Kida, Y.; Matsushita, Y.; Mizumatsu, S.; Hatano, M. Stereotactic radiosurgery and stereotactic radiotherapy for malignant skull base tumors. *Cureus* **2020**, *12*, e8401. [CrossRef]
11. Ho, J.C.; Phan, J. Reirradiation of Skull Base Tumors With Advanced Highly Conformal Techniques. *Curr. Oncol. Rep.* **2017**, *19*, 82. [CrossRef] [PubMed]
12. Ng, S.P.; Wang, H.; Pollard, C., 3rd; Nguyen, T.; Bahig, H.; Fuller, C.D.; Gunn, G.B.; Garden, A.S.; Reddy, J.P.; Morrison, W.H.; et al. Patient Outcomes after Reirradiation of Small Skull Base Tumors using Stereotactic Body Radiotherapy, Intensity Modulated Radiotherapy, or Proton Therapy. *J. Neurol. Surg. B Skull Base* **2020**, *81*, 638–644. [CrossRef] [PubMed]
13. Agarwal, A.; Flickinger, J.C.; Lunsford, D.; Kondziolka, D. Gamma knife radiosurgery for skull base chordomas: A 13 year review from a single institution. *Int. J. Radiat. Oncol. Biol. Phys.* **2002**, *54*, 248. [CrossRef]
14. Desai, R.; Rich, K.M. Therapeutic Role of Gamma Knife Stereotactic Radiosurgery in Neuro-Oncology. *Mo. Med.* **2020**, *117*, 33–38.
15. Cheng, Y.; Lin, Y.; Long, Y.; Du, L.; Chen, R.; Hu, T.; Guo, Q.; Liao, G.; Huang, J. Is the CyberKnife® radiosurgery system effective and safe for patients? An umbrella review of the evidence. *Future Oncol.* **2022**, *18*, 1777–1791. [CrossRef] [PubMed]
16. Joseph, B.; Supe, S.S.; Ramachandra, A. Cyberknife: A double edged sword? *Rep. Pract. Oncol. Radiother.* **2010**, *15*, 93–97. [CrossRef]
17. Kuo, J.S.; Yu, C.; Petrovich, Z.; Apuzzo, M.L.J. The CyberKnife Stereotactic Radiosurgery System: Description, Installation, and an Initial Evaluation of Use and Functionality. *Neurosurgery* **2003**, *53*, 1235–1239. [CrossRef] [PubMed]
18. Biston, M.C.; Dupuis, P.; Gassa, F.; Grégoire, V. Do all the linear accelerators comply with the ICRU 91's constraints for stereotactic body radiation therapy treatments? *Cancer/Radiothérapie* **2019**, *23*, 625–629. [CrossRef] [PubMed]
19. Chen, Q.; Rong, Y.; Burmeister, J.W.; Chao, E.H.; Corradini, N.A.; Followill, D.S.; Li, X.A.; Liu, A.; Qi, X.S.; Shi, H.; et al. AAPM Task Group Report 306: Quality control and assurance for tomotherapy: An update to Task Group Report 148. *Med. Phys.* **2023**, *50*, e25–e52. [CrossRef]
20. Rong, Y.; Welsh, J.S. Dosimetric and clinical review of helical tomotherapy. *Expert. Rev. Anticancer. Ther.* **2011**, *11*, 309–320. [CrossRef]
21. Frick, M.A.; Chhabra, A.M.; Lin, L.; Simone, C.B., 2nd. First Ever Use of Proton Stereotactic Body Radiation Therapy Delivered with Curative Intent to Bilateral Synchronous Primary Renal Cell Carcinomas. *Cureus* **2017**, *9*, e1799. [CrossRef] [PubMed]
22. Simone, C.B.; Lin, L. Proton SBRT is ready to move past uncertainties and towards improved clinical outcomes. *J. Radiosurg SBRT* **2023**, *9*, 3–6. [PubMed]
23. Chen, W.Z.; Xiao, Y.; Li, J. Impact of dose calculation algorithm on radiation therapy. *World J. Radiol.* **2014**, *6*, 874–880. [CrossRef] [PubMed]

24. Lechner, W.; Primeßnig, A.; Nenoff, L.; Wesolowska, P.; Izewska, J.; Georg, D. The influence of errors in small field dosimetry on the dosimetric accuracy of treatment plans. *Acta Oncol.* **2020**, *59*, 511–517. [CrossRef]
25. Malicki, J. The importance of accurate treatment planning, delivery, and dose verification. *Rep. Pract. Oncol. Radiother.* **2012**, *17*, 63–65. [CrossRef]
26. Diao, K.; Nguyen, T.P.; Moreno, A.C.; Reddy, J.P.; Garden, A.S.; Wang, C.H.; Tung, S.; Wang, C.; Wang, X.A.; Rosenthal, D.I.; et al. Stereotactic body ablative radiotherapy for reirradiation of small volume head and neck cancers is associated with prolonged survival: Large, single-institution, modern cohort study. *Head Neck* **2021**, *43*, 3331–3344. [CrossRef]
27. Gogineni, E.; Zhang, I.; Rana, Z.; Marrero, M.; Gill, G.; Sharma, A.; Riegel, A.C.; Teckie, S.; Ghaly, M. Quality of Life Outcomes Following Organ-Sparing SBRT in Previously Irradiated Recurrent Head and Neck Cancer. *Front. Oncol.* **2019**, *9*, 836. [CrossRef]
28. Paddick, I.; Lippitz, B. A simple dose gradient measurement tool to complement the conformity index. *J. Neurosurg.* **2006**, *105*, 194–201. [CrossRef]
29. Duggar, W.N.; Morris, B.; Fatemi, A.; Bonds, J.; He, R.; Kanakamedala, M.; Rey-Dios, R.; Vijayakumar, S.; Yang, C. Gamma Knife(®) icon CBCT offers improved localization workflow for frame-based treatment. *J. Appl. Clin. Med. Phys.* **2019**, *20*, 95–103. [CrossRef]
30. Xu, A.Y.; Wang, Y.F.; Wang, T.J.C.; Cheng, S.K.; Elliston, C.D.; Savacool, M.K.; Dona Lemus, O.; Sisti, M.B.; Wuu, C.S. Performance of the cone beam computed tomography-based patient positioning system on the Gamma Knife Icon™. *Med. Phys.* **2019**, *46*, 4333–4339. [CrossRef]
31. Elekta, A.B. High Definition Motion Management—Enabling stereotactic Gamma Knife® Radiosurgery with Non-Rigid Patient Fixations. Elekta White Paper 2015, Stockholm, Sweden. Available online: https://www.elekta.com/medical-affairs/bibliographies/High%20Definition%20Motion%20Management%20-%20enabling%20stereotactic%20Gamma%20Knife%C2%AE%20radiosurgery%20with%20non-rigid%20patient%20fixations%20white%20paper.pdf (accessed on 30 January 2025).
32. Knutson, N.C.; Hawkins, B.J.; Bollinger, D.; Goddu, S.M.; Kavanaugh, J.A.; Santanam, L.; Mitchell, T.J.; Zoberi, J.E.; Tsien, C.; Huang, J.; et al. Characterization and validation of an intra-fraction motion management system for masked-based radiosurgery. *J. Appl. Clin. Med. Phys.* **2019**, *20*, 21–26. [CrossRef] [PubMed]
33. Akino, Y.; Sumida, I.; Shiomi, H.; Higashinaka, N.; Murashima, Y.; Hayashida, M.; Mabuchi, N.; Ogawa, K. Evaluation of the accuracy of the CyberKnife Synchrony™ Respiratory Tracking System using a plastic scintillator. *Med. Phys.* **2018**, *45*, 3506–3515. [CrossRef] [PubMed]
34. Petti, P.L.; Rivard, M.J.; Alvarez, P.E.; Bednarz, G.; Daniel Bourland, J.; DeWerd, L.A.; Drzymala, R.E.; Johansson, J.; Kunugi, K.; Ma, L.; et al. Recommendations on the practice of calibration, dosimetry, and quality assurance for gamma stereotactic radiosurgery: Report of AAPM Task Group 178. *Med. Phys.* **2021**, *48*, e733–e770. [CrossRef]
35. Hu, Y.-H.; Hickling, S.V.; Qian, J.; Blackwell, C.R.; McLemore, L.B.; Tryggestad, E.J. Characterization and commissioning of a Leksell Gamma Knife ICON system for framed and frameless stereotactic radiosurgery. *J. Appl. Clin. Med. Phys.* **2022**, *23*, e13475. [CrossRef] [PubMed]
36. Sharma, S.C.; Ott, J.T.; Williams, J.B.; Dickow, D. Commissioning and acceptance testing of a CyberKnife linear accelerator. *J. Appl. Clin. Med. Phys.* **2007**, *8*, 119–125. [CrossRef] [PubMed]
37. Dieterich, S.; Cavedon, C.; Chuang, C.F.; Cohen, A.B.; Garrett, J.A.; Lee, C.L.; Lowenstein, J.R.; d'Souza, M.F.; Taylor, D.D., Jr.; Wu, X.; et al. Report of AAPM TG 135: Quality assurance for robotic radiosurgery. *Med. Phys.* **2011**, *38*, 2914–2936. [CrossRef]
38. Klein, E.E.; Hanley, J.; Bayouth, J.; Yin, F.F.; Simon, W.; Dresser, S.; Serago, C.; Aguirre, F.; Ma, L.; Arjomandy, B.; et al. Task Group 142 report: Quality assurance of medical accelerators. *Med. Phys.* **2009**, *36*, 4197–4212. [CrossRef]
39. Hanley, J.; Dresser, S.; Simon, W.; Flynn, R.; Klein, E.E.; Letourneau, D.; Liu, C.; Yin, F.F.; Arjomandy, B.; Ma, L.; et al. AAPM Task Group 198 Report: An implementation guide for TG 142 quality assurance of medical accelerators. *Med. Phys.* **2021**, *48*, e830–e885. [CrossRef]
40. Arjomandy, B.; Taylor, P.; Ainsley, C.; Safai, S.; Sahoo, N.; Pankuch, M.; Farr, J.B.; Yong Park, S.; Klein, E.; Flanz, J.; et al. AAPM task group 224: Comprehensive proton therapy machine quality assurance. *Med. Phys.* **2019**, *46*, e678–e705. [CrossRef]
41. Farr, J.B.; Moyers, M.F.; Allgower, C.E.; Bues, M.; Hsi, W.C.; Jin, H.; Mihailidis, D.N.; Lu, H.M.; Newhauser, W.D.; Sahoo, N.; et al. Clinical commissioning of intensity-modulated proton therapy systems: Report of AAPM Task Group 185. *Med. Phys.* **2021**, *48*, e1–e30. [CrossRef]
42. Madle, N. Versatility is the key for the future of radiotherapy linear accelerators. *J. Radiother. Pract.* **2007**, *6*, 59–61. [CrossRef]
43. Podgorsak, E.B. Treatment machines for external beam radiotherapy. In *Review of Radiation Oncology Physics: A Handbook for Teachers and Students*; IAEA: Vienna, Austria, 2005; pp. 103–132.
44. Da Silva Mendes, V.; Reiner, M.; Huang, L.; Reitz, D.; Straub, K.; Corradini, S.; Niyazi, M.; Belka, C.; Kurz, C.; Landry, G.; et al. ExacTrac Dynamic workflow evaluation: Combined surface optical/thermal imaging and X-ray positioning. *J. Appl. Clin. Med. Phys.* **2022**, *23*, e13754. [CrossRef] [PubMed]
45. Perrett, B.; Ukath, J.; Horgan, E.; Noble, C.; Ramachandran, P. A Framework for Exactrac Dynamic Commissioning for Stereotactic Radiosurgery and Stereotactic Ablative Radiotherapy. *J. Med. Phys.* **2022**, *47*, 398–408. [CrossRef]

46. Paxton, A.; Sarkar, V.; Price, R.G.; St. James, S.; Dial, C.; Poppe, M.M.; Salter, B.J. CT-on-Rails Utilization for Image Guidance and Plan Adaptation at a Single-Room Proton Therapy Center. *Int. J. Radiat. Oncol. Biol. Phys.* **2023**, *117*, e704. [CrossRef]
47. Nguyen, D.; Farah, J.; Barbet, N.; Khodri, M. Commissioning and performance testing of the first prototype of AlignRT InBore™ a Halcyon™ and Ethos™-dedicated surface guided radiation therapy platform. *Phys. Medica* **2020**, *80*, 159–166. [CrossRef]
48. González-Sanchis, A.; Brualla-González, L.; Fuster-Diana, C.; Gordo-Partearroyo, J.C.; Piñeiro-Vidal, T.; García-Hernandez, T.; López-Torrecilla, J.L. Surface-guided radiation therapy for breast cancer: More precise positioning. *Clin. Transl. Oncol.* **2021**, *23*, 2120–2126. [CrossRef]
49. Al-Hallaq, H.A.; Cerviño, L.; Gutierrez, A.N.; Havnen-Smith, A.; Higgins, S.A.; Kügele, M.; Padilla, L.; Pawlicki, T.; Remmes, N.; Smith, K.; et al. AAPM task group report 302: Surface-guided radiotherapy. *Med. Phys.* **2022**, *49*, e82–e112. [CrossRef]
50. Liu, X.; Li, Z.; Yin, Y. Clinical application of MR-Linac in tumor radiotherapy: A systematic review. *Radiat. Oncol.* **2023**, *18*, 52. [CrossRef]
51. Wang, H.; Yang, J.; Lee, A.; Phan, J.; Lim, T.Y.; Fuller, C.D.; Han, E.Y.; Rhee, D.J.; Salzillo, T.; Zhao, Y.; et al. MR-guided stereotactic radiation therapy for head and neck cancers. *Clin. Transl. Radiat. Oncol.* **2024**, *46*, 100760. [CrossRef]
52. Shirvani, S.M.; Huntzinger, C.J.; Melcher, T.; Olcott, P.D.; Voronenko, Y.; Bartlett-Roberto, J.; Mazin, S. Biology-guided radiotherapy: Redefining the role of radiotherapy in metastatic cancer. *Br. J. Radiol.* **2021**, *94*, 20200873. [CrossRef]
53. Surucu, M.; Ashraf, M.R.; Romero, I.O.; Zalavari, L.T.; Pham, D.; Vitzthum, L.K.; Gensheimer, M.F.; Yang, Y.; Xing, L.; Kovalchuk, N.; et al. Commissioning of a novel PET-Linac for biology-guided radiotherapy (BgRT). *Med. Phys.* **2024**, *51*, 4389–4401. [CrossRef] [PubMed]
54. Cui, T.; Nie, K.; Zhu, J.; Danish, S.; Weiner, J.; Chundury, A.; Ohri, N.; Zhang, Y.; Vergalasova, I.; Yue, N.; et al. Clinical Evaluation of the Inverse Planning System Utilized in Gamma Knife Lightning. *Front. Oncol.* **2022**, *12*, 832656. [CrossRef] [PubMed]
55. Wieczorek, D.J.; Kotecha, R.; Hall, M.D.; Tom, M.C.; Davis, S.; Ahluwalia, M.S.; McDermott, M.W.; Mehta, M.P.; Gutierrez, A.N.; Tolakanahalli, R. Systematic evaluation and plan quality assessment of the Leksell® gamma knife® lightning dose optimizer. *Med. Dosim.* **2022**, *47*, 70–78. [CrossRef] [PubMed]
56. Schüler, E.; Lo, A.; Chuang, C.F.; Soltys, S.G.; Pollom, E.L.; Wang, L. Clinical impact of the VOLO optimizer on treatment plan quality and clinical treatment efficiency for CyberKnife. *J. Appl. Clin. Med. Phys.* **2020**, *21*, 38–47. [CrossRef]
57. Paddick, I. A simple scoring ratio to index the conformity of radiosurgical treatment plans. Technical note. *J. Neurosurg.* **2000**, *93* (Suppl. S3), 219–222. [CrossRef]
58. Feuvret, L.; Noël, G.; Mazeron, J.-J.; Bey, P. Conformity index: A review. *Int. J. Radiat. Oncol. Biol. Phys.* **2006**, *64*, 333–342. [CrossRef]
59. Chou, C.-Y.; Tsai, T.-S.; Huang, H.-C.; Wang, C.-C.; Lee, S.-H.; Hsu, S.-M. Utilizing collimated aperture with proton pencil beam scanning (PBS) for stereotactic radiotherapy. *J. Appl. Clin. Med Phys.* **2024**, *25*, e14362. [CrossRef]
60. Feng, H.; Holmes, J.M.; Vora, S.A.; Stoker, J.B.; Bues, M.; Wong, W.W.; Sio, T.S.; Foote, R.L.; Patel, S.H.; Shen, J.; et al. Modelling small block aperture in an in-house developed GPU-accelerated Monte Carlo-based dose engine for pencil beam scanning proton therapy. *Phys. Med. Biol.* **2024**, *69*, 035003. [CrossRef]
61. Hickling, S.V.; Corner, S.; Kruse, J.J.; Deisher, A.J. Design and characterization of an aperture system and spot configuration for ocular treatments with a gantry-based spot scanning proton beam. *Med. Phys.* **2023**, *50*, 4521–4532. [CrossRef]
62. Holmes, J.; Shen, J.; Shan, J.; Patrick, C.L.; Wong, W.W.; Foote, R.L.; Patel, S.H.; Bues, M.; Liu, W. Technical note: Evaluation and second check of a commercial Monte Carlo dose engine for small-field apertures in pencil beam scanning proton therapy. *Med. Phys.* **2022**, *49*, 3497–3506. [CrossRef]
63. Wang, H.; Yang, J.N.; Zhang, X.D.; Li, J.; Frank, S.J.; Zhao, Z.X.; Luo, D.S.; Zhu, X.R.; Wang, C.J.; Tung, S.; et al. Treatment-Plan Comparison of Three Advanced Radiation Treatment Modalities for Fractionated Stereotactic Radiotherapy to the Head and Neck. *Int. J. Med. Phys. Clin. Eng. Radiat. Oncol.* **2019**, *8*, 106–120. [CrossRef]
64. Bagheri, H.; Soleimani, A.; Gharehaghaji, N.; Mesbahi, A.; Manouchehri, F.; Shekarchi, B.; Dormanesh, B.; Dadgar, H.A. An overview on small-field dosimetry in photon beam radiotherapy: Developments and challenges. *J. Cancer Res. Ther.* **2017**, *13*, 175–185. [CrossRef]
65. Fracchiolla, F.; Engwall, E.; Janson, M.; Tamm, F.; Lorentini, S.; Fellin, F.; Bertolini, M.; Algranati, C.; Righetto, R.; Farace, P.; et al. Clinical validation of a GPU-based Monte Carlo dose engine of a commercial treatment planning system for pencil beam scanning proton therapy. *Phys. Med.* **2021**, *88*, 226–234. [CrossRef] [PubMed]
66. Shan, J.; Feng, H.; Morales, D.H.; Patel, S.H.; Wong, W.W.; Fatyga, M.; Bues, M.; Schild, S.E.; Foote, R.L.; Liu, W. Virtual particle Monte Carlo: A new concept to avoid simulating secondary particles in proton therapy dose calculation. *Med. Phys.* **2022**, *49*, 6666–6683. [CrossRef] [PubMed]
67. Bosse, C.; Narayanasamy, G.; Saenz, D.; Myers, P.; Kirby, N.; Rasmussen, K.; Mavroidis, P.; Papanikolaou, N.; Stathakis, S. Dose Calculation Comparisons between Three Modern Treatment Planning Systems. *J. Med. Phys.* **2020**, *45*, 143–147. [CrossRef]
68. De Martino, F.; Clemente, S.; Graeff, C.; Palma, G.; Cella, L. Dose Calculation Algorithms for External Radiation Therapy: An Overview for Practitioners. *Appl. Sci.* **2021**, *11*, 6806. [CrossRef]

69. Manco, L.; Vega, K.; Maffei, N.; Gutierrez, M.V.; Cenacchi, E.; Bernabei, A.; Bruni, A.; D'Angelo, E.; Meduri, B.; Lohr, F.; et al. Validation of RayStation Monte Carlo dose calculation algorithm for multiple LINACs. *Phys. Med.* **2023**, *109*, 102588. [CrossRef]
70. Pantelis, E.; Logothetis, A.; Zoros, E.; Pappas, E.P.; Papagiannis, P.; Paddick, I.; Nordström, H.; Kollias, G.; Karaiskos, P. Dosimetric accuracy of the Convolution algorithm for Leksell Gamma Plan radiosurgery treatment planning: Evaluation in the presence of clinically relevant inhomogeneities. *J. Appl. Clin. Med. Phys.* **2023**, *24*, e13903. [CrossRef]
71. Schmitt, D.; Blanck, O.; Gauer, T.; Fix, M.K.; Brunner, T.B.; Fleckenstein, J.; Loutfi-Krauss, B.; Manser, P.; Werner, R.; Wilhelm, M.L.; et al. Technological quality requirements for stereotactic radiotherapy: Expert review group consensus from the DGMP Working Group for Physics and Technology in Stereotactic Radiotherapy. *Strahlenther. Onkol.* **2020**, *196*, 421–443. [CrossRef]
72. Mesko, S.; Wang, H.; Tung, S.; Wang, C.; Pasalic, D.; Chapman, B.V.; Moreno, A.C.; Reddy, J.P.; Garden, A.S.; Rosenthal, D.I.; et al. Estimating PTV Margins in Head and Neck Stereotactic Ablative Radiation Therapy (SABR) Through Target Site Analysis of Positioning and Intrafractional Accuracy. *Int. J. Radiat. Oncol. Biol. Phys.* **2020**, *106*, 185–193. [CrossRef]
73. Younkin, J.E.; Morales, D.H.; Shen, J.; Ding, X.; Stoker, J.B.; Yu, N.Y.; Sio, T.T.; Daniels, T.B.; Bues, M.; Fatyga, M.; et al. Technical Note: Multiple energy extraction techniques for synchrotron-based proton delivery systems may exacerbate motion interplay effects in lung cancer treatments. *Med. Phys.* **2021**, *48*, 4812–4823. [CrossRef] [PubMed]
74. Diwanji, T.P.; Mohindra, P.; Vyfhuis, M.; Snider, J.W., 3rd; Kalavagunta, C.; Mossahebi, S.; Yu, J.; Feigenberg, S.; Badiyan, S.N. Advances in radiotherapy techniques and delivery for non-small cell lung cancer: Benefits of intensity-modulated radiation therapy, proton therapy, and stereotactic body radiation therapy. *Transl. Lung Cancer Res.* **2017**, *6*, 131–147. [CrossRef] [PubMed]
75. Hsu, S.M.; Lai, Y.C.; Jeng, C.C.; Tseng, C.Y. Dosimetric comparison of different treatment modalities for stereotactic radiotherapy. *Radiat. Oncol.* **2017**, *12*, 155. [CrossRef] [PubMed]
76. Kumar, S.S.; Hall, L.; Li, X.; Downes, L.; Shearer, A.; Shelton, B.J.; Gerring, S.; McGarry, R.C. Comparison of outcomes of stereotactic body radiation therapy delivered with three different technologies to the lung. *J. Radiosurg SBRT* **2018**, *5*, 209–216. [PubMed]
77. Aljabab, S.; Vellayappan, B.; Vandervoort, E.; Bahm, J.; Zohr, R.; Sinclair, J.; Caudrelier, J.M.; Szanto, J.; Malone, S. Comparison of four techniques for spine stereotactic body radiotherapy: Dosimetric and efficiency analysis. *J. Appl. Clin. Med. Phys.* **2018**, *19*, 160–167. [CrossRef]
78. Cao, H.; Xiao, Z.; Zhang, Y.; Kwong, T.; Danish, S.F.; Weiner, J.; Wang, X.; Yue, N.; Dai, Z.; Kuang, Y.; et al. Dosimetric comparisons of different hypofractionated stereotactic radiotherapy techniques in treating intracranial tumors > 3 cm in longest diameter. *J. Neurosurg.* **2020**, *132*, 1024–1032. [CrossRef]
79. Seppälä, J.; Suilamo, S.; Tenhunen, M.; Sailas, L.; Virsunen, H.; Kaleva, E.; Keyriläinen, J. Dosimetric Comparison and Evaluation of 4 Stereotactic Body Radiotherapy Techniques for the Treatment of Prostate Cancer. *Technol. Cancer Res. Treat.* **2017**, *16*, 238–245. [CrossRef]
80. Phan, J.; Pollard, C.; Brown, P.D.; Guha-Thakurta, N.; Garden, A.S.; Rosenthal, D.I.; Fuller, C.D.; Frank, S.J.; Gunn, G.B.; Morrison, W.H.; et al. Stereotactic radiosurgery for trigeminal pain secondary to recurrent malignant skull base tumors. *J. Neurosurg.* **2019**, *130*, 812–821. [CrossRef]
81. Behrends, C.; Bäumer, C.; Verbeek, N.G.; Wulff, J.; Timmermann, B. Optimization of proton pencil beam positioning in collimated fields. *Med. Phys.* **2023**, *50*, 2540–2551. [CrossRef]

Disclaimer/Publisher's Note: The statements, opinions and data contained in all publications are solely those of the individual author(s) and contributor(s) and not of MDPI and/or the editor(s). MDPI and/or the editor(s) disclaim responsibility for any injury to people or property resulting from any ideas, methods, instructions or products referred to in the content.

MDPI AG
Grosspeteranlage 5
4052 Basel
Switzerland
Tel.: +41 61 683 77 34

Cancers Editorial Office
E-mail: cancers@mdpi.com
www.mdpi.com/journal/cancers

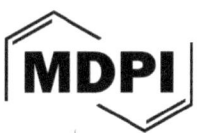

Disclaimer/Publisher's Note: The title and front matter of this reprint are at the discretion of the Guest Editors. The publisher is not responsible for their content or any associated concerns. The statements, opinions and data contained in all individual articles are solely those of the individual Editors and contributors and not of MDPI. MDPI disclaims responsibility for any injury to people or property resulting from any ideas, methods, instructions or products referred to in the content.

www.ingramcontent.com/pod-product-compliance
Lightning Source LLC
LaVergne TN
LVHW072348090526
838202LV00019B/2499